Gallstone Disease

Pathophysiology and Therapeutic Approaches

Editors
W. Swobodnik, H. Ditschuneit, and R. D. Soloway

With 99 Figures and 43 Tables

Springer-Verlag Berlin Heidelberg New York
London Paris Tokyo Hong Kong

Swobodnik, W.
Abteilung Innere Medizin II, Gastroenterologie und Ernährungswissenschaften, Universitätsklinikum Ulm, Robert-Koch-Straße 8, D-7900 Ulm, FRG

Soloway, R. D.
Division of Gastroenterology, 4.106 McCullough, G-64, University of Texas Medical Branch at Galveston, Galveston TX 77550, USA

Ditschuneit, H.
Abteilung Innere Medizin II, Gastroenterologie und Ernährungswissenschaften, Universitätsklinikum Ulm, Robert-Koch-Straße 8, D-7900 Ulm, FRG

ISBN-13:978-3-540-50965-3 e-ISBN-13:978-3-642-74619-2
DOI: 10.1007/978-3-642-74619-2

2127/3321-543210 – Printed on acid-free paper

Preface

The nonsurgical management of gallstone disease has drawn widespread clinical interest during the last decade as ultrasound surveys have indicated that cholelithiasis is predominantly an asymptomatic condition and much more prevalent than previously thought. This book presents an overview of the pathophysiologic and pathobiochemical principles of gallstone formation and the consequences for clinical therapeutic regimens. New information concerning the balance between vesicular and micellar transport of cholesterol, early cholesterol nucleation, and the influence of inhibiting and promoting compounds for cholesterol nucleation as well as information concerning the effects of changes in gallbladder motility and gallbladder mucosal function is reviewed. In order to make further progress in developing treatments which facilitate gallstone dissolution and in preventing disease, it is necessary to integrate this new data into our thinking.

Methods of treatment such as systemic litholysis of cholesterol gallbladder stones with bile acid preparations and mechanical fragmentation of stones either by extracorporal shock waves or intracorporal laser systems are carefully described and separate discussions of direct contact litholysis of cholesterol stones with ether preparations and the local litholytic treatment of calcified pigment stones are included. New therapeutic applications of HMG-CoA-reductase inhibitors and nonsteroidal anti-inflammatory drugs are also critically reviewed. Finally, for the interested reader an evaluation of prophylactic treatment against stone recurrence after successful conservative treatment and an appraisal of alternative management strategies supplement the information on the conservative treatment of gallstones.

Contents

Systemic Litholysis with Bile Acids

Extracorporeal Schock-Wave-Lithotripsy

Laser Lithotripsy

Local Litholysis

New Therapeutic Trends

Contributors

Ashby, B. S.
Department of Surgery, Southend Hospital, Prittlewell Chase, Southend, SS0 0RY, U.K.

Bender, C. E.
Division of Gastroenterology, Mayo Clinic, Rochester, MN 55905, USA

von Bergmann, K.
Abteilung Klinische Pharmakologie, Medizinische Klinik, Universität Bonn, Sigmund-Freud-Straße 25, 5300 Bonn 1, FRG

Bertolini, E.
Institute of Internal Medicine, University of Milan, Via Pace 9, 20122 Milan, Italy

Carey, M. C.
Department of Medicine, Brigham and Women's Hospital, 75 Francis Street, Boston, MA 02115, USA

Crosignani, A.
Institute of Internal Medicine, University of Milan, Via Pace 9, 20122 Milan, Italy

Demling, L.
Medizinische Klinik I mit Poliklinik, Universität Erlangen-Nürnberg, Krankenhausstraße 12, 8520 Erlangen, FRG

Ditschuneit, H.
Abteilung Innere Medizin II, Gastroenterologie und Ernährungswissenschaften, Universitätsklinikum Ulm, Robert-Koch-Straße 8, 7900 Ulm, FRG

Domschke, W.
Medizinische Klinik I mit Poliklinik, Universität Erlangen-Nürnberg, Krankenhausstraße 12, 8520 Erlangen, FRG

Dowling, R. H.
Gastroenterology Unit, Guy's Hospital, Guy's Tower, London SE1 9RT, UK

Draese, K.
Chirurgische Klinik, Krankenhaus Bad Oeynhausen, Wielandstraße 28, 4970 Bad Oeynhausen, FRG

Ell, C.
Medizinische Klinik I mit Poliklinik, Universität Erlangen-Nürnberg, Krankenhausstraße 12, 8250 Erlangen, FRG

Faust, U.
Institut für Biomedizinische Technik der Universität Stuttgart, Seidenstraße 36, 7000 Stuttgart 1, FRG

Fischer, S.
Abteilung Innere Medizin II, Gastroenterologie und Ernährungswissenschaften, Universitätsklinikum Ulm, Robert-Koch-Straße 8, 7900 Ulm, FRG

Floth, A.
Urologische Klinik, Universität Mainz, Langenbeckstraße 1, 6500 Mainz, FRG

Frenzel, F.
Abteilung für Gastroenterologie, Ferdinand-Sauerbruch-Klinikum, Arrenberger Straße 20–56, 5600 Wuppertal 1, FRG

Fromherz, P.
Abteilung für Biophysik der Universität Ulm, Oberer Eselsberg, 7900 Ulm, FRG

Gaisano, H. Y.
Gastroenterology Research Unit., Mayo Clinic and Foundation, Rochester, MN 55905, USA

Goebel, M.
Radiologische Klinik, Universität Mainz, Langenbeckstraße 1, 6500 Mainz, FRG

Grandinetti, G.
Institute of Internal Medicine, University of Milan, Via Pace 9, 20122 Milan, Italy

Greiner, L.
Abteilung für Gastroenterologie, Ferdinand-Sauerbruch-Klinikum, Arrenberger Straße 20–56, 5600 Wuppertal 1, FRG

Hahn, E. G.
Medizinische Klinik I mit Poliklinik, Universität Erlangen-Nürnberg, Krankenhausstraße 12, 8520 Erlangen, FRG

Harvey, P. R. C.
Department of Surgery and Research Institute, Mount Sinai Hospital, University of Toronto, 600 University Ave., Toronto, Ontario M5G 1X5, Canada

Heinemann, T.
Abteilung Klinische Pharmakologie, Medizinische Klinik, Universität Bonn, Sigmund-Freud-Straße 25, 5300 Bonn 1, FRG

Hochberger, J.
Medizinische Klinik I mit Poliklinik, Universität Erlangen-Nürnberg, Krankenhausstraße 12, 8520 Erlangen, FRG

Hohenfellner, R.
Urologische Klinik, Universität Mainz, Langenbeckstraße 1, 6500 Mainz, FRG

Holl, J.
Medizinische Klinik II, Universität München, Klinikum Großhadern, Marchioninistraße 15, 8000 München 70, FRG

Jakobeit, C.
Abteilung für Gastroenterologie, Ferdinand-Sauerbruch-Klinikum, Arrenberger Straße 20–56, 5600 Wuppertal 1, FRG

Janowitz, P.
Abteilung Innere Medizin II, Gastroenterologie und Ernährungswissenschaften, Universitätsklinikum Ulm, Robert-Koch-Straße 8, 7900 Ulm, FRG

Jazrawi, R. P.
Department of Biochemical Medicine, St. George's Hospital Medical School, Cranmer Terrace, London SW17 0RE, UK

Junginger, T.
Chirurgische Klinik, Universität Mainz, Langenbeckstraße 1, 6500 Mainz, FRG

Kerzel, M.
Medizinische Klinik I mit Poliklinik, Universität Erlangen-Nürnberg, Krankenhausstraße 12, 8520 Erlangen, FRG

Klüppelberg, U. G.
Gastroenterology Research Unit, Mayo Clinic and Foundation, Rochester, MN 55905, USA (present address: Innere Medizin II, Klinikum Großhadern der Universität München, Marchioninistraße 15, 8000 München 70, FRG)

Kurz, W.
Medizinische Klinik 1, Zentralkrankenhaus Reinkenheide, Postbrookstraße, 2850 Bremerhaven, FRG

LaMont, J. T.
Section of Gastroenterology, University Hospital, Boston University Medical Center, Boston, MA 02118, USA

Leibl, B.
Abteilung für Allgemeine Chirurgie, Universität Ulm, Steinhövelstraße 9, 7900 Ulm, FRG

LeRoy, A. J.
Division of Gastroenterology, Mayo Clinic, Rochester, MN 55905, USA

Lugli, R.
Patologia Speciale Medica, Universitá di Modena, Viale Vittorio Veneto 9, 41100 Modena, Italy

Lütjohann, D.
Abteilung Klinische Pharmakologie, Medizinische Klinik, Universität Bonn, Sigmund-Freud-Straße 25, 5300 Bonn 1, FRG

Malfertheiner, P.
Abteilung Innere Medizin II, Universität Ulm, Robert-Koch-Straße 8, 7900 Ulm, FRG

Martin, S.
Chirurgische Klinik, Krankenhaus Bad Oeynhausen, Wielandstraße 28, 4970 Bad Oeynhausen, FRG

McCullough, J. E.
Division of Gastroenterology, Mayo Clinic, Rochester, MN 55905, USA

Meier, T.
Institut für Lasertechnologien in der Medizin, Universität Ulm, Helmholtzstraße 12, 7900 Ulm, FRG

Merz, B.
Abteilung für Gastroenterologie, Ferdinand-Sauerbruch-Klinikum, Arrenberger Straße 20–56, 5600 Wuppertal 1, FRG

Meyer zum Büschenfelde, K.-H.
I. Medizinische Klinik und Poliklinik, Universität Mainz, Langenbeckstraße 1, 6500 Mainz, FRG

Mildenberger, P.
Radiologische Klinik, Universität Mainz, Langenbeckstraße 1, 6500 Mainz, FRG

Miller, L. J.
Gastroenterology Research Unit, Mayo Clinic and Foundation, Rochester, MN 55905, USA

Molero, X.
Gastroenterology Research Unit, Mayo Clinic and Foundation, Rochester, MN 55905, USA

Northfield, T. C.
Department of Biochemical Medicine, St. George's Hospital Medical School, Cranmer Terrace, London SW17 0RE, UK

Oettinger, W.
Abteilung für Allgemeine Chirurgie, Universität Ulm, Steinhövelstraße 9, 7900 Ulm, FRG

Orth, K.
Abteilung für Allgemeine Chirurgie, Universität Ulm, Steinhövelstraße 9, 7900 Ulm, FRG

Paumgartner, G.
Medizinische Klinik II, Universität München, Klinikum Großhadern, Marchioninistraße 15, 8000 München 70, FRG

Pellati, M.
Patologia Speciale Medica, Universitá di Modena, Viale Vittorio Veneto 9, 41100 Modena, Italy

Petersen, B. T.
Division of Gastroenterology, Mayo Clinic, Rochester, MN 55905, USA

Petroni, M. L.
Institute of Internal Medicine, University of Milan, Via Pace 9, 20122 Milan, Italy

Podda, M.
Chair of Internal Medicine, University of Milan, Via A. di Rudini 8, 20142 Milan, Italy

Rambow, A.
I. Medizinische Klinik und Poliklinik, Universität Mainz, Langenbeckstraße 1, 6500 Mainz, FRG

Sackmann, M.
Medizinische Klinik II, Universität München, Klinikum Großhadern, Marchioninistraße 15, 8000 München 70, FRG

Salvioli, G.
Patologia Speciale Medica, Universitá di Modena, Viale Vittorio Veneto 9, 41100 Modena, Italy

Sauerbruch, T.
Medizinische Klinik II, Universität München, Klinikum Großhaderm, Marchioninistraße 15, 8000 München 70, FRG

Schneider, H. T.
Medizinische Klinik I mit Poliklinik, Universität Erlangen-Nürnberg, Krankenhausstraße 12, 8520 Erlangen, FRG

Schopohl, J.
Chirurgische Klinik, Krankenhaus Bad Oeynhausen, Wielandstraße 28, 4970 Bad Oeynhausen, FRG

Smith, B. F.
Section of Gastroenterology and Hepatology, Boston City Hospital, Boston University Medical Center, 818 Harrison Avenue, Boston, MA 021118, USA

Soloway, R. D.
Division of Gastroenterology, 4.106 McCullough, G-64, University of Texas Medical Branch at Galveston, Galveston TX 77550, USA

Staritz, M.
I. Medizinische Klinik und Poliklinik, Universität Mainz, Langenbeckstraße 1, 6500 Mainz, FRG

Steiner, R.
Institut für Lasertechnologien in der Medizin, Universität Ulm, Helmholtzstraße 12, 7900 Ulm, FRG

Stiehl, A.
Medizinische Klinik, Klinikum der Universität Heidelberg, Bergheimer Straße 58, 6900 Heidelberg 1, FRG

Strasberg, S. M.
Department of Surgery and Research Institute, Mount Sinai Hospital, University of Toronto, 600 University Ave., Toronto, Ontario M5G 1X5, Canada

Swobodnik, W.
Abteilung Innere Medizin II, Gastroenterologie und Ernährungswissenschaften, Universitätsklinikum Ulm, Robert-Koch-Straße 8, 7900 Ulm, FRG

Thelen, M.
Radiologische Klinik, Universität Mainz, Langenbeckstraße 1, 6500 Mainz, FRG

Thistle, J. L.
Division of Gastroenterology, Mayo Clinic, Rochester, MN 55905, USA

Tudyka, J.
Abteilung Innere Medizin II, Gastroenterologie und Ernährungswissenschaften, Universitätsklinikum Ulm, Robert-Koch-Straße 8, 7900 Ulm, FRG

Wechsler, J. G.
Abteilung Innere Medizin II, Gastroenterologie und Ernährungswissenschaften, Universitätsklinikum Ulm, Robert-Koch-Straße 8, 7900 Ulm, FRG

Wenzel, H.
Abteilung für Gastroenterologie, Ferdinand-Sauerbruch-Klinikum, Arrenberger Straße 20–56, 5600 Wuppertal 1, FRG

Wu, J. G.
Department of Chemistry, Beijing University, Beijing 100871, People's Republic of China

Xu, D. F.
Section of Polymer Chemistry, Sinica Academica, Beijing 100871, People's Republic of China

Zöckler, C. E.
Chirurgische Klinik, Krankenhaus Bad Oeynhausen, Wielandstraße 28, 4970 Bad Oeynhausen, FRG

Zuin, M.
Institute of Internal Medicine, University of Milan, Via Pace 9, 20122 Milan, Italy

Pathobiochemistry and Pathophysiology of Gallstone Development: Importance for Clinical Decision Processes

Increased Biliary Lithogenicity Through Cholesterol Supersaturation

M.C. Carey

Department of Medicine, Brigham and Women's Hospital, 75 Francis Street, Boston, MA 02115 USA

Introduction

Cholesterol monohydrate (ChM) is the major organic component of most gallbladder stones in Western populations [1]. An essential thermodynamic prerequisite for the precipitation of cholesterol (Ch) from bile is that bile becomes supersaturated with Ch [2]. Although Ch is virtually insoluble in water, it is present in high concentrations in the hepatic and gallbladder biles of adult human beings [2], where it is solubilized in thermodynamically stable bile salt (BS) and BS-phospholipid (PL) micelles and dispersed in a thermodynamically metastable state by unilamellar PL-Ch vesicles [3]. Hepatic secretion of vesicles appears to be the principal conduit for PL and Ch secretion into bile [4]. Since the transhepatic flux of BS drives PL-Ch secretion, i.e., vesicle exocytosis [5], the origin of supersaturated bile must perforce lie in the hypersecretion of Ch-enriched vesicles in the face of normal BS secretion or the normal secretion of Ch-enriched vesicles in the face of BS hyposecretion [6].

This chapter will review briefly the metabolic origins and physical-chemical consequences of the defective lipid coupling that causes biliary Ch supersaturation. Because hepatic Ch and PL synthesis, hepatic uptake of Ch and PL from peripheral tissues and diet, and the BS flow through the hepatocytes are fluctuant [7], it is normal for bile to be supersaturated (i.e., vesicle-containing) in most adults during low BS fluxes through the enterohepatic circulation, i.e., during fasting, and unsaturated during high BS fluxes, particularly following dietary intake [8]. There is clear evidence, nonetheless, that, while all Ch gallstone patients have increased biliary lithogenicity through either relative (to BS) or absolute Ch supersaturation of their secreted biles, several other defects must be present simultaneously to make Ch crystallization and agglomeration of Ch crystals kinetically possible [9]. These factors will not be discussed in this chapter.

Pathophysiology of Ch Supersaturation

Origins of Hepatic Ch Pools

There are only three possible sources for supplying the cellular pool(s) of Ch available to the liver for its various metabolic, structural, and secretory needs [10, 11]. These sources are (1) Ch absorbed from the diet and delivered to the liver in chylomicron remnants, (2) Ch synthesized in extrahepatic tissues and delivered to the liver, principally through hepatic uptake of plasma low density lipoproteins (LDL), and (3) CH synthesized within the liver itself. It is clear that neither the mass of Ch returning to the liver from earlier secretion of lipoproteins – high density lipoproteins (HDL) or very low density lipoproteins (VLDL) – nor the fraction of biliary Ch absorbed from the small intestine represents net acquisition [11].

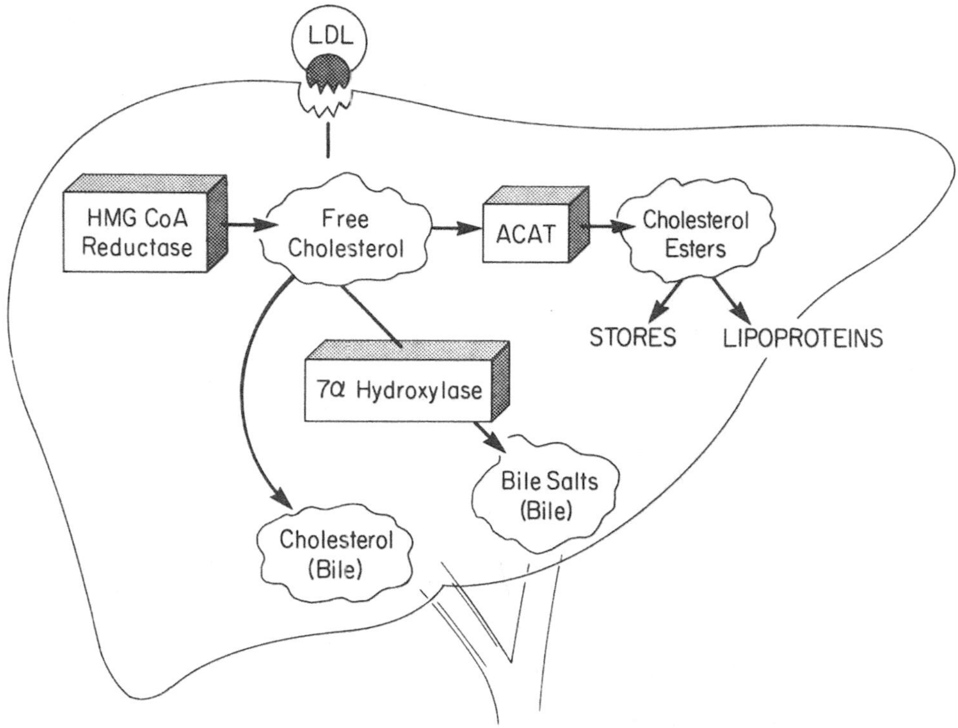

Fig. 1. Intracellular regulation of hepatic cholesterol flux. The major source of hepatocellular cholesterol is low density lipoproteins (*LDL*) of plasma. The single copy of apolipoprotein B-100 (*shaded*) on each LDL particle is the ligand that is recognized by apo B/E receptors, which trigger internalization of the whole lipoprotein particle. Not shown here is that chylomicron remnants, enriched with dietary and biliary cholesterol, are also endocytosed by the liver via different receptors that recognize only apolipoprotein E. Intracellularly, the hydrolysis of the cholesterol ester core of LDL releases free cholesterol molecules. A minor contribution to the hepatic free cholesterol pool is via de novo synthesis from acetate; the rate-controlling enzyme is HMG CoA reductase. The principal fates of excess free cholesterol molecules are: (1) re-esterification under the influence of microsomal enzyme acyl-coenzyme A cholesterol acyltransferase (*ACAT*): newly synthesized cholesterol esters may be stored in cytosolic oil droplets or between the constituent lipid monolayers of intracellular membranes, but most is used in assembling the core lipid of newly formed hepatic lipoproteins, principally VLDL, (2) de novo bile salt synthesis (rate-controlling enzyme is microsomal cholesterol 7α-hydroxylase), ≈500 mg/dl, (3) direct secretion of intact cholesterol molecules into bile. The homeostatic control of the levels of free cholesterol within the liver cell is maintained in a finely tuned state. Supersaturated bile represents a derangement in one or more of the mechanisms shown. (Reprinted from Ref. 9 with permission).

Hepatic Disposition of Ch Pools

There are several homeostatic mechanisms that maintain hepatic Ch pools constant which are kept under tight control when physiological conditions are normal [11]. Free Ch molecules must be solubilized among the phospho- and glycolipids of plasma membranes or intracellular organelles [12]. It has been estimated that about 90% of free Ch in human fibroblasts and 80–85% of free Ch in hepatocytes are in the plasma membranes and not in intracellular membranes [13, 14]. This occurs because intracellular membranes are relatively Ch deficient (Ch/PL ratio ≈ 0.1), whereas plasma membranes are relatively enriched (Ch/PL ≈ 0.3) [15]. Since any level of change in the Ch to PL ratio of cellular membranes can have quite marked effects on membrane function, it is not yet clear what tolerances are allowed pathophysiologically [16]. It seems, however, that the expansion of the recruitable pool of free Ch destined for bile possibly lies in the microsomal (SER) compartment [10, 11]. The liver disposes of Ch in the following ways (Fig. 1):

1. *Esterification to form Ch esters* (CE) [17]. Intracellular esterification is controlled by the microsomal acyl coenzyme A cholesterol acyltransferase (ACAT) enzyme system. Because of the lack of clear-cut molecular polarity, CEs have little solubility in membranes [15] and are either stored as cytoplasmic droplets or re-exported from the cell as newly synthesized lipoproteins, particularly VLDL [17]. Under basal conditions in the rat, the ratio of free to esterified Ch molecules in liver cells is 9:1 [10]. Curiously, in human beings and, especially, in gallstone patients, this simply measured ratio is not known. Cytoplasmic stores of CE are increased during the delivery of physiological levels of Ch to the liver or in any hepatic Ch overproduction states [10]. It is likely that the size of this biliary precursor pool could be rapidly modified through the combined influences of hepatic ACAT and, perhaps, cholesteryl ester hydrolase (CEH) enzymes [11, 18].
2. *Synthesis of primary BS* controlled by the microsomal rate-limiting enzyme, Ch 7α-hydroxylase [19]. As far as is known, this enzyme in human beings is principally under negative feedback control by secondary (i.e., more hydrophobic) bile acids in the returning limb of the enterohepatic circulation [20]; it appears that the enzyme is not tightly controlled by the availability of Ch substrate, as it is in some laboratory animals [11].
3. *Direct secretion of free Ch into bile* [11]. The Ch molecules probably form a functionally distinct pool destined for bile (in association with PL molecules) in the form of vesicles. There is little critical evidence that there are any major hormonal, motor, or even functional abnormalities of the enterohepatic circulation or BS pool, or appreciable qualitative or quantitative changes in the BS pattern that may be responsible for absolute or relative hypersecretion of biliary Ch in human beings [9, 10]. Current concepts suggest that absolute hypersecretion of biliary Ch occurs because a functional pool of free Ch molecules becomes available for recruitment into bile via the normal transhepatic flux of BS in the enterohepatic circulation [10].

Causes of an Expanded and Recruitable Hepatic Pool of Biliary Ch

The causes of an expanded and recruitable hepatic pool of biliary Ch may be divided into pathophysiological conditions associated with increased hepatic uptake, increased synthesis, or decreased catabolic mechanisms of Ch that lead to the expansion of an intracellular pool of Ch that is recruitable by BS [21]. Changes in the absolute flux of BS or their relative hydrophobicity are now considered insufficient in most cases to account for the great excess of Ch that appears in bile when it is supersaturated with Ch in human beings and in lithogenic animal models [9, 10]. The identified biochemical causes are listed in Fig. 2. They include:

1. Increased activity or number of LDL receptors, particularly caused by estrogens, in normal women, women taking oral contraceptives, and men on sex-steroid therapy [21–23].

2. Increased uptake of Ch from the diet via chylomicron remnants (not displayed in Fig. 2) [24, 25].
3. Increased Ch synthesis through the increased activity of both hepatic and extrahepatic HMG coenzyme A (CoA) reductase, such as in human obesity and any hypertriglyceridemic state [26–28].
4. Decreased Ch esterification as a result of the diminished activity of ACAT; thereby, less free Ch is shunted into CE stores or de novo lipoprotein formation. This occurs during therapy with progestational agents, during pregnancy, and with the ingestion of lipid-lowering "fibrates" [9, 21].
5. Decreased catabolism of Ch to bile acids, which may occur in chronic liver disease and as a result of aging or constitutional and congenital factors [9, 21].

It would be expected, therefore, that as the expanded free Ch pool becomes available for recruitment into bile, there would be one or more reciprocal phenomena, such as a decrease in Ch esterification, decreased secretion of VLDL particles, and decreased BS synthesis, some of which have been observed in experimental animals [29–31].

Biochemistry	Causes
1. Apo B/E Receptors ↑	Constitutional Estrogens
2. HMGCoA Reductase ↑	Obesity Hypertriglyceridemia
3. 7α Hydroxylase ↓	Constitutional Increasing Age
4. ACAT ↓	Progestogens 'Fibrates'

Fig. 2. Hypersecretion of biliary cholesterol: biochemistry and principal causes

Physical Chemistry of Ch Supersaturation

Several lines of evidence now suggest that the most plausible hypothesis of biliary lipid secretion is the hepatocellular export of biliary Ch and PL (with perhaps some BS) as unilamellar vesicles [32]. The remainder of the hepatocellular flux of BS exits via electrodiffusion through a specific protein transporter on the canalicular membranes [33]. Interactions between BS and vesicles are not instantaneous, and physical-chemical remodeling of vesicles by BS, both below and above their CMC values, continues all along the intrahepatic and the extrahepatic biliary tree to form simple BS–Ch micelles, mixed BS–PL–Ch micelles, and Ch–PL vesicles. Even at the level of the gallbladder, the physical state of biliary lipids has not yet achieved true equilibrium. In fact, equilibration of Ch–PL vesicles in the presence of saturated micelles would mean the formation of ChM crystals [9] (Fig. 3).

Hepatocellular, Sinusoidal, and Intrahepatic Biliary Tree

An old observation, repeatedly confirmed, is that, when bile becomes enriched with Ch, there is a parallel enrichment with PL [34]. Hence, the most likely site for the putative assembly of biliary vesicles destined for bile is the SER (microsomes) [5]. From this site, vesicles most likely move via the Golgi apparatus to join part of the BS flux across the hepatocytes [35] and then along a microtubular network [32] to fuse with specific regions

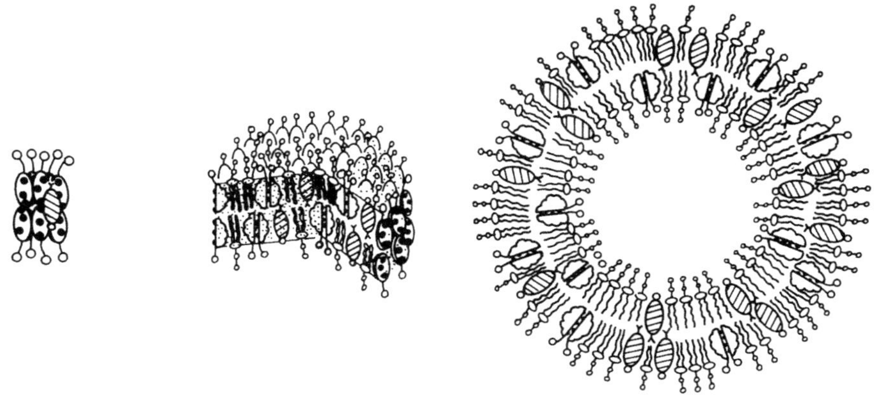

Fig. 3. Biliary lipid aggregates, the principal binders and solubilizers of calcium, bilirubinate (UCB), and cholesterol (Ch) in bile. Molecules of each biliary lipid are represented by symbols to display their space-filling shape. = cholesterol; = lecithin (L); = bile salt (BS). diners. Simple BS–Ch micelles coexist with BS–L–Ch mixed micelles in Ch unsaturated biles. In Ch supersaturated biles, supramicellar concentrations of Ch are solubilized by unilamellar L–Ch vesicles that may contain small amounts of BS. In "black" pigment stone biles, there are no vesicles since nearly all such biles are Ch unsaturated; these biles are likely to be supersaturated with $Ca(HUCB)_2$ due to the absence of vesicles for binding Ca^{2+} and solubilizing $HUCB^-$. The quantitative importance of each heteroassembly in binding/solubilizing calcium, UCB and, possibly, calcium UCB salts is not fully defined. In bile, proteins such as albumin and glycoproteins, bile salt monomers, and conjugated bilirubin also bind calcium but are quantitatively less important than the lipid particles. (Reprinted from Ref. 7 with permission).

of the canalicular membrane. This is followed by exocytosis into bile, by mechanisms which are unknown. Since PL is also secreted in excess and since the vesicles normally seen in the canalicular lumen of hepatocyte couplets [36] are the same size as those in supersaturated bile ($\approx$600 Å in diameter) [37], then quantitatively more vesicles must be secreted into bile in Ch lithogenic states.

Aqueous phase BS may be present as monomers or as micelles within the canalicular lumen [38]. Even at concentrations well below their CMC values, BS partition preferentially into the vesicular PL bilayer, provided it is not saturated with Ch [39]. In the vicinity of the CMC, vesicles are transformed into rod-like fragments (of a hexagonal liquid-crystalline phase) [38, 40]. At still higher BS concentrations, these rod-like fragments become progressively transformed into mixed micelles [38–40]. However, in the lithogenic state, the BS concentration may be insufficient to convert all vesicles via rods to micelles and vesicles persist, becoming enriched with Ch and even reaching Ch/PL ratios as high as 2 [38, 39]. This occurs via micellar dissolution of PL, but not Ch, from vesicles by Ch saturated micelles. It has also been shown that, if the micellar BS to PL–Ch ratio is sufficient to dissolve all vesicles into supersaturated micelles with the passage of time, a new population of Ch-rich vesicles will form from the supersaturated mixed micelles [40]. Because of the well-known negative curvilinear relationship between the Ch saturation index and BS secretion rate [7], bile is principally vesicular at low BS secretion rates and principally micellar at high BS secretion rates [8]. In this example, physiologically defective coupling provides strong independent evidence for the continued hepatic secretion of Ch-rich vesicles even when BS secretion rates are suboptimal for complete solubilization.

Extrahepatic Biliary Tree and Gallbladder

Both pigment stones of noninfectious origin (trivially known as "black" pigment stones) and Ch stones form only in the gallbladder [9, 41]. Infectious pigment stones (trivially known as "brown" pigment stones) generally form in the extrahepatic biliary tree and, very rarely, intrahepatically [41]. Hence, the gallbladder is crucial for the formation of most gallstones, which result solely from subtle physical-chemical and biochemical imbalances in sterile bile. Nucleation in the gallbladder probably involves a train of physical-chemical events that are likely to be intimately involved with vesicles [42]; Ch-rich PL unilamellar vesicles pre-exist in Ch lithogenic bile, since the cholesterol saturation indices of these biles are greater than 1. Following fusion and growth of the vesicles, Ch crystals may eventually form. In contrast, in calcium pigment lithogenic biles, vesicles are usually absent since the cholesterol saturation indices are generally less than 1 [41]. Nevertheless, intact PL is found in these stones [43], suggesting that when calcium monohydrogen bilirubinate ($Ca(HUCB)_2$) nucleates, it does so by simultaneously removing PL from micelles to lower the otherwise unfavorable interfacial tension between the hydrophobic calcium salt and bile, as also occurs in Ch stone disease [44]. In black pigment gallstones, there is more Ch at the center of the stones than on the periphery, whereas in Ch stones there is more $Ca(HUCB)_2$ at the center than on the periphery [41]. This probably reflects the fact that either pre-existing or de novo formed vesicles in bile are not only solubilizers of Ch but are potentially potent binders of Ca ions and unconjugated bilirubinate (UCB) [41]. The involvement of vesicle fusion in the initial stages of formation of both types of gallstones would explain the presence of Ch molecules and $Ca(HUCB)_2$ at the centers of the purest black pigment and Ch stones, respectively.

Summary

Our understanding of increased biliary lithogenicity through Ch supersaturation of bile is slowly falling into place. From both the pathophysiological and physical-chemical viewpoints, the paradigms have radically changed from previously held beliefs. There appears to be no clear-cut abnormality in the enterohepatic cycling of BS to which Ch supersaturation of bile in the otherwise normal Western adult can now be directly attributed; rather, there is absolute biliary hypersecretion of Ch made possible by the expansion of an intrahepatic Ch pool derived from diet, plasma, or de novo synthesis that is recruitable for secretion into bile by the normal transhepatic flux of BS. In fact, in conditions where there is uncompensated intestinal loss of BS from the enterohepatic circulation, the patient appears to be at risk for $CaCO_3/Ca(HUCB)_2$ gallstones and not Ch gallstones [45]. The principal physical-chemical correlation of hypersecretion of biliary Ch is that bile contains more Ch-enriched PL vesicles than can be solubilized by BS. These vesicles are kept Ch-enriched by the ability of BS micelles, that may already be saturated with Ch but unsaturated with PL, to continuously dissolve vesicle PL. Vesicles are key solubilizers of excess Ch in bile, but also are involved in binding Ca^{2+} ions and UCB. Hence, vesicles appear to be intrinsically involved in the earliest stages of both Ch and pigment gallstones, explaining the appearance of Ch at the center of the purest pigment stones and Ca pigment at the center of the purest Ch stones.

References

1. Carey MC, O'Donovan MA (1984) Gallstone disease: current concepts on the epidemiology, pathogenesis and management. In: Petersdorf RG et al. (eds) Harrison's principles of internal medicine. Update V. McGraw-Hill, New York, pp 139–168
2. Carey MC, Small DM (1978) Physical-chemistry of cholesterol solubility in bile. Relationship to gallstone formation and dissolution in man. J Clin Invest 61:998–1026
3. Carey MC, Cohen DE (1987) Biliary transport of cholesterol in vesicles, micelles and liquid crystals. In: Paumgartner G, Stiehl A, Gerok W (eds) Bile acids and the liver. MTP Press, Lancaster, pp 287–300
4. Cohen DE, Angelico M, Carey MC (1989) Quasielastic light scattering evidence for vesicular secretion of biliary lipids. Am J Physiol 20:G1–G8
5. Mazer NA, Carey MC (1984) Mathematical model of biliary lipid secretion: a quantitative analysis of physiological and biochemical data from man and other species. J Lipid Res 25:932–953
6. Hofmann AF (1988) Pathogenesis of cholesterol gallstones. J Clin Gastroenterol 10:S1–S11
7. Carey MC, Cahalane MJ (1988) Enterohepatic circulation. In: Arias IM, Jacoby WB, Popper H, Schacter D, Shafritz D (eds) The liver: biology and pathobiology, 2nd ed. Raven, New York, pp 573–616
8. Pattinson NR, Chapman BA (1986) Distribution of biliary cholesterol between mixed micelles and non-micelles in relation to fasting and feeding in humans. Gastroenterology 91:697–702
9. Carey MC (1989) Formation of cholesterol gallstones: the new paradigms. In: Paumgartner G, Stiehl A, Gerok W (eds) Trends in bile acid research. Kluwer, Dordrecht, pp 259–281
10. Bilhartz LE, Spady DK, Dietschy JM (1989) Inappropriate hepatic cholesterol synthesis expands the cellular pool of sterol available for recruitment by bile acids in the rat. J Clin Invest 84:1181–1187
11. Turley SD, Dietschy JM (1988) The metabolism and excretion of cholesterol by the liver. In: Arias IM, Jacoby WB, Popper H, Schacter D, Shafritz D (eds) The liver: biology and pathobiology, 2nd ed. Raven, New York, pp 617–641
12. Small DM (1968) A classification of biologic lipids based upon their interaction in aqueous systems. J Am Oil Chem Soc 45:108–119
13. Lange Y, Swaisgood MH, Ramos BV, Steck TL (1989) Plasma membranes contain half the phospholipid and 90% of the cholesterol and sphingomyelin in cultured human fibroblasts. J Biol Chem 264:3786–3793
14. Lange Y, Ramos BV (1983) Analysis of the distribution of cholesterol in the intact cell. J Biol Chem 258:15130–15134
15. Small DM (1977) Liquid crystals in living and dying systems. J Colloid Interface Sci 58:581–602
16. Yeagle PL (1988) Biology of cholesterol. CRC Press, Boca Raton
17. Clarke CF, Edwards PA, Fogelman AM (1987) Cellular regulation of cholesterol metabolism. In: Gotto AM Jr (ed) Plasma lipoproteins. Elsevier, Amsterdam, pp 261–276
18. Myant NB (1981) The biology of cholesterol and related steroids. Heinemann, London, p 275
19. Fears R, Sabine JR (eds) (1986) Cholesterol 7α-hydroxylase (7α-monooxygenase). CRC Press, Boca Raton, pp 3–204
20. Scheibner J, Stange EF (1989) Elimination of secondary bile acids by colectomy induces bile acid synthesis in the rat. In: Paumgartner G, Stiehl A, Gerok W (eds) Trends in bile acid research. Kluwer, Dordrecht, pp 67–73
21. Einarsson K, Angelin B (1988) Pathogenesis of cholesterol gallstone disease: the secretory defect. In: Northfield T, Jazrawi R, Zentler-Munro P (eds) Bile acids in health and disease. Kluwer, Dordrecht, pp 99–116
22. Eriksson M, Berglund L, Rudling M, Henriksson P, Angelin B (1989) Effects of estrogen on low density lipoprotein metabolism in males. J Clin Invest 84:802–810
23. Henriksson P, Einarsson K, Eriksson A, Kelter U, Angelin B (1989) Estrogen-induced gallstone formation in males. J Clin Invest 84:811–816
24. DenBesten L, Connor WE, Bell S (1973) The effect of dietary cholesterol on the composition of human bile. Surgery 73:266–273
25. Lee DWT, Gilmore CJ, Bonorris G, Cohen H, Marks JW, Cho-Sue M, Meiselman M, Schoenfield LJ (1985) Effect of dietary cholesterol on biliary lipids in patients with gallstones and normal subjects. Am J Clin Nutr 42:414–420

26. Angelin B, Backman L, Einarsson K, Eriksson L, Ewerth S (1981) Hepatic cholesterol metabolism in obesity: activity of microsomal 3-hydroxy 3-methylglutaryl coenzyme A reductase. J Lipid Res 23:770–773
27. Miettinen TA (1970) Cholesterol production in obesity. Circulation 44:842–850
28. Ahlberg J, Angelin B, Björkhem I, Einarsson K, Leijd B (1979) Hepatic cholesterol metabolism in normo- and hyperlipidemic patients with cholesterol gallstones. J Lipid Res 20:107–115
29. Nervi F, Marinovic I, Rigotti A, Ulloa N (1988) Regulation of biliary cholesterol secretion: functional relationship between the canalicular and sinusoidal cholesterol secretory pathways in the rat. J Clin Invest 82:1818–1825
30. Nervi F, Bronfman M, Allalón W, Depiereux E, DelPozo R (1984) Regulation of biliary cholesterol secretion in the rat: role of hepatic cholesterol esterification. J Clin Invest 74:2226–2237
31. Stone BG, Erickson SK, Craig WY, Cooper AD (1985) Regulation of rat biliary cholesterol secretion by agents that allow intrahepatic cholesterol metabolism: evidence for a distinct biliary precursor pool. J Clin Invest 76:1773–1781
32. Coleman R, Rahman K, Bellringer ME, Carrella M (1988) Biliary lipid secretion and its control. In: Northfield T, Jazrawi R, Zentler-Munro P (eds) Bile acids in health and disease. Kluwer, Dordrecht, pp 43–60
33. Meier PJ (1989) The bile salt secretory polarity of hepatocytes. J Hepatol 9:124–129
34. Van der Linden W, Bergman F (1977) Formation and dissolution of gallstones in experimental animals. Int Rev Exp Pathol 17:173–233
35. Lamri Y, Roda A, Dumont M, Feldman G, Erlinger S (1988) Immunoperoxidase localization of bile salts in rat liver cells. Evidence for a role of the Golgi apparatus in bile salt transport. J Clin Invest 82:1173–1182
36. Möckel GM, Gorti S, Tanaka T, Carey MC (1988) Microscope laser light scattering of bile formation. Hepatology 8:1367 (Abst)
37. Sömjen GJ, Gilat T (1986) Changing concepts of cholesterol solubility in bile. Gastroenterology 91:772–775
38. Cohen DE, Carey MC (1990) Alteration of hepatic lipids in bile ducts and gallbladder. Hepatology (Suppl), in press
39. Cohen DE (1986) Studies of biliary lipid secretion and aggregation in model and native biles. PhD dissertation, Harvard University, pp 10–207
40. Cohen DE, Angelico M, Carey MC (1990) Structural alterations in lecithin-cholesterol vesicles following interactions with monomeric and micellar bile salts: physical-chemical basis for subselection of biliary lecithin species and aggregative states of biliary lipids during bile formation. J Lipid Res, in press
41. Cahalane MJ, Neubrand MW, Carey MC (1988) Physical-chemical pathogenesis of pigment gallstones. Semin Liver Dis 8:317–328
42. Holzbach RT, Barnhart RL, Nader JM (1988) Pathogenesis of cholesterol gallstone disease: the physico-chemical defect. In: Northfield T, Jazrawi R, Zentler-Munro P (eds) Bile acids in health and disease. Kluwer, Dordrecht, pp 117–133
43. Robins SJ, Fasulo JM, Patton GM (1982) Lipids of pigment gallstones. Biochim Biophys Acta 712:21–25
44. Mazer NA, Carey MC (1983) Quasielastic light scattering studies of aqueous biliary lipid systems. Cholesterol solubilization and precipitation in model bile solutions. Biochemistry 22:426–442
45. Magnuson TH, Lillemoe KD, Pitt HA (1989) The relationship of clinical risk factors to gallstone composition. Hepatology 10:738 (Abst)

Nucleation and Aggregation of Cholesterol Crystals in the Early Phase of Gallstone Genesis

G. Salvioli, R. Lugli, and M. Pellati

Patologia Speciale Medica, Università di Modena, Viale Vittorio Veneto 9, 41100 Modena, Italy

Introduction

Lipid composition does not seem to be a good criteria for discriminating between the bile of healthy subjects and that of patients with cholesterol gallstones (Table 1). About 30%–70% of healthy persons have bile supersaturated in cholesterol [37] and transported in varying proportions as mixed micelles (completely saturated only with cholesterol or 50% saturated with lecithin) and vesicles [60] having a larger size and greater ratio of cholesterol to phospholipids (Ch/PL ratio) than micelles [77]. Mixed micelles are frequently metastable, i.e., in a state of incomplete and unstable crystallinity which can drop to a lower free-energy level over time with the formation of different phases [76]. Vesicles have a greater cholesterol-solubilizing capacity (Ch/PL molar ratio approximately 1) than mixed micelles and can remain stable for a long time [18]. Therefore bile, like other biological systems, is thermodynamically unstable until its free energy reaches the minimum [29].

The phase diagram of human bile is presented in Fig. 1. The micellar zone contains an isotropic phase delimitated by the "tie line" connecting the points corresponding to the two equilibrium compositions. Micelles represent the most important form of cholesterol transport [16], but vesicles are normally present above all in hepatic bile and in diluted samples [77–79]. When the cholesterol content in bile exceeds that which can be solubilized by micelles, the excess is dispersed in vesicles having a high Ch/PL molar ratio and low concentration of bile salts.

It seems that cholesterol monohydrate (ChM) crystals arise from vesicles and to a lesser extent from mixed micelles [32, 54, 44]. This process is termed nucleation. The

Table 1. Composition of bile

	Control	Cholesterol stone
Cholesterol saturation index [95]	0.98	1.28[a]
Total lipid concentration (g%) [95]	10.1	9.0
Bile salts (molar %)	74.4	71.5
Phospholipids (molar %)	18.6	18.8
Cholesterol (molar %)	7.0	9.7[a]
Proteins (mg/ml) [95]	5.3	5.0
Glycoproteins [64]	0.55	1.60[a]
Hexosamine (μg/ml) [69]	83	137[a]
Viscosity (relative) [10]	2.85	3.24[a]
pH [81]		5.6–8.0

[a] $p<0.05$

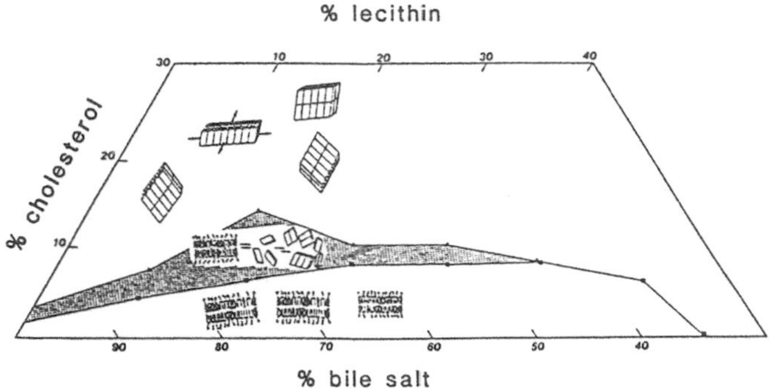

Fig. 1. Supersaturation in cholesterol in the zone above the micellar zone is metastable; it leads to spontaneous formation of vesicles which become more saturated in cholesterol, increasing both the ratio of bile salt to lecithin and the total lipid concentration of bile [39]. The nucleation of ChM is a phase change due to the appearance of a new phase (crystals). The more hydrophobic (deoxycholate and chenodeoxycholate) bile salts induce a greater proportion of mixed micelles to simple micelles and a wider micellar zone

interaction between a large number of particles and their clustering is the crucial point in ChM nucleation. A large interfacial area is a source of free energy, and further stabilization may be reached by decreasing this area [26, 44]; its driving force is the difference in solubility of cholesterol between different particles.

The process of nucleation can be evaluated by the nucleation time (NT), which furnishes a good discrimination between subjects with or without stones [36] than the cholesterol saturation index (CSI). Besides lipid content, biliary proteins may also play an important role in the nucleation process; the presence of protein-lipid complexes [46] or the possibility that the proteins normally present in bile are adsorbed onto the surface of the various particles can promote or inhibit the formation and growth of cholesterol crystals. This has been demonstrated for calcium salt crystals.

The growth of initial ChM crystals retained in the gallbladder constitutes the second phase in stone formation. The kinetics of crystal growth is complex; a better understanding of stone morphology should lead to a greater knowledge about this process. It is possible that the apparent growth is not actually growth per se, but a sort of stimulated renucleation.

Vesicles

The preparation of vesicles involves the input of a large amount of energy, but they can also be prepared by the dialysis of mixed micelles (or removing the detergents by other methods). Their diameter is greater than 200 Å and changes in relation to the lipid content [82].

The hydration of lipids determines some physiological properties [21], such as their density and their tendency to aggregate and to fuse [92]. Fusion and aggregation are terms frequently used together, but these processes are quite different. Liposomes and vesicles are stable structures that do not fuse spontaneously but have the tendency to aggregate by van der Waals attraction [92]. Even when vesicles are clustered in stable aggregates, another barrier must be overcome before the membranes of the vesicles come into close contact and fuse. The cause of the repulsive forces is the presence of the so-called hydration forces in the strongly hydrated polar groups of phospholipid molecules [66]. The bridging between opposed vesicles requires the disruption of "a wall of water" normally keeping the membranes separate [66], with the establishment of hydrophobic contact [42].

In general, the more fluid that is in the bilayers, the greater is the range of repulsive forces. Some molecules can be adsorbed onto or dissolved in the lipid bilayer; proteins are the most commonly represented and can exert an inhibiting or promoting effect on the process of aggregation-fusion. For example, insulin facilitates the fusion (exchange of lipid components) of vesicles, displacing the membrane-bound water through the interactions of vesicle surface-bound insulin [45]. The fusion is accomplished solely by lipid–lipid interactions between areas devoid of membrane proteins; this follows local destabilization of the normal bilayer [40].

Whereas negatively charged components (fatty acids are present in bile and may be incorporated into the vesicles) and counterions (such as Ca^{2+}) induce an attraction which overcomes the other repulsive forces, inducing adhesion and fusion [61], cholesterol increases the hydration of phosphatidylcholine molecules on the plane of the bilayer, exercising a marked ordering influence on bilayer lipids [40]; its presence can inhibit the fusion process induced, for example, by insulin [45]. Cholesterol content in biliary vesicles may be very high – native bile is rich in vesicles with a Ch/PL ratio over 1 [77] – and bare lipid patch formation could be a sufficient condition for the formation of large clustering [92]. The precipitation of ChM crystals from supersaturated vesicles is an important step [18, 40], and the growth of ChM crystals on or around vesicle aggregates has been demonstrated by light microscopy [32].

It should be noted that cholesterol is more soluble in water (10^{-8} *M*) than are phospholipids (10^{-10} *M*) [71]. Its desorption from bilayers increases with the molar percentage of cholesterol in vesicles [55, 56]. Moreover, the curvature of the lipid–water interface and the diameter of the particles modulate the process. The factors influencing the behavior of vesicles include: hydration, dehydration, repulsion, aggregation, fusion, cholesterol, calcium, high fluidity, charged phospholipids, fatty acids, pH, insulin, glycoproteins. Its transfer between vesicles may be an important stage in ChM crystal formation. Cholesterol monomers diffuse and may be adsorbed onto the hydrophobic domain of the mucin gel [17], which becomes the backbone for the nucleation process. Monomers of phospholipids diffuse faster into the water phase from mixed micelles than from vesicles [59]; bile salts (dihydroxy more than trihydroxy) reduce phospholipid stability in the bilayer and increase the rate of intervesicular phospholipid transfer. Therefore the composition of the bile acid pool could play a role in facilitating the process of cholesterol and phospholipid exchange occurring between particles, which might anticipate the crystallization.

The most important steps anticipating the appearance of ChM crystals are the following:

- Excess cholesterol not solubilized by the micelles is dispersed in larger vesicles (250–1300 Å) containing few bile salts [54].
- Aggregation and fusion of vesicles bring about birefringent crystalline droplets (>8000 Å) [54] which can be detected by light microscopy.
- Divalent cations ($Ca^{2+} > Mg^{2+}$) bind lecithin vesicles, reducing the repulsion between them [52].
- Vesicles with a Ch/PL ratio higher than 1 aggregate more easily, and ChM crystals can appear.
- When the phospholipid molar percentage is low (ratio of bile salts/phospholipids >5), nucleation occurs more rapidly; in these situations the vesicles are supersaturated in cholesterol and are unstable.
- In each case the formation of small vesicular aggregates anticipate the appearance of ChM crystals.

Cholesterol Monohydrate Crystals

ChM crystals are composed of regularly repeated blocks of unit structure having a triclinic growth system, indicating symmetry of the lattice. Each sheet of parallel cholesterol molecules contains molecules in a particular array (head:tail-tail:head-head-tail, etc.) [19]. Hydroxy groups are hydrogen bound to each other as well as to water molecules. The first single ChM crystals (not visible by light microscopy and not removed completely by ultracentrifugation), may be heterogeneous foci able to arise the crystallization rate until the crystal cluster reaches the critical size for nucleation [75] (see Fig. 2).

Crystals aggregate to one another to form large particles that become echogenic when their size is greater than 50 µm. The density of ChM (1.045 g/ml) is very close to that of micellar solutions, and their distribution in the centrifuge tube is not always at the bottom. Vesicles are lighter than micelles, and the density of gallbladder bile ranges from 1.040 g/ml at the bottom to 1.020 at the top (gallstone density ranges from 1.040 to 1.080 g/ml). This parameter is largely dependent on the ionic content and the Ch/PL molar ratio. Thureborn's data show that the upper part of the gallbladder contains particles with the highest Ch/PL molar ratio [84].

The presence of ChM crystals in bile is important if associated with evaluation of the NT of bile samples. This importance is due to the following:

- ChM crystals are present in the gallbladder bile of 74%–100% of gallstone subjects but are absent in normal subjects [68, 73].
- Gallbladder bile of subjects with cholesterol gallstones has ChM crystals or develops them within 48 h, whereas the bile of stone-free subjects does not, in spite of supersaturation [73].
- NT is shorter when the bile sample has (a) a high total lipid concentration; (b) a high molar ratio of bile salt to lecithin and a high CSI [32, 33] (these factors increase cholesterol transport in the vesicular phase); and (c) a high content of mucin [49, 51].
- Heterogeneous nucleation requires large particles as nuclei approximately (100–1000 Å), much larger than proteins and glycoproteins secreted by the liver [75].
- Gallbladder bile of subjects with cholesterol gallstones added to control bile reduces its nucleation rate [12].

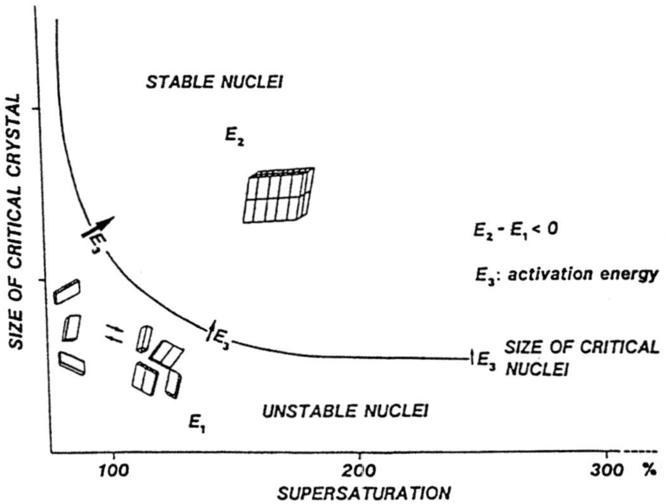

Fig. 2. Relationship between supersaturation and critical size of cholesterol crystals

Nucleation Time

NT is defined as the time necessary to observe the appearance of ChM crystals from a clear isotropic bile obtained after ultracentrifugation or ultrafiltration and incubated at 37 °C. The procedure for evaluating NT by light microscopy is the isotropic interphase of bile samples obtained by ultracentrifugation at 37 °C (100 000 *g* for 2 h) and incubated at 37 °C (in sterile tubes, under nitrogen). The samples are checked every day by polarized light microscopy; the appearance of visible (>1 μm) crystals indicates that nucleation has occurred. Airfuge allows the rapid preparation of samples for microscopic examination. Problems related to the determination of NT include:

- Failure of ultracentrifugation and ultrafiltration to remove very small crystals which allow heterogeneous nucleation.
- The optical method is specific but not sensitive.
- Sedimented materials adsorb lecithin.
- The materials used in the incubation set can influence the results.
- Coulter counter is not accurate enough to evaluate the size of ChM crystals since they have an anisometric shape
- Duodenal bile is not useful for NT determination since it contains less phospholipid [87].

The NT determined by light microscopy is a cumulative index either for true nucleation (process with submicroscopic dimension) or for the first phase of the growth process. Artificial bile has a lower NT (80- to 100-fold) than does human bile, indicating a higher metastability [41]. In both types of bile, the NT decreases when either the CSI or the Ch/PL molar ratio of vesicles is increased [33].

Factors influencing NT include the following:

- The bile salt/phospholipid ratio [44] and the calcium ion concentration [85] alter both the NT of model bile and the number of vesicles.
- Apolipoproteins A-I and A-II are antinucleating agents at very low concentrations [38].
- Crude preparations of biliary proteins may inhibit cholesterol nucleation [38], but inhibitors and promoters of nucleation may coexist in the same sample [13].
- Mucin has a nucleating effect only at high concentrations (>2 mg/ml) [51], but no difference in amount or composition of mucus was found in gallbladder bile from patients with or without gallstones [69, 90]. However the ratio of glycoprotein to protein in bile is increased in gallstone bile [64].
- Bilirubinate and calcium shortens NT, but the reduction of Ca^{2+} concentration in bile with EDTA does not change NT [27].
- Mucin probably does not have a potent concanavalin A binding, nucleation-promoting activity since it contains mannose or glucose and is resistant to pronase. Moreover, it is active at concentrations below 50 μg/ml [31].

It seems, however, that cholesterol gallstone bile contains potent nucleating factors; the greatest dilution that induces a significant shortening of NT of a supersaturated model bile (CSI = 1.20) indicates the nucleation-promoting activity titer [23]. The process of nucleation requires energy; moreover, the molecules of cholesterol should diffuse well and must be in sufficient number to reach the critical size. An important point is that the free energy to reach the critical size decreases increasing the CSI. All particles larger than critical size grow, while those smaller dissolve [28].

Nucleation may be influenced by foreign material surfaces in the form of nonspecific localized material or by the presence of a sufficent number of molecules fixed in relative positions corresponding to lattice sites (epitaxial growth) [28].

Surface defects are fundamental for deposition to occur, and the presence of nucleating and antinucleating factors play an important modulating role. Under physiological conditions, first small ChM crystals are emptied into the intestine during each meal, but on the condition that gallbladder motility is in the normal range, and that the bile has a normal viscosity.

The rheological properties of bile influences its flow behavior. Hepatic bile viscosity is less than that of gallbladder bile [10], and gallstone bile has a higher viscosity than normal bile [10]. The concentration of bile during its stay in the gallbladder and the presence of mucous substances produced by the gallbladder wall are the major factors regulating the viscosity of bile. When a low-viscosity fluid, such as hepatic bile, pushes a high-viscosity fluid, such as gallbladder bile, a fluid instability occurs and interfacial phenomena appear. Concentrated biles emit a high-intensity spin echo signal whereas hepatic bile produces a low-intensity signal. After gallbladder emptying, dilute hepatic bile settles on top of the concentrated bile the two emitting signals, of different intensity [7, 41].

Hepatic bile rich in vesicles does not mix homogeneously and rapidly with the denser bile of gallbladder. A phenomenon referred to as stratification occurs inducing a higher concentration of solute in the lower region of the glallbladder [83, 84], whereas the upper fractions, as reported above, contain particles with a high Ch/PL ratio; these are more unstable and can induce ChM crystal formation after their adhesion and fusion (Fig. 3). In Table 2 NT values obtained by various authors are listed.

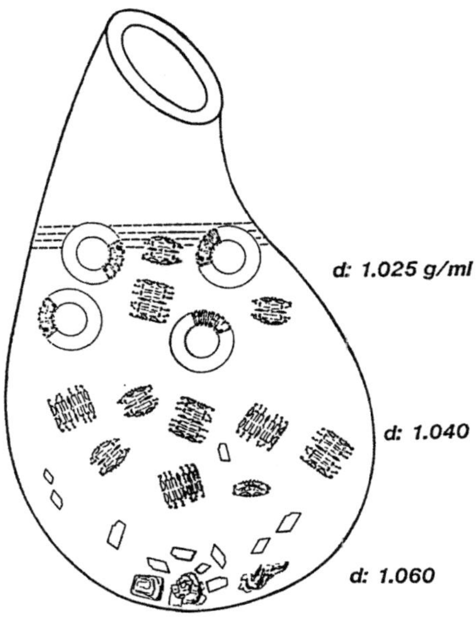

Fig. 3. Stratification of bile within the gallbladder indicates that the less dense bile is discharged first; in fact, the layers of lowest specific gravity reside near the neck and cystic duct [58]. Fluid instability occurs when a less viscous fluid flows into the more viscous fluid with formation of viscous fingers [22, 93]. In these low-density layers, large particles are characterized by high Ch/PL molar ratio; the lower layers also have a greater content of very detergent bile salts (DCA) [58]. The gallbladder wall produces mucin, a polymer containing 75%–80% carbohydrates; above 2 mg/ml mucin aggregates forming a gel [74]

Table 2. Nucleation time in unseeded biles

Reference	Bile samples	NT (days)	CSI
Holan et al. [36]	GB controls	3–21	0.86
	GB-GS	2–4	1.13
Gollish et al. [30]	GB-controls	14.0	ND
	GB-GS	1.88	ND
	H-GS	7–31	ND
Harvey et al. [34]	GB-controls	14.8	ND
	GB-GS	2.6	ND
Whiting and Watts [89]	GB-controls	6–21	0.90
	GB-GS	2–10	1.70

GB, Gallbladder; GS, gallstone; H, hepatic; ND, no data.

Table 3. Distribution of cholesterol between micellar and vesicle phases in bile

Reference	Bile	Method	% of cholesterol in	
			Vesicles	Micelles
Sömjen and Gilat [78]	GB	Column [a]	24–57	11–55
Peled et al. [63]	GB	Column [a]	11.1	88.9
	H		30.9	69.1
Pattinson and Chapman [62]	H	Ult [c]	35–65	35–65
Lee et al. [50]	GB	Column [b]	31.8	68.2
	H	Ult [d]	71.6	28.4

GB, gallbladder bile; H, Hepatic bile; Ult, ultracentrifugation.
[a] Sephacryl eluted with buffer containing taurocholate 10 m*M*
[b] Sephadex G-75 eluted with 1.75 m*M* taurodeoxycholate
[c] Ultracentrifugation in sucrose gradient
[d] Ultracentrifugation in CsCl density gradient

Particles Promoting Cholesterol Monohydrate Crystals

The percentage of cholesterol transported by vesicles increases when the CSI rises, and when the total lipid concentration decreases [39] (see Table 3). Peled et al. [63] showed that the percentage of cholesterol carried by vesicles increases with the Ch/PL molar ratio in bile. Comparing the NT of vesicles and that of micelles, the same authors demonstrated that vesicles nucleate more rapidly than micelles [63]; this result accords with the data of Lee et al. [48]. The Ch/PL ratio of vesicles rises with the bile salt/phospholipid ratio of model biles: similarly, the NT of solutions declines [32].

Proteins (about 5% of biliary constituents by dry weight) are associated with biliary lipids [47, 95]; during gel chromatography of gallbladder bile, cholesterol, phospholipids and bile salts are coeluted with apolipoproteins A-I and A-II [38]. The partition of proteins between vesicles and micelles is a very important point, considering the possible influence on NT. Proteins may be incorporated into the liposomal bilayers during the transition from micelle to bilayer [94]. But adsorption of proteins (such as apolipoproteins) to the lecithin monolayer changes with their composition and is influenced by the addition of cholesterol [45, 67].

Bile acids have different detergencies [deoxycholic acid (DCA) > chenodeoxycholic acid (CDCA) > cholic acid (CA) > ursodeoxycholic acid (UDCA)] and this influences the percentages of particles (single and mixed micelles, vesicles) present in bile [72]. Vesicles contain low concentrations of bile salt which bind exclusively to the outer membrane leaflet, since their transbilayer movement (flip-flop) is slow [14]. The binding of most hydrophilic bile salts, such as UDCA, to the bilayer is lower than that of hydrophobic bile acid, such as deoxycholate [74]. UDCA induces a very slow solubilization of phosphatidylcholine liposomes [70] in comparison to the other bile salts. Moreover, the phase diagram of tauroursodeoxycholate almost completely lacks the phase 2 region [70]. Therefore, the bile acid composition of the biliary pool should play a role either influencing cholesterol saturation or favoring the formation of supersaturated and metastable vesicles; the detergency of the bile salt pool also modulates the interactions between lipid and proteins on the surface of particles, as does bile viscosity, modifying the threshold of its sol-gel transition [74].

Although Groen et al. [31] did not observe variations in NT when hydrophilic bile salts were replaced with the most detergent ones, Hofmann et al. [35] found that bile CSI of male patients with gallstones is positively correlated with DCA percentage in bile and negatively correlated with CDCA. Our data (Table 4) confirm these data; however, the DCA percentage shows the greatest correlation with CSI of bile. Ahlberg et al. [2] reported a high proportion of DCA in the bile of subjects at risk of developing gallstones. Our data on artificial biles show that DCA-rich bile nucleates faster than UDCA-rich bile, having the same value for cholesterol saturation (160%). The prevalence of ursodeoxycholate makes less hydrophobic the biliary pool so that liposomes are easily formed [70].

Table 4. Lipid composition of bile in healthy subjects and cholesterol gallstone patients

	Controls ($n=23$)	Cholesterol gallstones ($n=48$)
TLC (g/dl)	12.4 ±2.6	11.7 ±3.1
Ch (molar %)	7.7 ±1.7	9.9 ±2[a]
PL (molar %)	20.6 ±3.1	20.8 ±2.7
BS (molar %)	71.6 ±4.2	69.1 ±4.4[b]
CSI	1.09±0.2	1.39±0.2[a]
LCA (molar %)	2.2 ±0.7	1.8 ±0.7
DCA (molar %)	18.9 ±8.0	31.6 ±8.6[a]
CDC (molar %)	38.7 ±4.6	36.6 ±7.7
CA (molar %)	39.5 ±7.3	29.5 ±5[a]

[a] $p<0.001$
[b] $p<0.027$
LCA, Lithocolic acid; DCA, deoxycolic acid; CDCA chenodeoxycholic acid; CA, cholic acid; TLC, total lipid concentration. Values indicate the percentages evaluated by gas liquid chromatography.

Other Factors Influencing Nucleation

Cholesterol stones seldom contain other materials such as carbonate and phosphate. At very low concentrations (under 4%) they do not modify the radiolucency of cholesterol gallstones [86].

Calcium precipitation in bile is believed to be important in the initiation of pigmented and also of cholesterol gallstones. Calcium salts may represent a nidus on which cholesterol precipitates from supersaturated bile [85]. The precipitation of calcium salts on the surface of cholesterol stones occurs spontaneously or during bile acid therapy. In the presence of ionized Ca^{2+} many anions (carbonate, phosphate, bilirubinate, fatty acids) are precipitable when the solubility product of a given salt is exceeded; the particles produced (10–100 nm in diameter) reduce the free energy required for critical nucleus formation. Calcium induces interparticle binding whereas other cations may facilitate the aggregation by charge neutralization of the polar groups present on the surfaces of vesicles. Ca^{2+} induces the fusion of charged vesicles [61] but also that of bilayers [52], reducing the repulsive forces between them.

Vesicles and liposomes have been used as models for understanding calcium salt precipitation. Bile salts behave as Ca^{2+} ionophores in artificial membranes [1, 76]. Toor et al. [85] demonstrated a great influence of calcium on the growth rate of ChM crystals. Ca^{2+} binding to a neutral lipid monolayer is weak but induces a conformational change in the lecithin phosphatidylcholine polar group: one calcium molecule coordinates with two phosphatidylcholine molecules [5]. Moreover, sonication in the presence of CA^{2+} induces the formation of vesicles smaller than those formed in the absence of Ca^{2+}, with high cuvature coupled with high membrane fluidity and disorder; under these conditions their fusion is easier [15].

The presence of phosphate lowers by three- to fourfold the concentration of calcium required for the fusion of charged vesicles [26] or of vesicles containing low percentages of charged lipids; vesicle fusion occurs when calcium phosphate precipitation is initiated, suggesting that crystal nucleation on the vesicle surface is the initial event. Calcium forms complexation products with some carbohydrates influencing the physicochemical properties of some biliary glycoproteins [6].

Radiolucent stones containing high relative amounts of calcium bilirubinate (7% of weight) and calcium carbonate (7%) in the outer layer are frequently resistant to medical dissolution therapy [3]. The problem is determining whether these components enter the stones before or after their formation.

Cholesterol Crystal Growth

Whereas the first crystals of ChM have an ordered structure, the growth process leads to more complex structures depending on the aggregation of the first particles, a process proceeding cluster by cluster or with deposition of individual particles [8, 43]. While NT can be defined as the earliest time required for the detection of solid crystals of cholesterol, the growth time is the time necessary to double the initial number of ChM in seeded bile [88, 89].

Ultrafiltered bile is mixed with 100 µl ChM suspension (previously prepared by sonication), and then incubated at 37 °C. The number of crystals is checked at the beginning and then each day using a hemacytometer and polarized light microscopy in order to count the number of crystals [88, 89]. The observation ends when the number of ChM crystals found is twice the initial value. The problems are that (a) neither ultracentrifugation nor ultrafiltration completely eliminates the submicroscopic solid ChM crystals from bile, and (b) the aggregation of crystals may induce counting errors. The size of ChM crystals can be evaluated by a Coulter counter, but this method does not distinguish between crystals and other particles. Whiting and Watts proposed the isolation by filtration of labeled ChM crystals; this method allows the evaluation of cholesterol mass precipitated over time and the time lag in different situations [88]. These authors found that the mass of cholesterol formed is great at low bile salt/phospholipid ratios and is reduced with an increasing molar proportion of phospholipids [90].

Some bile samples from normal subjects show a growth time similar to that of gallstone patients [89]. From this observation Whiting and Watts infer that stone-free bile lacks a nucleating agent. The same authors demonstrated that the CSI of bile supporting crystal growth is usually greater than 0.8 [89]. Other authors have studied the growth of cholesterol crystal in seeding conditions measuring the amount of ChM formed after the addition of nucleating agents such as calcium bilirubinate, hydroxyapatite, and $CaCO_3$: the cholesterol produced in 24 h was 1640, 1440, and 1120 μg respectively (800 μg in unseeded condition) [91].

ChM crystal growth is slower than that of ionic crystals. In vivo the rate of stone growth was 1–4 mm per year [57]. Important questions include: why crystal agglomerates adapt close packing, why some continue to grow, and why others stop. It is possible that the coherence of particles in the stones is a function of the surface and shape of the solid-phase particles; moreover, the presence of an organic matrix in the stones could play an important role. Surface characteristics probably favor further precipitation, whereas calcium rim formation makes the stones resistant to possible changes in shape and size. Transport and diffusion of individual cholesterol molecules regulate the growth of ChM crystals; these properties are influenced by bile viscosity [22], high viscosity slowing the movement of molecules reducing crystal growth rate. Therefore, mucin should slow the growth of crystals.

The kind of nucleator (in the case of heterogeneous nucleation) can modify both the rate of crystallization and the pattern of crystals grown [8]. In general, crystal growth may follow different models, such as spiral growth, water adsorption layer, and polynuclear. The rate of crystal growth is not a simple or linear function of the supersaturation. This favors the screw dislocation model of growth, but the rheological properties of bile may induce local supersaturation areas with consequent modification of the shape of the crystal and of the stones. An ellipsoid shape is characteristic of conditions in which a plethora of dislocations occur, such as in diffusion-controlled growth; if diffusion is destroyed by stirring, there is a uniform deposition, and the shape becomes more spherical.

The antinucleating agents should also be active in this phase of stone formation, as occurs in urine where certain mucopolysaccharides, such as heparin, inhibit the aggregation of calcium oxalate. The adsorption of antinucleating agents on the crystal could inhibit its growth, producing a barrier between the crystal surface and solution molecules and thereby reducing the rate of crystal propagation.

Relationships Between Biliary Proteins and Nucleation/Growth Processes

The concentration of protein in the gallbladder bile of patients with gallstones is similar to that in control subjects [39, 95], but the glycoprotein/protein ratio is greater in the former (Table 1). Glycoproteins speed up the nucleation of cholesterol [50], but filtration through a 300 000 dalton cutoff ultrafilter removes large proteins without affecting NT [80]. The crucial point seems to be: (a) the nature of biliary proteins, (b) their partition between particles present in bile, and (c) their activity (promoting or inhibiting) on nucleation and growth processes.

Biliary proteins are represented by transport and enzymatic proteins, immunoglobulins, enzymes associated with hepatocyte membrane, hormones, and glycoproteins [47]. Albumin is present in bile and solubilizes small amounts of cholesterol [71]. Glycoproteins have been studied in depth; they have a great water-binding capacity (in particular the glycosylated chains of mucin). The increased secretion of mucus by the gallbladder wall (an early event in the study of experimental gallstones) also explains the reduced acidification of gallbladder bile observed in gallbladder subjects [20] due to its H^+ ion buffering capacity; others, however, have not confirmed this result [53]. Carey and Cahalane [17] point out the importance of the gel matrix of bile as an inducer of nucleation/growth of ChM crystals. The role of mucin as a stone inducer is not clear: Whiting and Watts did not find a correlation between NT and the hexosamine content of the gallbladder bile [90]. However the inhibition of glycoprotein synthesis with anti-inflammatory drugs reduced stone formation during fasting in obese patients [11].

Some biological fluids are multicomponent solutions in which competitive adsorption may occur. When proteins are adsorbed onto the surface of the early crystals, they may concentrate and bind sufficient ions or other compounds favoring the nucleation on their surface. For example, urate crystals bind albumin accelerating the nucleation process in vitro [65]. However this does not seem to be the case for ChM crystals.

Some proteins promoting the nucleation/growth of crystals are β-sheet structured and rich in aspartic acid [25]; their adsorption on crystal nuclei can exert an inhibitory effect changing the curvature of the surface [25]. The antifreeze polypeptide is a single α-helix alanine-rich protein with a flexible rod conformation, binding to the faces of ice nuclei. It is able to destroy any long-range order. The antinucleating agents are active in the solid phase, the solution phase, and the solid-liquid interphase.

Unfortunately no clear data are available about the nature of biliary proteins influencing cholesterol nucleation. The efficacy of their activity could be prevented by binding to other components of bile; for example, phospholipids are sometimes the physiological binding site for proteins [67].

Apolipoprotein A-I at very low concentrations, resembling those of human bile, influences the transition of micelles to vesicles upon dilution [24]. This physicochemical behavior could explain the antinucleating effect of high-density apolipoproteins [24].

Conclusions

The problems in understanding nucleation/growth processes of cholesterol in bile are many and are related to the knowledge of risk factors for the development of cholelithiasis [9].

The steps in cholesterol stone formation are:

1. Formation of vesicles very rich in cholesterol.
2. Aggregation and fusion of these at a rate influenced by promoting and inhibiting factors (which must be defined). These are probably proteins or polypeptides binding lipids in different ways.
3. Departure of cholesterol from liposomes to form crystals when the initial cluster reaches a critical size (which is influenced by the CSI).
4. The intervention of a gel matrix is probable, particularly when hypersecretion of mucus and bile stasis induce the entrapment of particulate matter from bile (biliary sludge) [48].
5. The kinetics of ChM crystal growth is not a clarified process. It is regulated by surface phenomena leading to the formation of stones having solely a round or a faceted shape and variable size. The factors conditioning different solidification patterns are un-

known, but these are certainly influenced by surface structure, degree of supersaturation of bile, and the diffusion onto the surface of the solute.

References

1. Abramson JJ, Shamoo AE (1979) Anionic detergents as divalent cation ionophores across black lipid membranes. J Membr Biol 50:241–255
2. Ahlberg J, Angelin B, Einarsson K (1980) Biliary lipid composition in normo- and hyperlipoproteinemia. Gastroenterology 79:90–94
3. Alvisi V, Bigi A, Marchetti F, Pazzi P, Roversi N (1988) Structural and chemical characterization of gallstones resistant to dissolution therapy. J Inorg Biochem 3:109–116
4. Armstrong MJ, Carey MC (1982) The hydrophobic-hydrophilic balance of bile salts. Inverse correlation between reverse-phase high performance liquid chromatographic mobilities and micellar cholesterol-solubilizing capacities. J Lipid Res 23:70–80
5. Attenbach C, Seeling J (1984) Ca^{2+} binding to phosphatidylcholine bilayers as studied by deuterium magnetic resonance. Evidence for the formation of a Ca^{2+} complex with two phospholipid molecules. Biochemistry 23:3913–3920
6. Austgen M, Ferber E, Trendelenburg F (1983) Die Phospholipide im Sekret der zentralen Atemwege. Prax Klin Pneumol 37:751–752
7. Bakan DA, Barnhart JL (1988) Determination of parameters affecting proton relaxation of hepatic and gallbladder biles in dogs. Hepatology 8:341–346
8. Barone JP, Svrjcek D, Nancollas GH (1983) The crystal growth of barium fluoride in aqueous solutions. J Crystal Growth 62:27–33
9. Bennion LJ, Grundy SM (1978) Risk factors for the development of cholelithiasis in man. N Engl J Med 299:1161–1167
10. Bouchier IDA, Cooperband SR, El Kodsi BM (1985) Mucous substances and viscosity of normal and pathological human bile. Gastroenterology 49:343–353
11. Broomfield PH, Chopra R, Sheinbaum RC, Bonorris CG, Silverman A, Schoenfield LJ, Marks JW (1988) Effects of ursodeoxycholic acid and aspirin on the formation of lithogenic bile and gallstones during loss of weight. N Engl J Med 319:1567–1572
12. Burnstein MJ, Ilson RG, Petrunka CN, Taylor RD, Strasberg SM (1983) Evidence for a potent nucleating factor in the gallbladder bile of patients with cholesterol gallstones. Gastroenterology 85:801–807
13. Busch N, Matrinck NY, Cottle A, Mancuso DJ, Tokumo H, Holzbach RT (1988) Inhibiting and promoting effects on cholesterol crystal nucleation are found in protein fractions from normal human gallbladder bile (GBB) Hepatology 8:88 (abstr)
14. Cabral DJ, Small DM, Lilly HS, Hamilton JA (1987) Transbilayer movement of bile ends in model membranes. Biochemistry 26:1801–1804
15. Calbow K, Avramovic-Zikic O, Wessel S (1981) The effect of divalent cations on the interaction of dipalmitoyl phosphatidylcholine vesicles. J Coll Interface Sci 82:233–239
16. Carey MC, Small DM (1978) The physical chemistry of cholesterol solubility in bile. J Clin Invest 61:988–1026
17. Carey MC, Cahalane MJ (1988) Whither biliary sludge? Gastroenterology 95:508–523
18. Collins JJ, Phillips MC (1982) The stability and structure of cholesterol-rich codispersion of cholesterol and phosphatidylcholine. J Lipid Res 23:291–298
19. Craven BM (1976) Crystal structure of cholesterol monohydrate. Nature 260:727–729
20. Crawford N, Brooke BN (1955) The pH buffering power of human bile. Lancet 1:1096–1097
21. Crowe JH, Crowe LM (1988) Factors affecting the stability of dry liposomes. Biochim Biophys Acta 939:327–334
22. Cussler EL, Evans DF, De Palma RG (1970) A model for gallbladder function and cholesterol gallstone formation. Proc Natl Acad Sci USA 67:400–407
23. Drapers JAG, Groen AK, Stout JPJ, Noordam C, Hoek FJ, Jansen PLM, Tytgat GNJ (1987) Quantification of cholesterol nucleation promoting activity in human gallbladder bile. Clin Chim Acta 165:295–302
24. Donovan JM, Benedek GB, Carey MC (1987) Formation of mixed micelles and vesicles of human apolipoproteins A-I and A-II with synthetic and natural lecithins and the bile salts sodium taurocholate: quasi-elastic light scattering studies. Biochemistry 26:8125–8133

25. Feeney RE, Burcham TS (1986) Antifreeze glycoproteins from polar fish blood. Ann Rev Biophys Biophys Chem 15:59–78
26. Fraley R, Wilschut J, Düzgünes N, Smith C, Papahadjopoulos D (1980) Studies on the mechanism of membrane fusion: role of phosphate in promoting calcium ion fusion of phospholipid vesicles. Biochemistry 19:6021–6029
27. Gallinger S, Harvey PRC, Petrunka CN, Strasberg SM (1986) Effect of binding of ionised calcium on the in vitro nucleation of cholesterol and calcium bilirubinate in human gallbladder bile. Gut 27:1382–1386
28. Garside J (1982) Nucleation. In: Nancollas GH (ed) Biological mineralization and demineralization. Dahlem Konferenzen. Springer, Berlin Heidelberg New York, pp 23–35
29. Gibbs JW (1961) The scientific papers, Vol 1. Dover, New York
30. Gollish SH, Burnstein MJ, Ilson RG, Petrunka CN, Strasberg SM (1983) Nucleation of cholesterol monohydrate-crystals from hepatic and gallbladder bile of patients with cholesterol gallstones. Gut 24:836–844
31. Groen AK, Stout JPJ, Drapers JAG, Hoek FJ, Grijm R, Tytgat GNJ (1988) Cholesterol nucleation-influencing activity in T-tube bile. Hepatology 8:347–352
32. Halpern Z, Dudley MA, Kibe A, Lynn MP, Breuer AC, Holzbach RT (1986) Rapid vesicle formation and aggregation in abnormal human biles. A time-lapse video-enhanced contrast microscopy study. Gastroenterology 90:875–885
33. Halpern Z, Dudley MA, Lynn MP, Nader JM, Breuer AC, Holzbach RT (1986) Vesicle aggregation in model systems of supersaturated bile: relation to crystal nucleation and lipid composition of the vesicular phase. J Lipid Res 27:295–306
34. Harvey PCR, Rupar CA, Gallinger S, Petrunka CN, Strasberg SN (1986) Quantitative and qualitative comparison of gallbladder mucus glycoprotein from patients with or without gallstones. Gut 27:374–381
35. Hofmann AF, Grundy SM, Lachin JM, Lan SP, Baum RA, Hanson RF, Hersh T, Hightower NC Jr, Marks JW, Mekhijan H, Shaefer RA, Soloway RD, Thistle JL, Thomas FB, Tyor MP, National Cooperative Gallstone Study Group (1982) Pretreatment biliary lipid composition in white patients with radiolucent gallstones in the National Cooperative Gallstone Study. Gastroenterology 83:738–752
36. Holan KR, Holzbach RT, Hermann RE, Cooperman AM, Claffey NJ (1979) Nucleation time: key factor in the pathogenesis of cholesterol gallstone disease. Gastroenterology 77:611–617
37. Holzbach RT, Marsh M, Olszewski M, Holan K (1973) Cholesterol solubility in bile: evidence that supersaturated bile is frequent in healthy man. J Clin Invest 52:1457–1479
38. Holzbach RT, Kibe A, Thiel E, Howell JH, Marsh M, Hermann RE (1984) Biliary proteins. Unique inhibitors of cholesterol crystal nucleation in human gallbladder bile. J Clin Invest 73:35–45
39. Holzbach RT (1984) Metastability behaviour of supersaturated bile. Hepatology 4:1559–1589
40. Horn RG (1984) Direct measurement of the force between two lipid bilayers and observation of their fusion. Biochim Biophys Acta 778:224–228
41. Hricak H, Filly RA, Margulis AR, Moon KL, Crooks LE, Kaufman L (1983) Work in progress: nuclear magnetic resonance imaging of the gallbladder. Radiology 147:481–484
42. Israelachvili JN, McGuiggan PM (1988) Forces between surfaces in liquids. Science 241:795–800
43. Kahlweit M (1975) Ostwald ripening of precipitates. Adv Colloid Interf Sci 5:1–35
44. Kibe A, Dudley MA, Halpern Z, Lynn MP, Breuer AC, Holzbach RT (1985) Factors affecting cholesterol monohydrate crystal nucleation time in model systems of supersaturated bile. J Lipid Res 26:1102–1111
45. Lai JY, Chow DD, Hwang KJ (1988) Effect of lipid composition on insulin-mediated fusion of small unilamellar liposomes: a kinetic study. J Pharm Sci 77:432–437
46. Lairon DH, La Font H, Hauton JC (1972) Lack of mixed micelles bile salt-lecithin-cholesterol in bile and the presence of a lipoproteic complex. Biochimie 54:529–530
47. La Russo NF (1984) Proteins in bile: how they get there and what they do. Am J Physiol 247:G199–G205
48. Lee SP, Nicholls JF (1986) Nature and composition of biliary sludge. Gastroenterology 90:677–686
49. Lee TJ, Smith BF (1987) Gallbladder mucin accelerates cholesterol crystal nucleation from cholesterol; enriched vesicles in model bile. Gastroenterology 92:1748 (abstr)

50. Lee SP, Park HZ, Madani H, Kaler EW (1987) Partial characterization of a non micellar system of cholesterol solubilization in bile. Am J Physiol 252:375–383 G
51. Levy PF, Smith BF, La Mont JT (1984) Human gallbladder mucin accelerates nucleation of cholesterol in artificial bile. Gastroenterology 87:270–275
52. Lis LJ, Lis WT, Parsegian VA, Rand RP (1981) Adsorption of divalent cations to a variety of phosphatidylcholine bilayers. Biochemistry 20:1771–1777
53. Magnuson TH, Lillemoe KD, Zarkin BA, Pitt HA (1988) Patients with gallstones acidify bile normally. Hepatology 8:1224 (abstr)
54. Mazer NA, Carey MC (1983) Quasi elastic light scattering studies of aqueous biliary lipid systems cholesterol solubilization and precipitation in model bile solutions. Biochemistry 22:426–442
55. Mc Lean LR, Phillips MC (1982) Cholesterol desorption from cluster of phosphatidylcholine and cholesterol in unilamellar vesicle bilayers during lipid transfer or exchange. Biochemistry 21:4053–4059
56. Mc Lean LR, Phillips MC (1984) Cholesterol transfer from small and large unilamellar vesicles. Biochim Biophys Acta 776:21–26
57. Mok HYI, Druffel ERM, Rampone WM (1986) Chronology of cholelithiasis. Dating gallstones from atmospheric radiocarbon produced by nuclear bomb explosions. N Engl J Med 314:1075–1077
58. Nakayama F, van der Linden W (1975) Stratification of bile in the gallbladder and gallstone formation. Surg Gynecol Obstet 141:587–590
59. Nichols JW (1988) Phospholipid transfer between phosphatidylcholine-taurocholate mixed micelles. Biochemistry 27:3925–3931
60. Olszewski MF, Holzbach RT, Saupe A, Brown GH (1973) Liquid crystals in human bile. Nature 242:336–337
61. Ortiz A, Gomez-Fernandez JC (1988) Calcium-induced aggregation of phosphatidylcholine vesicles containing free oleic-acid. Chem Phys Lipids 46:256–266
62. Pattinson NR, Chapman BA (1986) Distribution of biliary cholesterol between mixed micelles and nonmicelles in relation to fasting and feeding in humans. Gastroenterology 91:697–702
63. Peled Y, Halpern Z, Baruch R, Goldman G, Gilat T (1988) Cholesterol nucleation from its carrier in human bile. Hepatology 8:914–918
64. Perdigoto R, Yamazaki K, La Russo NF (1988) Biliary glycoproteins: quantitative differences in subjects with and without gallstones. Hepatology 8:1257 (abstr)
65. Perl-Treves D, Addadi L (1988) A structural approach to pathological crystallizations. Gout: the possible role of albumin in sodium urate crystallization. Proc R Soc Lond [Biol] p 235:145–159
66. Rand RP (1981) Interacting phospholipid bilayers: measured forces and induced structural changes. Annu Rev Biophys Bioengin 10:277–314
67. Rossi JD, Wallace BA (1983) Binding of fibronectin to phospholipid vesicles. J Biol Chem 258:3327–3331
68. Sahlin S, Ahlberg J, Angelin B, Ewerth S, Nilsell K, Reihnér E (1988) Occurrence of cholesterol monohydrate crystals in gallbladder and hepatic bile in man: influence of bile acid treatment. Eur J Clin Invest 18:386–390
69. Sahlin S, Danielson A, Angelin B, Reihnér E, Henriksson R, Einarsson K (1988) Mucin in gall bladder bile of gall stone patients: influence of treatment with chenodeoxycholic and ursodeoxycholic acid. Gut 29:1506–1510
70. Salvioli G, Igimi H, Carey MC (1983) Cholesterol gallstone dissolution in bile. Dissimilar kinetics of crystalline cholesterol monohydrate by conjugated chenodeoxycholate-lecithin and conjugated ursodeoxycholate-lecithin mixtures: dissimilar phase equilibria and dissolution mechanisms. J Lipid Res 24:701–720
71. Salvioli G, Lugli R, Pradelli JM (1987) Solubilization of cholesterol by high density lipoproteins. Atherosclerosis Rev 16:87–94
72. Schubert R, Schmidt KH (1988) Structural changes in vesicle membranes and mixed micelles in various lipid compositions after binding of different bile salts. Biochemistry 27:8787–8794
73. Sedaghat A, Grundy SM (1980) Cholesterol crystals and the formation of cholesterol gallstones. N Engl J Med 302:1274–1277
74. Shiau YF, Reed M (1986) Phase transition of mucus. Gastroenterology 90:1631 (abstr)

75. Small DM (1981) The staging of cholesterol gallstones with respect to nucleation and growth. In: Paumgartner G, Stiehl A, Gerok W (eds) Bile acids and lipids. MTP Press, Lancaster, pp 291–300
76. Smallwood RA, Restall CJ, Chapman D (1981) Bile salts interactions: the effect of sodium taurocholate (NaTC) on the permeability of lipid bilayer to water and urea. In: Paumgartner G, Stiehl A, Gerok W (eds) Bile acids and lipids. MTP Press, Lancaster, pp 171–180
77. Sömjen GJ, Gilat T (1983) A non-micellar mode of cholesterol transport in human bile. FEBS Lett 156:265–268
78. Sömjen GJ, Gilat T (1985) Contribution of vesicular and micellar carriers to cholesterol transport in human bile. J Lipid Res 26:699–704
79. Sömjen GJ, Harvey PRC, Rosenberg R, Werbin N, Strasberg SM, Gilat T (1988) Quantitation of phospholipid vesicles and their cholesterol content in human bile by quasi-elastic light scattering. Biochim Biophys Acta 963:265–270
80. Strasberg SM, Harvey PCR, Gallinger S (1984) Cholesterol nucleation in gallstone patients. In: Paumgartner G, Stiehl A, Gerok W (eds) Enterohepatic circulation of bile acids and sterol metabolism. MTP Press, Lancaster, pp 299–304
81. Sutor DJ, Wilkie LI (1976) Diurnal variations of the pH of pathological gallbladder bile. Gut 17:971–974
82. Szoka F Jr, Papahadjopoulos D (1980) Comparative properties and methods of preparation of lipid vesicles (liposomes). Ann Rev Biophys Bioengin 9:467–508
83. Tera H (1960) Stratification of human gallbladder in vivo. Acta Chir Scand [Suppl] 256:1–85
84. Thureborn E (1966) On the stratification of human bile and its importance for the solubility of cholesterol. Gastroenterology 50:775–780
85. Toor EN, Evans DF, Cussler EL (1978) Cholesterol monohydrate growth in model bile solutions. Proc Natl Acad Sci USA 75:6230–6234
86. Trotman BW, Petrella EJ, Soloway RD, Sanchez HM, Morris TA III, Miller WT (1975) Evaluation of radiographic lucency or opaqueness of gallstones as a means of identifying cholesterol or pigment stones. Correlation of lucency or opaqueness with calcium and mineral. Gastroenterology 68:1563–1566
87. van der Linden W, Nakayama F (1982) Hepatic versus duodenal bile. Scand J Gastroenterol 11:487–502
88. Whiting MJ, Watts JM (1983) Cholesterol crystal formation and growth in model solutions. J Lipid Res 24:861–868
89. Whiting MJ, Watts JM (1984) Supersaturated bile from obese patients without gallstones supports cholesterol crystal growth but not nucleation. Gastroenterology 86:243–248
90. Whiting MJ, Watts JM (1985) Cholesterol gallstone pathogenesis: a study of potential nucleating agents for cholesterol crystal formation in bile. Clin Sci 68:589–596
91. Williamson BWA, Trainer M (1986) Gallstone pathogenesis: physicochemical factors which control the nucleation of cholesterol by compounds in gallstones. Gut 27:A 1005 (abstr)
92. Wilschut J, Hoekstra D (1984) Membrane fusion from liposomes to biological membranes. TIBS 9:479–485
93. Witten TA, Cates ME (1986) Tenuous structures from disorderly growth processes. Science 232:1607–1612
94. Wrigglesworth M (1988) Incorporation of membrane proteins into liposomal bilayers. Mol Aspects Med 10:223–232
95. Yamazaki K, Powers SP, La Russo NF (1988) Biliary proteins: assessment of quantitative techniques and comparison in gallstone and nongallstone subjects. J Lipid Res 29:1055–1063

Modulation of the Edge Tension of Lipid Membranes by Cholate and Cholesterol and the Micelle-Vesicle Transition in Model Bile Systems*

P. Fromherz

Abteilung Biophysik der Universität Ulm, Oberer Eselsberg, D-7800 Ulm, FRG

Introduction

Let us consider a cut across a lipid membrane (Fig. 1). Hydrocarbon is exposed to water. The work per unit length required to create an open edge is denoted as edge tension. We attribute the existence and stability of closed – edge-free – membranes to a high level of edge tension, which prevents spontaneous fragmentation: "Membranes hate edges" [1]. Fragmentation of a membrane, for example, in digestion, requires the reduction of edge tension to a very low level. We can suppose that chemicals such as bile salts bind to the open edge and shield the hydrocarbon from water due to their amphiphilic character [2, 3].

The present paper discusses the way in which this classical idea of solubilization may be put in a physicochemical framework. The goal of this approach is a quantitative characterization, on the one hand, of the activity of bile salts with respect to solubilization of lipid and, on the other, of the resistance of lipid to solubilization. To determine the edge tension we consider the process of vesicle formation as it occurs after dilution of dispersions of lipid and bile salt. The effect of cholesterol with respect to membrane stability is considered on the basis of the limit of solubilization.

Edge Activity of Bile Salt

It is generally assumed that bile salts adsorb to edges of membranes [2, 3]. They are said to be "edge active" [4–7]. We describe the drop in edge tension as induced by the "edge actants" by a Gibbs isotherm [4] in analogy to the change in interfacial tension by surfactants in a macroscopic oil/water system. The edge tension (γ_E) decreases with the free concentration cholate in water (C_W) according to Eq. 1 [4]:

$$\gamma_E = \gamma_E^0 - kT \cdot \bar{n}_E \cdot K_{WE} \cdot C_W \tag{1}$$

γ_E^0 is the intrinsic edge tension, $\bar{n}_E$ is the density of binding sites, K_{WE} is the binding constant, and kT is the thermal energy. The linear relation holds for low concentrations ($C_W \cdot K_{WE} \ll 1$). The edge tension vanishes at a critical free concentration of cholate, ($C_W = C_W^*$), as expressed by Eq. 2:

$$C_W^* = \gamma_E^0 / kT \cdot \bar{n}_E \cdot K_{WE} \tag{2}$$

Vanishing edge tension initiates spontaneous fragmentation of the membrane. The concept of edge activity provides a physical interpretation of the well-known solubilization of lipid by bile salts above a threshold concentration.

---

* This research was supported by the Deutsche Forschungsgemeinschaft (Schwerpunkt „Biophysik der Zelle," Fr349/4 and Sonderforschungsbereich 239, D7)

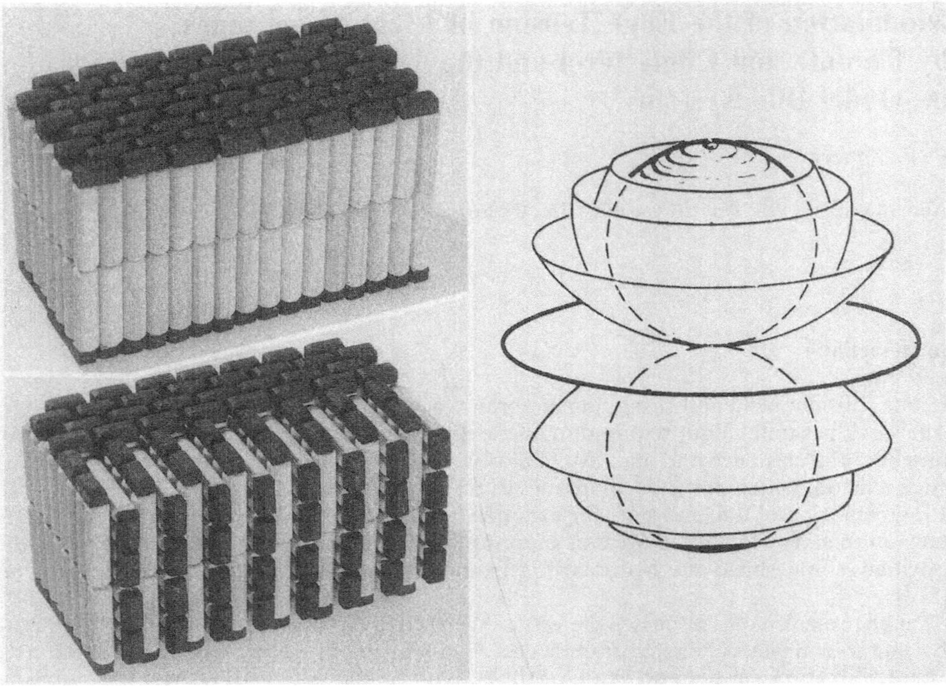

Fig. 1. *Left*, molecular models of the open edge of a bilayer. Hydrocarbon chains are *light*; head-groups are *dark*. *Upper*, unperturbed packing of bilayer; *lower*, micellar splay in block architecture [18]. *Right*, Shape transition of a fluid membrane from a disk with open edge to a closed vesicle [4]

Such an interpretation of the phase limit of micellization, however, is justified only if it is possible to observe the continuous decrease in edge tension at subthreshold levels of the concentration of bile salt. As a probe we use the mechanical instability of planar disks of membranes with respect to bending up to spherical vesicles (Euler instability).

Disk-Vesicle Instability

In an open discoid membrane the edge energy is reduced by bending which reduces the perimeter of edge (Fig. 1). A spheroidal deformation of a disk, however, gives rise to an elastic energy of curvature. If the maximal edge energy (of planar disk) exceeds the maximal elastic energy (of closed shell), spontaneous closure may occur [8]. The transitions disk-to-vesicle and vesicle-to-disk exhibit hysteresis [4]. The threshold of the radius for closure of a disk (R_D^*) is expressed by Eq. 3, where the bending elasticity is characterized by an elastic modulus (k_{EL}) [9, 10]. The larger the disk, the smaller is the edge tension required for closure:

$$\gamma_E = \frac{8 \cdot k_{EL}}{R_D^*} \tag{3}$$

The critical radius is a measure of the edge tension at a given elastic modulus. The elastic bending modulus has been studied in great detail [11]. We may determine the edge-tension in a given solution of bile salt by observing the size of disks which close spontaneously. We apply the "tensiometer" defined by Eq. 3 for dispersions of lecithin in solutions of variable free concentration of bile salt which controls edge tension, according to Eq. 1.

Dilution of a Lecithin/Cholate Dispersion

In a dispersion of lipid the total concentration of bile salt (C_T) is higher than the free concentration as bile salt binds to the plane of a membrane [12]. C_T and C_W are related according to Eq. 4, where C_L is the lipid concentration, and K_{WM} is the binding constant:

$$C_T = C_W \cdot (1 + K_{WM} \cdot C_L) \tag{4}$$

The total concentration required for fragmentation (to mixed micelles) – at the critical free concentration ($C_W = C_W^*$) – is given by: $C_W^* \cdot (1 + K_{WM} \cdot C_L) = \mathrm{CFC}$ (i.e., critical fragmentation concentration). At higher concentrations the free concentration remains constant at a level of $C_W^* = \mathrm{IMC}$ (i.e., intermicellar concentration). Also the bound concentration is invariant, as $C_W^* \cdot K_{WM} \cdot C_L$. The surplus ($C_T - \mathrm{CFC}$) is adsorbed to the edges promoting solubilization to smaller and smaller micelles. From a micellar solution (with $C_T > \mathrm{CFC}$) we may cross the CFC line – i.e., we may enter the regime of finite edge tension – by dilution at a constant ratio of lipid to cholate ($q_L = C_L/C_T$). The more we dilute, the lower is the free concentration (Eq. 4), the higher is the edge tension (Eq. 1), and the smaller is the radius of the disks which close to vesicles (Eq. 3).

Let us consider the dilution of a micellar solution of egg lecithin and sodium cholate at a molar ratio $q_L = 0.7$. We characterize the dispersion by quasielastic light scattering [12, 13]. The particles grow after dilution to a stationary value within 5–20 min. From the values of the first and second cumulant in the stationary state an effective radius of disks (R_D^e) is calculated [7]; this is plotted in Fig. 2 versus the total concentration of

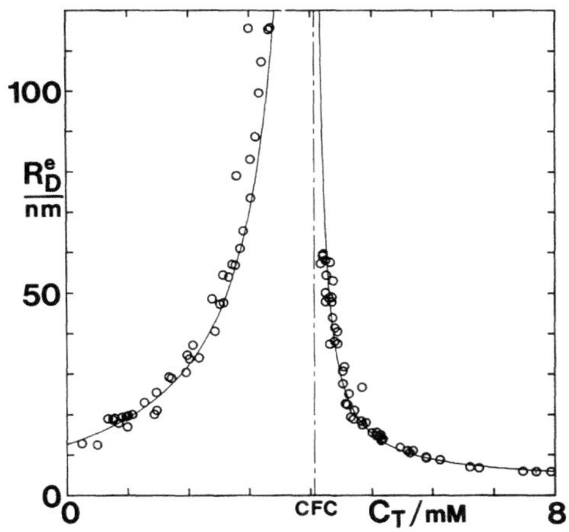

Fig. 2. Size of lipid aggregates as expressed by the effective radius of disks (R_D^e) versus total concentration of cholate (C_T) after dilution of lecithin/cholate dispersions (molar ratio lecithin/cholate = 0.7; salt concentration 420 m*M* NaCl, 25 °C) [7]. The critical fragmentation concentration (*CFC*) is marked. The micellar branch (*right*) is fitted by a modified "mixed disk model" [7, 12]. The vesicular branch (*left*) is fitted by the Euler-Gibbs model of disk-vesicle transition in the limit of a linear Gibbs isotherm [7]

cholate [7, 14]. Above the threshold concentration for (C_T>CFC) the effective radius diverges as the system approaches the phase limit (right branch in Fig. 2). We attribute this effect to a growth of micellar disks as due to the reduced surplus of cholate which stabilizes edges [12]. At subthreshold concentrations (C_T<CFC) the effective radius diverges towards the threshold as well. The particles in the stationary state are vesicles of a diameter which equals the effective radius of disks as seen by electron microscopy [7].

We attribute the saturation of growth and the formation of vesicles to the transformation of open disks to closed vesicles. The observed radius is identified with the critical radius of disks ($R_D^e = R_D^*$). The divergence in the size of closing disks is attributed to vanishing edge tension near the phase limit (Eqs. 1, 2). The modulated size of vesicles near the phase limit is compatible with a disk-vesicle transition as controlled by a modulated edge tension. However, to justify the evaluation of an edge-tension (using Eq. 3) an independent confirmation of a transformation of shape is required.

Birefringence of a Lecithin/Cholate Dispersion

Membrane disks of lecithin and cholate are anisotropic with respect to their static electrical polarizability due to the anisotropic electrical double layer [15, 16]. An electrical field may orient the disks. The orientation may be observed by birefringence as the disks are anisotropic with respect to their optical polarizability. The structural anisotropy of a dispersion in an electrical field is characterized by the Kerr constant [15, 16].

Let us consider a dilution of a micellar solution of lecithin and sodium cholate at a low salt concentration of 10 mM NaCl [17]. The effective radius of disks increases in time, as shown in Fig. 3; the Kerr constant increases dramatically – correlated with growth. We attribute this effect to the increasing anisotropy of polarizability of larger disks. The Kerr constant of the dispersion drops suddenly at the time at which the growth of particles tends to saturate. The drop in anisotropy at constant size of particles is compatible only with a shape transition within the colloidal dispersion from anisotropic particles to isotropic particles, i.e., from disks to vesicles.

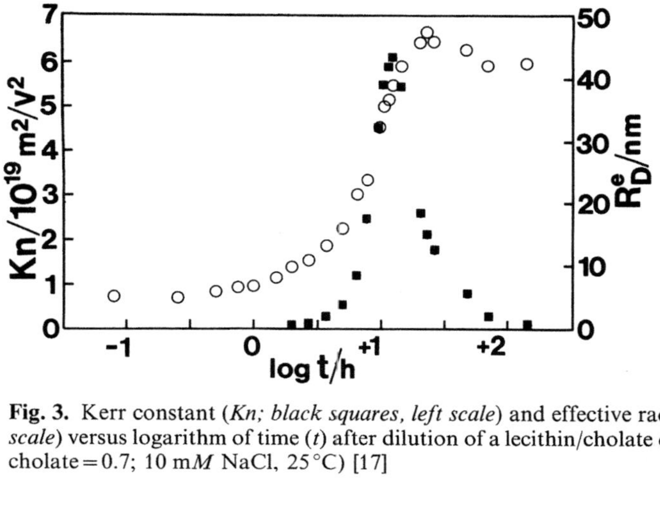

Fig. 3. Kerr constant (*Kn; black squares, left scale*) and effective radius of disks (R_D^e) (*circles, right scale*) versus logarithm of time (t) after dilution of a lecithin/cholate dispersion (molar ratio lecithin/cholate = 0.7; 10 mM NaCl, 25 °C) [17]

Edge Tension of Lecithin

Presuming on the actual occurrence of the shape transformation disk-to-vesicle, we evaluate the edge tension from the size of vesicles as observed after dilution of the cholate/lecithin dispersion.

The effective radii as shown in Fig. 2 are evaluated in terms of the edge tension according to Eq. 3. The total concentrations of cholate are evaluated in terms of the free concentration according to Eq. 4. The results are plotted in Fig. 4 [7]. An elastic modulus of $k_{EL} = 2.2 \cdot 10^{-19}$ J and a binding constant of $K_{WM} = 0.22$ mM^{-1} are used in the evaluation [7]. The edge tension decreases with the free concentration of cholate, as shown in Fig. 4. The drop in edge tension is compatible with the linear approximation of a Gibbs isotherm according to Eq. 1. The limit of vanishing edge tension is attained at a free concentration of cholate of $C_W^* = 2.5$ mM. This value for C_W^* is identical with that obtained from the limit of the micellar phase using the relationship, $\mathrm{CFC} = C_W^* \cdot (1 + K_{WM} \cdot C_L)$, The coincidence provides strong support that the solubilization of lipid by bile salt may indeed be considered as a result of vanishing edge tension.

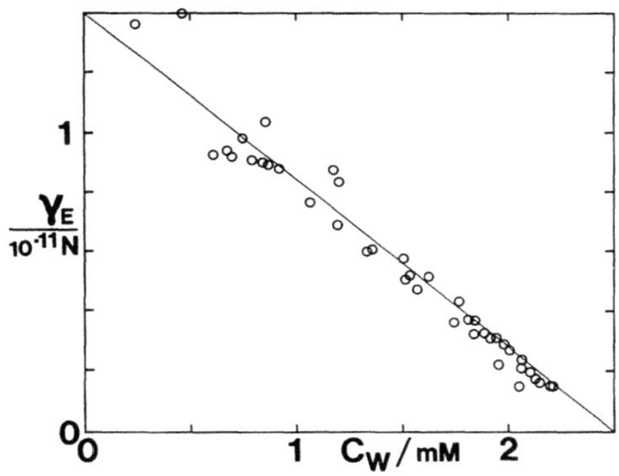

Fig. 4. Edge tension (γ_E) of egg lecithin in a solution of sodium cholate versus the free concentration of cholate (C_W) [7]

Cholesterol and Edge Tension

The total concentration of bile salt ($C_T = \mathrm{CFC}$) required to solubilize a given amount of lipid is governed by the critical free concentration (Eq. 4). The level of C_W^* is governed by the intrinsic edge tension of the lipid (Eq. 2). Thus a high intrinsic edge tension is the origin of a high concentration of bile salt required for solubilization.

The edge tension of egg lecithin – $\gamma_E^0 = 1.4 \cdot 10^{-20}$ J/nm, as evaluated above (Fig. 4) – is distinctly lower than the hydrophobic energy of the exposed hydrocarbon: $\gamma_E^{HC} = 7 \cdot 10^{-20}$ J/nm [4]. The stabilization of the edge may be assigned to a reorganization of the bulky headgroups of lecithin at the edge by micellar splay (Fig. 1) [18]. A lipid molecule with a small headgroup – of "inverted cone shape" [19] – may release the mutual repulsion of bulky headgroups within the membrane. For this energetic reason it tends to avoid the edge. Such a solute with "negative adsorption" enhances the edge tension according to the Gibbs isotherm [4]. Cholesterol is usually considered to be a lipid of inverted cone shape [20]. We postulate that cholesterol enhances the edge tension [4] and predict that the critical concentration of bile salt is enhanced by cholesterol.

The limit of solubilization of egg lecithin and cholesterol by taurocholate has been studied in great detail [21]. From the data, linear relations (CFC ~ C_L, see Eq. 5) may

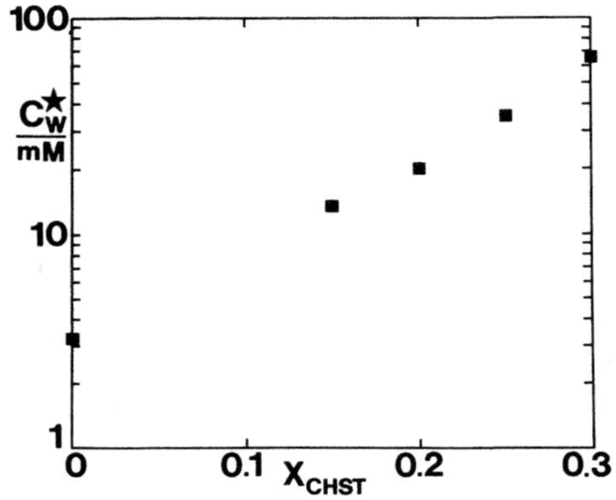

Fig. 5. Critical free concentration of taurocholate (C_W^*) versus molar fraction of cholesterol (x_{CHST}) in lipid (lecithin and cholesterol) as evaluated from the phase diagram (150 m*M* NaCl, 37 °C) [21, 22]

be interpolated between the concentration of bile salt and the concentration of total lipid (lecithin and cholesterol) at various molar fractions of cholesterol ($x_{CHST} = C_{CHST}/C_L$) in the membrane [22]. From an extrapolation to $C_L = 0$ the critical free concentrations are obtained (Eq. 5). The result is shown in Fig. 5. The critical concentration grows exponentially with the molar fraction. Within a linear approximation of the Gibbs isotherm [Eqs. 1, 2) such a relation would reflect an exponential increase in the intrinsic edge tension. In a previous paper, however, the phase limit of the lecithin/taurocholate system was described by the logarithmic approximation of the Gibbs isotherm – using the limit $C_W \cdot K_{WE} \gg 1$ for the adsorption of to the edge [6] – as expressed by Eq. 5:

$$\gamma_E^0 = kT \cdot \bar{n}_E \cdot \ln(K_{WE} \cdot C_W^*) \quad (5)$$

With this approximation the exponential increase in C_W^* with the molar fraction of cholesterol would reflect a linear relationship ($\gamma_E^0 \sim x_{CHST}$) between the intrinsic edge tension and the molar fraction of cholesterol. Such a relation seems to be more likely.

We attribute the high amount of bile salt required to solubilize cholesterol-rich lipid to a high edge tension. This gives rise to a high critical concentration of free bile salt which is the origin of a high intermicellar concentration and a high concentration of bile in the solubilized membrane. The biological function of cholesterol is generally attributed to a "stabilization" of membranes. We suggest that it is the enhancement of edge tension which provides this stabilization, and that it is the same enhancement which hinders solubilization.

Summary

The energy of the open edge of lipid bilayers controls the stability of membranes. The edge tension is controlled by the accumulation and depletion of solutes as described by a Gibbs isotherm. Cholesterol avoids the edge, enhances the edge tension, and stabilizes membranes. Bile salt accumulates at the edge, lowers the edge tension, and induces solubilization. The effect of cholesterol and bile salt in a three-component dispersion of lipid is antagonistic.

References

1. Gingell D, Ginsberg L (1978) Problems in the physical interpretation of membrane interaction and fusion. In: Poste G, Nicolson GL (eds) Membrane fusion. Elsevier/North Holland, Amsterdam, pp 791–833
2. Small DM (1967) Physicochemical studies of cholesterol gallstone formation. Gastroenterology 52:607–610
3. Small DM, Penkett SA, Chapman D (1969) Studies on simple and mixed bile salt micelles by nuclear magnetic resonance spectrosopy. Biochim Biophys Acta 176:178–189
4. Fromherz P (1983) Lipid vesicle structure: size control by edge-active agents. Chem Phys Lett 94:259–266
5. Fromherz P, Rüppel D (1985) Lipid vesicle formation: the transition from open disks to closed shells. FEBS Lett 179:155–159
6. Fromherz P, Röcker C, Rüppel D (1986) From disocoid micelles to spherical vesicles. The concept of edge activity. Faraday Discuss Chem Soc 81: 39–48
7. Fromherz P, Wiedenmann E (1990) The formation of lipid vesicles in lecithin/cholate dispersions and the concept of edge-activity. Biophys J (submitted)
8. Fergason JL, Brown GH (1968) Liquid crystals and living systems. J Am Oil Chem Soc 45:120–127
9. Helfrich W (1973) Elastic properties of lipid bilayers: theory and possible experiments. Z Naturforsch [C] 28:693–703
10. Helfrich W (1974) The size of bilayer vesicles generated by sonication. Phys Lett A 50:115–116
11. Bivas I, Hanusse P, Bothorel P, Lalanne J, Aguerre-Chariol O (1987) An application of the optical spectroscopy to the determination of the curvature elastic modulus of biological and model membranes. J Phys 48:855–867
12. Mazer NA, Benedek GB, Carey MC (1980) Quasielastic light-scattering of aqueous biliary lipid systems. Mixed micelle formation in bile-lecithin solutions. Biochemistry 19:601–615
13. Schurtenberger P, Mazer NA, Känzig W (1985) Micelle to vesicle transition in aqueous solutions of bile salt and lecithin. J Phys Chem 89:1042–1049
14. Wiedenmann E (1987) Untersuchung der Mizell-Vesikel Umwandlung mit quasielastischer Lichtstreuung. Diplomarbeit, University of Ulm
15. Fredericq E, Houssier C (1960) Electric dichroism and electric birefringence. Clarendon, Oxford
16. Hoffmann H, Schorr W (1985) Electro-optical properties of rodlike micelles. Ber Bunsenges Phys Chem 89:538–545
17. Lappöhn A (1988) Untersuchung der Mizell-Vesikel-Umwandlung mit elektrischer Doppelbrechung. Diplomarbeit, University of Ulm
18. Fromherz P (1984) The assembly of amphiphiles: molecular and phenomenological models. In: Luisi PL, Straub BE (eds) Reverse micelles. Plenum, New York
19. Haydon DA, Taylor J (1963) The stability and properties of bimolecular lipid leaflets in aqueous solution. J. Theor Biol. 4:281–296
20. Israelachvili JN, Marcelja S, Horn RG (1980) Physical principles of membrane organization. Q Rev. Biophys. 13:121–200
21. Carey MC, Small DM (1978) The physical chemistry of cholesterol solubility in bile. J. Clin. Invest. 61:988–1026
22. Fromherz P (1990) Does cholesterol stabilize lipid membranes by an enhancement of the edge-tension? (in preparation)

Pigment Gallstones and Secondary Calcification of Gallstones

R. D. Soloway [1], J. G. Wu [2], and D. F. Xu [3]

[1] Division of Gastroenterology, 4.106 McCullough, G-64, University of Texas Medical Branch at Galveston, Galveston TX 77550, USA
[2] Department of Chemistry, Beijing University, Beijing 100871, People's Republic of China
[3] Section of Polymer Chemistry, Sinica Academica, Beijing 100871, People's Republic of China

Types of Gallstones

For more than a century, biliary tract stones have been broadly identified by their gross characteristics [28]. In fact, this method has been remarkably accurate and has led to the correct classification of more than 90% of stones [29]. However, a number of subclassifications have been proposed which do not take full account of compositional characteristics and thus may not have any pathologic significance. Although subclassification may be important, the classification proposed at the NIH International Gallstone Workshop [30] is compatible with differences in clinical, biochemical, epidemiological, and compositional characteristics of stones that identify three groups with mutually exclusive pathogeneses: cholesterol, black pigment, and brown pigment stones. The accumulated information suggests that although some of the same compounds occur in different types of stones, there are distinguishing compositional differences that allow classification into these three groups in almost all cases. Such a classification clarifies discussion about pathogenesis. For example, the fact that pigmented centers and rings occur in cholesterol stones does not mean that all stones form on a pigment nidus, or the fact that both black and brown pigment stones contain calcium bilirubinate does not mean that the pathogenesis of these stone types is the same.

Cholesterol Gallstones

Stones composed of cholesterol display a great variety of sizes and shapes from patient to patient, but stones from the same patient are remarkably similar. On cross section, these stones display pigmented centers and rings indicating that similar conditions for stone growth have occurred throughout the gallbladder. However, these conditions have changed cyclically over time. Stones contain a spectrum of cholesterol from 50% to 100%, and so-called *solitaire* or pure cholesterol stones do not differ significantly in cholesterol content from many of the so-called combination cholesterol stones with pigmented centers and layers [17]. Rather, it appears that these stones form a compositional continuum [24]. Most cholesterol stones contain 80%–95% cholesterol, but a few contain only 50–70% cholesterol, and the noncholesterol components consist of some calcium salts but primarily macromolecules such as proteins.

Calcium bilirubinate is visually present, accounting for the pigmentation in cholesterol stones, but in the United States calcium hydroxyapatite has also been reported to be present [29, 24]. In Europe, calcium carbonate is reported frequently in cholesterol stones [26], but we have noted only infrequent stones containing calcium carbonate in the United States (personal experience, more than 400 sets of stones). In Bolivia, we have found an even smaller proportion of noncholesterol components, and gallstones there contain almost 100% cholesterol [18, 19]. The composition of cholesterol stones appears to differ with geography. This may be due to genetics, water hardness, diet, or other as yet unknown factors. We are presently examining cholesterol stone composition in a multiracial population in Texas with a similar diet. We are finding many fewer pigment gallstones in Galveston than in Philadelphia, reflecting the larger proportion of Hispanic patients at our hospital in the former. These differences and as yet unexplored regional differences in composition may explain the lower incidence of stone calcification during treatment with chenodeoxycholic acid and ursodeoxycholic acid in the United States compared to Europe.

Radio-opacity on plain films appears to require the presence of calcium hydroxyapatite or calcium carbonate [32], which, because of smaller anionic size, contain calcium to a greater proportion by weight than does calcium bilirubinate. This is supported by the observation that most brown pigment stones are radiolucent and, when present within the liver, may be missed on computerized axial tomography (CAT) scan because they are at tissue density. The use of CAT scans has detected calcium more frequently than that of plain films, perhaps because CAT scans may also detect calcium bilirubinate or have a lower threshold for detection of calcium. In addition, geographic differences in the proportions of cholesterol to noncholesterol components may provide confounding variables.

Use of scanning electron microscopy coupled with surface analysis techniques such as electron scanning for chemical analysis and energy-dispersive X-ray analysis has produced information concerning the composition and structure of cholesterol stone centers and rings [22]. Although centers are pigmented in most cholesterol stones, analysis of dissected centers indicates that the major component is cholesterol, thus distinguishing these from pigment stones in which cholesterol is aminor component [5, 13]. Only one of 67 centers that we examined had the ropelike structures which have been identified as characteristic of the fractured surfaces of pigment gallstones [13]. We have previously considered these forms to be microcrystals [12], but the ropelike configuration more closely represents a heterogeneous polymer with foci of crystallization resembling a number of artificial polymers (unpublished finding, D-F. Xu, August 1988).

In both centers and rings of cholesterol stones, increases in the non-cholesterol components changed the loose crystalline arrangement of rhomboid cholesterol crystals, separated by relatively wide spaces in the predominant cholesterol layers, to a progressively more sheetlike arrangement containing few or absent pores [13]. We concluded that these microscopic findings were compatible with the clinical observation that treatment with chenodeoxycholic acid often resulted in partial gallstone dissolution, and that such dissolution often stopped at pigmented layers [5]. We hypothesized that such layers presented a physical impedance to penetration by litholytic bile acids and retarded or arrested further stone dissolution if the proportion of protein and calcium salts was sufficient. Such layers can now be breached by lithotripsy.

Black Pigment Gallstones

These gallstones are much smaller than cholesterol stones, and their surfaces vary from very smooth to very irregular. Layers are not usually seen, but electron microprobe analysis reveals inhomogeneity in deposition. These stones contain less than 10% cholesterol and 20%–90% proteins and other macromolecules, with the remainder being various combinations of calcium salts. Calcium bilirubinates can vary between 20% and 80% [29, 24]. Calcium hydroxyapatite varies from 0% to 40% of stone weight, and in a few stones this may be the primary calcium salt [29, 24]. In some stones calcium carbonate predominates, but in 60% of black stones from the Philadelphia series it is absent [29, 24].

On fractured section, the resultant surface of one black stone, containing more than 90% calcium bilirubinate, was smooth and glasslike. When the surface was exposed to an argon beam, which differentially chips away the softer components of the surface at the rate of 50 Å per minute, microcrystals or polymers of calcium bilirubinate were demonstrated [12]. During this process, the calcium content of the surface, measured by electron scanning for chemical analysis, increased progressively [22]. We interpreted the enrichment of calcium together with the demonstration of rodlike structures to mean that calcium bilirubinate salts were selectively preserved while the intervening protein was chipped away. In other black stones, ropelike polymeric structures were noted to protrude from the fractured surface. Use of energy-dispersive X-ray analysis of the elements within a single polymeric strand demonstrated both calcium and phosphorus, indicating the presence of a calcium phosphate salt. Infrared spectroscopy identified the presence of calcium hydroxyapatite [13]. Calcium carbonate has not been identified in this form.

The stone that contained more than 90% calcium bilirubinate was also exposed to an oxygen plasma (O^-) environment which selectively oxidizes organic components. Increasing length of exposure demonstrated a progressively more prominent network where protein had been present. This appeared to interlace with a network of calcium salts because the surface once again contained progressively more calcium [22]. Since the rodlike structures were not demonstrated by this technique, we have concluded that the portions of the protein at a distance from the calcium salts were oxidized, and that continuing exposure oxidized protein closer to the calcium salts but not the portion just adjacent to the salts. The signals for deposition of calcium salts and for turning deposition off are not known. Presumably, since the process should be similar to bone formation and stone formation elsewhere in the body, because all involve the deposition of calcium phosphate salts, a change in the configuration of mucin proteins might predispose to calcium binding and calcium salt deposition, while deposition of a subsequent layer of protein might inhibit further crystallization by covering the microcrystals and preventing further crystal growth. The process would recommence when the same or other protein on the surface of the stone was altered, permitting calcium binding once again and formation of a subsequent layer.

Brown Pigment Stones

Brown stones contain 10%–30% cholesterol, 5%–15% proteins and macromolecules, 18%–80% calcium bilirubinate, little or no calcium, phosphate, and carbonate, and 12%–67% calcium salts of fatty acids [24]. These stones contain alternating layers which are comprised predominantly of calcium bilirubinate or calcium salts of fatty acids. Other layers contain various proportions of these components. The signals for changes in the composition of these layers are unknown. Presumably there are both "on" and "off" signals. Calcium bilirubinate appears to form through the action of bacterial or tissue β-glucuronidase [9, 27] while calcium salts of fatty acids reflect the composition of lecithin and are formed through the action of phospholipase on lecithin, presumably at the a_1 position of the glycerol backbone [20]. Again, the controls for variations in the activities of these two enzymes are unknown. Although these stones may contain as much bilirubin as black stones, it is in an alternate, nonpolymeric or crystalline form [12]. The stones are red-brown, most frequently, the color of calcium bilirubinate, and on exposure to an argon beam, the loose structure does not reveal a protein network or the presence of microcrystals or polymers of calcium bilirubinate or fatty acids. On exposure to the argon beam the structure of brown stones does not change, but the surface becomes more crumbly.

Epidemiology of Gallstones

The proportions of these three types of stones can be determined with certainty only at operation. Information from surgical series around the world indicates that the proportions in gallbladder stones vary quite remarkably. In Philadelphia, cholesterol stones account for 71% and black stones 29% [29], while brown stones are present in less than 1% of gallbladders. In the southwestern United States, among the Amerind populations, the incidence of cholesterol stones may approach 100%, but this has not been examined. In Bolivia, a population with a large Amerind admixture, cholesterol stones are the only type recovered [19]. This trend seems to be true of Amerind groups throughout the Western Hemisphere, although the Eskimos have not been examined, and the population in Chile, essentially European in origin, has a very high incidence of cholesterol stones. Factors in addition to diet must be important since there are great differences between the dietary intake of various Indian populations. For example, the Bolivians have a potato-based diet, while the Mexicans have a corn-based diet. Although blacks in the United States have the same proportions of gallstones as whites [5], in Africa, certain tribes such as the Masai have a 0% incidence. In northern India, there is a 75% incidence of cholesterol, 23% black, and 2% brown stones. The incidence of gallstone disease in China varies greatly depending on the diet, but in parts of China, brown stones account for 90%, cholesterol 5%, and black stones 5%. Mongolia is 800 miles from Beijing, but its population is largely a nomadic herding people and consume dairy products. They have a much higher incidence of cholesterol stones than in other parts of China that consume the more traditional vegetable, rice, and fish diet (personal communication, X.-S. Zhou, Beijing).

Japan has had the best documentation of the changes in gallstone frequency caused by changes in diet. Up to 1945, the Japanese followed their traditional diet, and the incidence was 21% cholesterol, 9% black, and 70% brown stones [35]. In 1978, the operative incidence was reexamined, and the frequency of stones had increased from 5% to 10%, and the incidence had become 70% cholesterol, 9% black, and 21% brown stones [6]. Interestingly, when Japanese or Chinese populations moved to Australia, Hawaii, or the mainland United States, the incidence of brown stones in the descendents was probably no different than in the general population, because informal polls indicated that surgeons in these areas detect brown stones only in immigrants, or in the common bile duct after cholecystectomy, as in patients of Western origin (personal communication). Clearly, environment and, presumably, diet plays a large role in the type of gallstone formed. In addition, however, genetics appears to influence stone type.

Comparisons Between Black and Brown Pigment Stones

The differences in geographic location and the effects of race have been discussed in the section on epidemiology. Black stones are predominantly located in the gallbladder, and those that form there do not recur after cholecystectomy [6]. Stones that form behind strictures in the common duct, which are not associated with infections such as in primary sclerosing cholangitis, are black stones, but these are quite small and contain high concentrations of protein. Brown stones that form primarily in the common bile ducts or in the intrahepatic radicles are almost uniformly associated with infection and recur frequently after stone removal, presenting a major source of morbidity among patients from Asia with this condition [14]. These stones can form in the absence of gallbladder stones, unlike black and cholesterol stones which form primarily in the gallbladder [14]. In Western countries, cholesterol stones are the most common type of common bile duct stone detected in the first 2 years after cholecystectomy, representing retained stones passed from the gallbladder into the common bile duct and missed at the time of cholecystectomy [11]. Brown stones predominate among common duct stones detected more than 2 years after cholecystectomy, suggesting that brown stones form primarily in the common bile duct in the West as well as the Orient. In contrast, black stones are found primarily in the gallbladder throughout the world.

Both black and brown stones are slightly more common in women than men; the ratio is 1.2:1 [6]. This ratio is significantly less than the 2.4:1 ratio frequently quoted for cholesterol stones. Both black and brown stones are present in older populations [31, 6].

Black stones are associated with hemolysis [24], cirrhosis [24], total parenteral nutrition [15], and primary sclerosing cholangitis but occur most frequently in the elderly with none of these conditions [29]. Brown stones are associated with bacterial and questionably with parasitic infections [24]. Scandinavian investigators have clearly demonstrated that brown stones are associated with stasis and infection accompanying paravaterian diverticuli of the duodenum [8].

Black stones have not been shown to be related to diet in man but are clearly related to diet in hamsters, prairie dogs, guinea pigs, and perhaps other animal models [10]. Brown stones are clearly related to diet in man. Rural Japanese hospitals in 1976–1978, when patients there were more likely to follow a traditional Japanese diet than in the cities, had a higher incidence of brown stones than did urban Japanese hospitals [6]. In Chinese Mongolia, where a meat and dairy diet is standard, cholesterol stones are more frequent than in the rest of China. Beijing has a larger proportion of cholesterol stones than does rural China. Black stones are cured by cholecystectomy despite continuing hemolysis or cirrhosis, while brown stones are frequently recurrent when removed from a dilated biliary ductal system.

Age has definite effects on the type of gallstone formed. In Philadelphia, among patients between the ages of 70 and 90, black stones outnumber cholesterol gallstones [31]. Similar data have been obtained in an operative series from Japan [6]. In an animal study, feeding an essential fatty acid deficient diet to weanling, 5-week-old hamsters led to cholesterol gallstone formation in 80% of animals. In 5-month-old, adolescent hamsters, the same diet produced cholesterol gallstones in 60% and black pigment stones in 20% [7], supporting the premise that age favors the formation of black stones through an as yet unknown mechanism.

Gallstone Pathogenesis

Although the physiochemical events in bile leading to the precipitation of cholesterol are known, the events leading to the precipitation of calcium salts have only been postulated. The initiating events involving proteins that occur in the mucus layer during stone nidation and the intermittent events that occur at the stone surface leading to stone growth are only postulated at this time. We believe that more definitive knowledge of this process, at the molecular level, can be determined using methods to define the three-dimensional structure of stone components, so that when such components are identified in stones, their sites of interaction can be identified, and changes in molecular configuration caused by their participation in stone formation can be more accurately determined. In addition, study of the microstructure of stones may help define the "on" and "off" signals for the formation of layers during stone growth.

Models of Calcium Bilirubinate Salts

Our research has focused on the use of Fourier transform infrared spectroscopy to determine the three-dimensional structure of the calcium bilirubinates. Since the exact

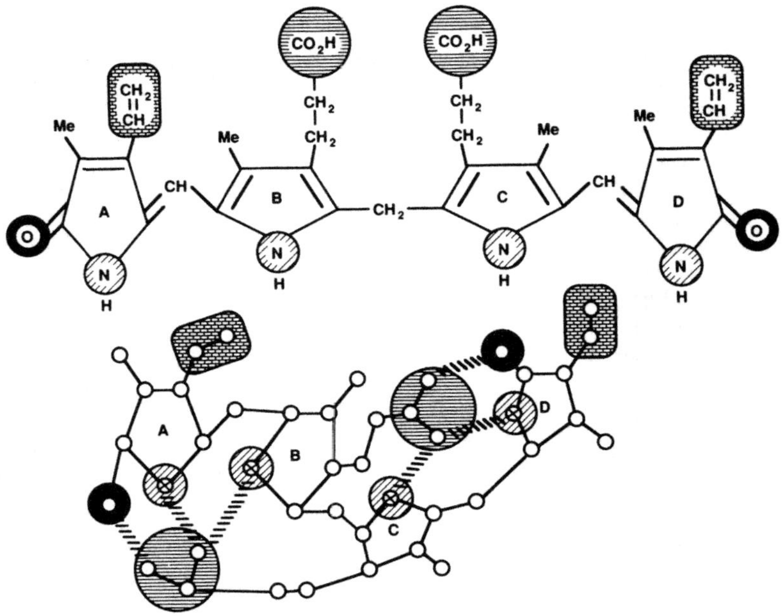

Fig. 1. The two-dimensional and three-dimensional structure of protonated bilirubin XIα based on the structure determined by Bonnett et al. [3] and modified from a review by Schmid with modification by Ostrow [16]

structure of the calcium bilirubinates has not been determined, because single crystals have not been produced allowing X-ray diffraction to be undertaken, we have developed a series of models of increasing complexity, based on infrared spectroscopy, which have reflected the evolution of our thinking as we have obtained more data from our studies.

In the absence of single crystals of calcium bilirubinate (a requirement for analysis by X-ray diffraction) atomic distances, interatomic angles, and atomic force constants cannot be determined, and therefore a three-dimensional structure cannot be definitively established, as has been done by Bonnett and his colleagues [3] for protonated bilirubin. In Figure 1, based on Bonnett's work, from a review by Schmid with modification by Ostrow [16], resides the explanation of the lack of water solubility for protonated bilirubin. Despite the presence of two carboxylic acid groups, the water insolubility is due to the presence of six strong intramolecular hydrogen bonds, three per carboxylic acid group, which folds the molecule into the form of a "ridge tile," so called because of the shape of the tile at the peak of a tile roof. The carboxylic acid groups are thus internally bound and are unavailable for interaction with water, in contrast to many dicarboxylic acids which are not internally hydrogen bound, such as diglucuronyl bilirubin, and therefore are highly water soluble.

A crystalline structure, based on X-ray diffraction for calcium bilirubinate, may never be established since the salt, as identified in stones, may always be heterogeneous because it is a variable mixture of the acid and neutral salts of calcium bilirubinate [2].

Sutor and Wilkie [25] called attention to the reduction in the infrared peak for protonated bilirubin at 1700 cm^{-1}, due to the carboxyl carbonyl group, when the acid salt of calcium bilirubinate was formed. In the acid salt, only one of the two carboxyl groups was associated with calcium while the other remained protonated. They also noted the deletion of the peak at 1700 cm^{-1} when the neutral salt was formed, and both carboxyl groups were associated with calcium. Based on these observations, we examined black pigment gallstones and standards and found that peak height at 1700 cm^{-1} could be used to determine the proportion of the acid and neutral salts of calcium bilirubinate in gallstones [1]. At that time, we constructed several diagrams to depict the acid and neutral salts (Fig. 2), similar to those recently published in a review by Carey and his associates [30].

The acid salt is formed in vitro between pH 6.5 and 7.5 and has a calcium to bilirubin ratio of 1:2 [2]. One calcium is connected to two molecules of bilirubin, forming a dimer. One carboxyl group from each bilirubin molecule remains protonated, but its spacial configuration was not considered. Mechanisms for forming branch polymers in the model are not obvious. We considered mixed polymers of calcium salts and proteins but could not account for the configuration of calcium bilirubinate in the rodlike structures that had been identified by scanning electron microscopy [12].

Our first conceptualizations of the three-dimensional structure of the neutral salt of calcium bilirubinate (Figs. 3, 4) are easier than that for the acid salt. The ratio of calcium to bilirubinate was 1:1, and both carboxyl groups were joined to calcium. Either two calciums were joined to two bilirubin molecules creating a dimer, or one calcium was joined to one bilirubin creating a monomer (Fig. 2). A linear polymer could also be formed through calcium bridging between bilirubin molecules forming a chain of bilirubin molecules connected by carboxyl groups. The arrangement of the rest of the molecule was not considered at that time.

On pursuing a detailed comparison of the partial infrared spectra of protonated bilirubin and the neutral salt of calcium bilirubinate, we realized that changes had taken place in the location of a number of peaks in addition to the 1700 cm^{-1} peak. In infrared spectroscopy, disappearance of peaks is most significant, followed by the extent of the shift in peak location in the infrared spectrum, measured per centimeter (wave numbers). Peak shifts and disappearance indicate that groups adjacent to the group producing the peak had changed in structure. In standards, peaks are sharp because the adjacent groups come from a small population of configurations since all of the molecules are identical. In complex mixtures of components such as gallstones, a proportion of groups responsible for the peaks may be adjacent to a number of different groups from dissimilar molecules, broadening the peak and changing the peak location. In addition, if the group responsible for the band is actually covalently bound to a heterogeneous group, the

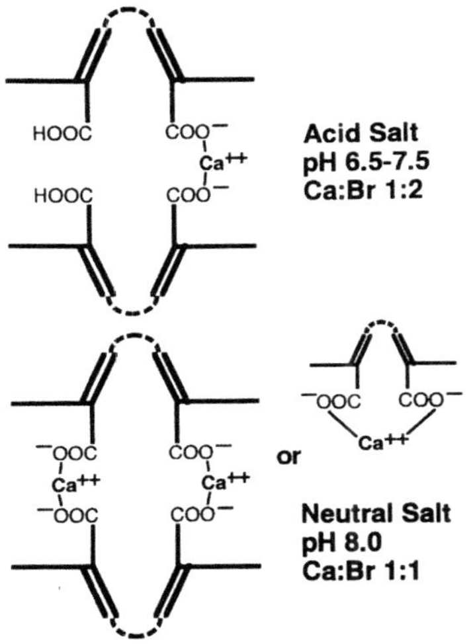

Fig. 2. Diagram showing possible configurations of the acid and neutral salts of calcium bilirubinate. The acid salt forms in vitro at pH 6.5–7.5 while the neutral salt forms at pH 8.0

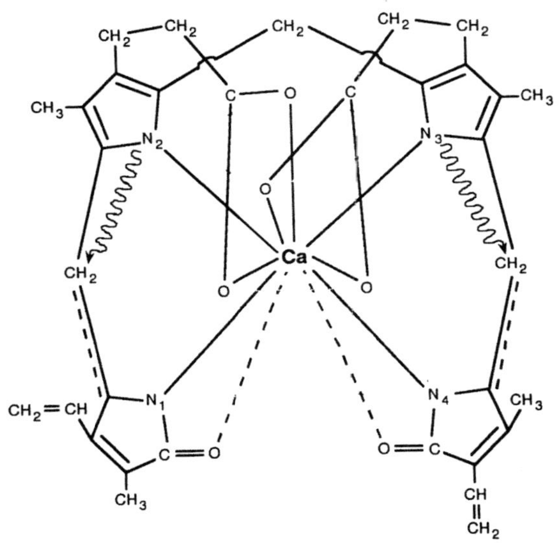

Fig. 3. First model for the three-dimensional coordination structure for the neutral salt of calcium bilirubinate. Calcium is coordinated with four nitrogens and four oxygens in an antiprism conformation. *Wavy line*, the partial transfer of the hydrogen from the pyrrole nitrogen to the methene bridge with partial loss of the double bond (*dashed line*). The lactam oxygens form a cap with the antiprism

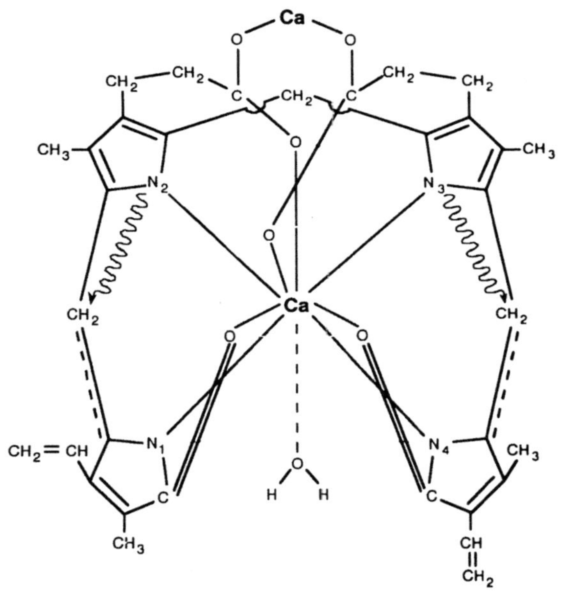

Fig. 4. Alternative model for the three-dimensional coordination structure for the neutral salt of calcium bilirubinate. The carboxyl oxygens are coordinated with two instead of one calcium ion, and the lactam oxygens have been coordinated

vibrations of the original group are greatly changed and may even disappear, as with the substitution of calcium for hydrogen during the formation of calcium bilirubinate. Binding of the protonated carboxyl group to a heterogeneous molecule such as a protein will lead to a shift in peak location. We therefore expanded our comparisons of protonated bilirubin and the salts of calcium bilirubinate to include the entire mid-infrared spectrum from 400 to 4000 cm^{-1}. Professor Wu pointed out that our previous models were incorrect since bonds between ionized calcium and bilirubinate are coordinate rather than ionic. Coordinate bonds are much stronger, accounting for the very small solubility of calcium bilirubinate in water at physiologic pH.

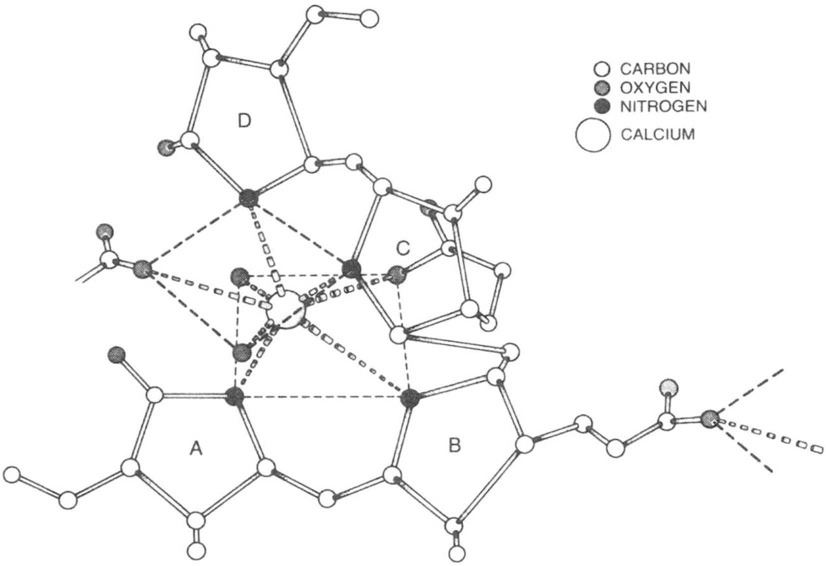

Fig. 5. Interim model (1989) for the three-dimensional structure for the neutral salt of calcium bilirubinate

Figure 3 shows calcium with eight coordinate rather than two ionic bonds, and, reflecting the identity of the groups responsible for the peak disappearances and large shifts noted in the infrared spectra, calcium is shown forming an antiprism with a ring of pyrroles and lactam nitrogens in an oblique plane with carboxyl oxygens coordinating above and below the plane. The features of this model that are likely to be wrong are that the lactam oxygens are coordinated near each other in the same plane, and that both oxygens from each carboxyl group are coordinated with the same calcium, both of which cause an unstable arrangement. As determined from the crystalline structure of lanthanum mucate, a homologous compound, only one oxygen of each carboxyl group is coordinated to the same metal ion [34]. There is no provision in this model for linear or branching polymerization. In addition, there was minimal change in the infrared peaks representing the lactam oxygens, indicating that they are not involved in the coordination structure, even though they are shown as only contributing as caps to the antiprism, making a coordination number of ten.

We have just constructed interim models of the neutral salt of calcium bilirubinate, based on our latest studies (Fig. 5). Calcium is located in the center and is coordinated in an antiprism with four nitrogens and four oxygens. For reasons of symmetry, the A and B ring nitrogens are located at one end of the antiprism while the C and D ring nitrogens are located at the other end. The rings are therefore arranged in an ascending helical fashion. One oxygen from each carboxyl group is also coordinated with the calcium, while carboxyl oxygens from neighboring bilirubin molecules and/or water of hydration (two for the neutral salt) may be coordinated or may form a cap at either end of the antiprism. Polymers are formed through the carboxyl groups coordinating with neighboring calcium ions. When both carboxyl groups are coordinated with neighboring calcium ions, and carboxyls from adjacent bilirubin molecules are coordinated with this calcium in their place, the possibility for a branching polymer exists.

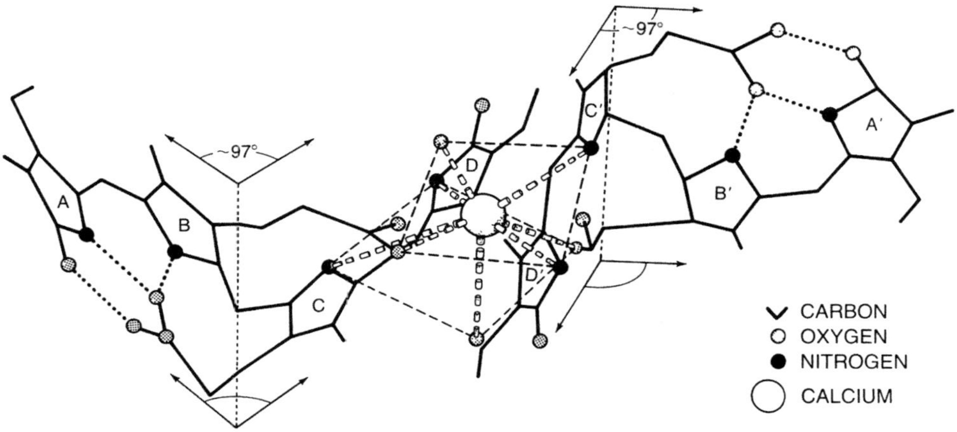

Fig. 6. Interim model (1989) for the three-dimensional structure for the acid salt of calcium bilirubinate

We have also constructed our first interim model for the acid salt of calcium bilirubinate (Fig. 6). This was more difficult to conceptualize because it requires a ratio of one calcium to two bilirubin molecules. Because each bilirubinate still contains one protonated carboxyl group, it is depicted in the classic "ridge tile" position (also see Fig. 1 for comparison) for one-half of the molecule and maintaining the 97° angle between the A-B and the C-D planes. At the same time, the C-D and the C′-D′ rings must be positioned to form the calcium antiprism, now formed by one-half of two molecules rather than from one molecule as with neutral calcium bilirubinate. The molecules have been placed in mirror and inverted positions so that one ionized carboxyl group can enter the top ring of the antiprism while the other carboxyl group from the second molecule can enter the bottom ring to preserve symmetry. Carboxyl groups from adjacent bilirubinate molecules and a water of hydration (one per dimer), must be included to complete the antiprism. Opportunity for branching takes place when carboxyl groups from three or four adjacent bilirubinate molecules are involved in forming a calcium antiprism.

Our view of the structure of the calcium salts is still evolving as we obtain additional data from our infrared studies. However, knowledge of the structures of gallstone components such as calcium bilirubinate will allow better understanding of its binding capabilities and will help to develop a complete picture of what takes place when calcium bilirubinate binds to a heterogeneous molecule such as glycoprotein.

References

1. Berman JM, Dabezies MA, Malet PF, Soloway RD (1985) Fourier transform infrared spectroscopy (FTIR) can identify and quantitate the acid and neutral salts of calcium bilirubinate (abstr). Gastroenterology 88:1711
2. Berman JM, Soloway RD (1986) Pigment gallstones contain both monoamniotic and dianionic calcium bilirubinate indicating formation at a higher pH than cholesterol gallstones (abstr). Gastroenterology 90:1785
3. Bonnett R, Davies JE, Hursthouse MB et al. (1978) The structure of bilirubin. Proc Soc Lond 202:249–268
4. Cahalane MJ, Neubrand MW, Carey MC (1988) Physical-chemical pathogenesis of pigment gallstones. Semin Liver Dis 8:317–328

5. Freilich HS, Malet PF, Schwartz JS, Soloway RD, and the National Cooperative Gallstone Study Group (1986) Chemical and morphologic characteristics of cholesterol gallstones which failed to dissolve on chenodiol. The National Cooperative Gallstone Study. Gastroenterology 91:713–718
6. Hikasa Y, Nagase M, Soloway RD, Tanimura H, Setoyama M, Kato H (1981) Gallstones in western Japan. 1. Epidemiologic factors affecting the type and location of gallstones. Arch J Surg 50:272–288
7. Hikasa Y, Nagase M, Tanimura H, Shioda R, Setoyama M, Kobayashi N, Mukaihara S, Kamata T, Maruyama K, Kato H, Mori K (1980) Epidemiology and etiology of gallstones. Arch Jpn Surg 49:555–571
8. Lotveit T, Osnes M (1984) Duodenal diverticula. Scand J Gastroenterol 19:579–581
9. Maki T (1966) Pathogenesis of calcium bilirubinate gallstone. Ann Surg 164:90–100
10. Malet PF (1985) Chapter 20: Animal models of gallstone formation. In: Cohen S, Soloway RD (eds) Contemporary issues in gastroenterology, vol 4. Gallstones. Churchill Livingstone, New York, pp 309–334
11. Malet PF, Dabezies MA, Huang GH, Long WB, Gadacz TR, Soloway RD (1988) Quantitative infrared spectroscopy of common duct gallstones. Gastroenterology 94:1217–1221
12. Malet PF, Takabayashi A, Trotman BW, Soloway RD, Weston NS (1984) Black and brown pigment gallstones differ in microstructure and microcomposition. Hepatology 4:227–234
13. Malet PF, Williamson CE, Trotman BW, Soloway RD (1986) Composition of pigment centers of cholesterol gallstones. Hepatology 6:477–481
14. Nagase M, Hikasa Y, Soloway RD, Tanimura H, Setoyama M, Kato H (1980) Gallstones in western Japan. Factors affects the prevalence of intrahepatic gallstones. Gastroenterology 78:684–690
15. O'Brien CB, Berman JM, Fleming CR, Malet PF, Soloway RD (1986) Total parenteral nutrition gallstones contain more calcium bilirubinate than sickle cell gallstones (abstr). Gastroenterology 90:1752
16. Ostrow JD (1986) Overview of bile pigment metabolism. In: Ostrow JD (ed) Bile pigments and jaundice: molecular, metabolic, and medical aspects. Marcel Dekker, New York, pp 1–6
17. AJ Harding Rains (1964) Gallstones. Causes and treatment. Thomas, Springfield
18. Rios-Dalenz J, Takabayashi A, Henson DE, Strom BL, Soloway RD (1983) The epidemiology of cancer of the extrahepatic biliary tract in Bolivia. Int J Epidemiol 12:1546–1560
19. Rios-Dalenz J, Takabayashi A, Henson DE, Strom BL, Soloway RD (1985) Cancer of the extrahepatic biliary tract in Bolivia. II. Suggestions concerning etiology. Am J Gastroenterol 80:371–375
20. Robins SJ, Fasulo JM, Patton GM (1982) Lipids of pigment gallstones. Biochim Biophys Acta 712:21–25
21. Sarva RP, Farivar S, Fromm H, Poller W (1981) Study of the sensitivity and specificity of computerized tomography in the detection of calcified gallstones which appear radiolucent by conventional roentgenography. Gastrointest Radiol 6:165–167
22. Soloway RD, Fayusal EB, Trotman BW, Weston NE, Ficca Jr JF (1982) Water which appear radiolucent by conventional roentgenography. Gastrointestinal content of gallstones: location and contribution to a hypothesis concerning stone structure. Hepatology 2:223–229
23. Soloway RD, Trotman BW (1985) Pigment gallstones, Chapter 22, 581–599. In: Ostrow JE (ed) Bile pigments and jaundice: molecular, metabolic and medical aspects. Marcel Dekker, New York
24. Soloway RD, Trotman BW, Maddrey WC, Nakayama F (1986) The influence of hemolysis, infection and stasis on the calcium salts in pigment gallstones. Dig Dis Sci 31:454–460
25. Sutor DJ, Wilkie LI (1977) The crystalline salts of calcium bilirubinate in human gallstones. Clin Sci Mol Med 53:101–103
26. Sutor DJ, Wooley SE (1969) X-ray diffraction studies of the composition of gallstones from English and Australian patients. Gut 10:618–619
27. Tabata M, Nakayama F (1981) Bacteria and gallstones. Etiological significance. Dig Dis Sci 26:218–224
28. Thudichum JLW (1863) Treatise on gallstones: their chemistry, pathology and treatment. Churchill, London
29. Trotman BW, Ostrow JD, Soloway RD (1974) Pigment vs cholesterol cholelithiasis: comparison of stone and bile composition. Am J Dig Dis 19:585–590

30. Trotman BW, Soloway RD (1982) Pigment gallstone disease: summary of the National Institutes of Health–International Workshop. Hepatology 2:879–884
31. Trotman BW, Soloway RD (1975) Pigment vs cholesterol cholelithiasis. Clinical and epidemiologic aspects. Am J Dig Dis 20:735–740
32. Trotman BW, Petrella EJ, Soloway RD, Sanchez HM, Morris III TA, Miller WT (1975) Evaluation of radiographic lucency or opaqueness of gallstones as a means of identifying cholesterol or pigment stones. Correlation of lucency or opaqueness with calcium and minerals. Gastroenterology 68:1563–1566
33. Wang J-F, Lin Y-H, Soloway RD, Wu J-G, Xu G-X (1988) Preparation and FT-IR spectra of calcium bilirubinate. Microchim Acta 1:53–55
34. Yang G-D, Fan Y-G, Liang H, Guo H, Wu J-G, Xu G-X (1988) Synthesis, properties and structure study of lanthanum 2,3,4,5-tetrahydroxy hexanedioate. Acta Scientiarum Naturalium 21:385–391
35. Miyake H, Kuwatsuka T, Tamesue N et al. (1963) Comparative studies on the chemical composition of gallstones in Japan, China and the United States. Fukuoka Igaku Zasshi 54:781–826

The Influence of the Gallbladder Epithelium on Gallstone Formation *

B. F. Smith

Section of Gastroenterology and Hepatology, Boston City Hospital, Boston University Medical Center, Boston, MA 02118, USA

Structure and Function of the Gallbladder Epithelium

Morphology of the Gallbladder Epithelium

The gallbladder has the simplest mucosal structure in the gastrointestinal tract. The surface epithelium of the gallbladder mucosa contains a single layer of monomorphic columnar cells which overlie the fibromuscular layers of the gallbladder wall. Unlike the other epithelia in the gastrointestinal tract, the gallbladder epithelium does not contain a submucosa. The surface epithelium is arranged into ridges and folds which effectively increase the surface area exposed to the gallbladder lumen. True glands are found only in the neck of the gallbladder, and these contain simple mucus-secreting cells. Ultrastructural studies of surface epithelial cells have identified intracytoplasmic vesicles which transport the secretory glycoprotein mucin from the Golgi apparatus to the apical surface where secretion takes place by exocytosis. In addition, during periods of active fluid absorption, dilatation of the lateral intracellular spaces can be observed.

Absorptive Function of the Gallbladder Epithelium

The only physiologic roles which have been identified for the gallbladder are the storage of bile during interprandial periods and the coordinate secretion of bile into the gut during feeding to facilitate nutrient absorption. Approximately 600 ml hepatic bile is produced per day, yet the capacity of the human gallbladder is only 40 ml. The ability of the gallbladder to efficiently concentrate and store bile is dependent on the absorption of water and electrolytes by the gallbladder epithelium. Active transport of sodium across the basolateral membrane of the epithelial cell, mediated most probably via Na^+/K^+ ATPase, forms an electrochemical gradient for sodium transport across the epithelium [1]. Sodium transport appears to be coupled to chloride transport, and electrolyte and water flux across the "leaky" gallbladder epithelium occurs by both a transcellular and a paracellular route. The resultant gallbladder bile is a concentrated yet isotonic solution which has a total lipid concentration three to five times greater than hepatic bile. The ability of the gallbladder to concentrate bile is not only important for efficient storage of bile but also facilitates the solubilization of biliary cholesterol by the concentration of lipid in gallbladder bile.

Transport of organic solutes across the gallbladder epithelium occurs during gallbladder obstruction, but organic solute absorption does not appear to be physiologically important. Nonpolar substances such as bilirubin and deconjugated bile acids can be

* This research was supported by NIH Research Grant DK39017

transported across the gallbladder epithelium, but these solutes are present in extremely small concentrations in bile under ordinary conditions.

Synthesis and Secretion of Gallbladder Mucus

The second major function of the gallbladder epithelium is the secretion of mucus. Concentrated gallbladder bile has the potential to injure the surface epithelium because of the detergent properties of the endogenous bile acids. It has been assumed that the mucus gel adherent to the surface of the gallbladder epithelium protects the mucosal lining cells although the mechanism by which mucus exerts this protective effect has not been elucidated. Very little information is available regarding the physiologic factors which regulate the synthesis and secretion of gallbladder mucin, the major organic component of mucus. This topic will be discussed in detail in a subsequent chapter (Smith/LaMont). The remainder of this chapter is devoted to summarizing the data which indicate that gallbladder mucin, the principal secretory product of the gallbladder epithelium, is a critical element in the pathophysiology of cholesterol gallstone formation.

Gallbladder Mucin: Structure and Function

Structure and Composition of Gallbladder Mucin

Gallbladder mucin is a secretory glycoprotein with an estimated molecular weight of 2×10^6 Da [2]. Branching oligosaccharide side chains are linked to a central peptide core via *O*-glycosidic bonds between *N*-acetylgalactosamine residues and the hydroxy amino acids serine and threonine. Five monosaccharides are present in mucin: *N*-acetyl-galactosamine, *N*-acetylglucosamine, *N*-acetylneuraminic acid, galactose, and fucose. These carbohydrates in aggregate account for approximately 75% of mucin weight, with the central peptide core contributing 17% of mucin weight. Mucins in general are the most densely glycosylated secretory glycoproteins. Gallbladder mucin also contains multiple sulfate residues which account for approximately 4% of mucin weight.

The central peptide core of mucin contains two functionally distinct domains. One domain contains an abundance of serine, threonine, and proline residues. This domain is densely glycosylated and resistant to proteolytic digestion. A second domain appears to be "naked," that is, nonglycosylated. The exposed peptide core in these domains contains hydrophobic binding regions for bilirubin and biliary lipids [2–4] and is sensitive to proteolysis by a variety of endopeptidases.

Viscoelastic and Gel-Forming Properties of Mucin

Mucus is a complex epithelial secretion found throughout the gastrointestinal tract as a viscous gel which is adherent to the mucosal surface. Mucin is the principal organic constituent of mucus and is present both in the mucus gel on the mucosal surface and as a sol in the bulk aqueous phase in the lumen. Other components identified in mucus are cellular debris, serum and membrane proteins, immunoglobulins, electrolytes, and water. Extensive polymerization of mucin appears to be responsible for the viscoelastic properties of mucus gel.

Debate still exists concerning the size of the mucin monomer and the manner by which mucin monomers polymerize to form the mucus gel. The large size of mucin and its tendency to aggregate in solution have made the study of mucin structure by the standard techniques of protein biochemistry quite difficult. We have recently studied mucin subunit interactions using quasielastic laser light scattering [5]. Our data indicate that mucin monomers aggregate above a concentration of 2 mg/ml resulting in a steep increase in viscosity with increasing mucin concentration. Aggregation appears to involve noncovalent hydrophobic and electrostatic associations between mucin subunits, although potential covalent interactions cannot be excluded at present. More detailed information regarding the structure of the mucin monomer will be required to further elucidate the physical properties of mucus gel not only in the gallbladder but throughout the gastrointestinal tract.

Gallbladder Mucin and Gallstone Formation

Animal Models of Gallstone Formation

Recent studies of cholesterol gallstone formation in several animal models have identified an important role for gallbladder mucus in the initial stages of stone formation. Lee et al. studied the evolution of cholesterol gallstone formation in the cholesterol-fed prairie dog [6]. These investigators examined the alterations in the physical chemistry of biliary lipids which occur in response to cholesterol feeding and correlated these findings with alterations in the synthesis and secretion of mucin by the gallbladder epithelium. Gallbladder bile became supersaturated with cholesterol after 5 days on the cholesterol diet and remained supersaturated during the remainder of the study period. Hypersecretion of mucus by the gallbladder epithelium occurred in response to cholesterol feeding and was associated with the accumulation of a thick mucus gel adherent to the mucosal surface of the gallbladder. Mucin synthesis and secretion by the gallbladder epithelium peaked at 5 days after introduction of the cholesterol diet at which time secretion was five times control values. Cholesterol crystals were visible microscopically within the mucus gel but not in the bulk aqueous phase of gallbladder bile. Mucin hypersecretion during gallstone formation occurred only in the gallbladder and could be prevented by cystic duct ligation, suggesting that the stimulus for hypersecretion was carried in lithogenic bile. Based on examination of the gallbladder bile of the cholesterol-fed prairie dogs, it appeared that mucus gel provided a nidus for cholesterol crystal nucleation during the initial stages of cholesterol gallstone formation in this model.

MacPherson et al. used scanning electron microscopy to detail the earliest events which occur on the gallbladder mucosal surface in response to cholesterol feeding in the ground squirrel, a model of gallstone formation similar to the prairie dog [7]. The cholesterol saturation index of gallbladder bile rose within 12 h of initiating cholesterol feeding in these animals. By 18 h a discontinuous layer of thickened mucus began to accumulate on the gallbladder mucosal surface. Hypersecretion of mucus clearly preceded the appearance of cholesterol monohydrate crystals, which were first observed in the mucus gel at 24 h. These investigators provided the first definitive demonstration that mucus gel accumulates on the gallbladder surface prior to the initial nucleation of cholesterol crystals from cholesterol-supersaturated bile. Taken in conjunction with the previous studies of Lee et al., these findings make apparent that gallbladder mucus plays a pivotal role in the earliest stage of gallstone formation, the nucleation of cholesterol crystals.

A subsequent study by Lee et al. further emphasized the importance of mucus for cholesterol crystal nucleation and examined the potential for pharmacologic inhibition of cholesterol gallstone formation [8]. These authors used aspirin, a known inhibitor of mucus secretion in the gut, to prevent hypersecretion of mucus during gallstone formation in the cholesterol-fed prairie dog. Even though aspirin did not change the time course or degree of cholesterol supersaturation of bile which occurred in response to cholesterol feeding, apsirin did inhibit mucin hypersecretion and prevented the formation of cholesterol crystals and stones in these animals. This further supports the hypothesis that mucus gel in the gallbladder lumen provides a nidus for the nucleation of cholesterol crystals from supersaturated bile. In the absence of this nidus for the heterogeneous nucleation of cholesterol crystals, gallbladder bile does not appear to reach the degree of supersaturation required to support the homogeneous nucleation of cholesterol crystals.

Mucin in Gallstone Structure

A second line of evidence which indicates the importance of mucus for gallstone formation has been developed from studies of human gallstone structure. Numerous investigators have noted that a majority of cholesterol gallstones contain a central pigmented nidus where growth of the stone presumably began. Glycoproteins have been repeatedly identified in the nidus of cholesterol gallstones by use of histochemical stains [9, 10]. Studies of gallstone ultrastructure by scanning electron microscopy have identified a fibrillar protein network associated with bile pigment at the center of gallstones which is intermeshed between plates of cholesterol crystals [11, 12]. This noncrystalline component of gallstones has been termed the gallstone matrix and appears to represent the glue which binds plates of cholesterol crystals into stones.

Our laboratory has recently reported that a macromolecular complex of mucin and bilirubin is a major structural component of the gallstone matrix [13]. Analysis of the pigments in the gallstone matrix revealed that approximately 85% was unconjugated bilirubin and 15% was monoconjugated bilirubin. This distribution of bilirubin conjugates is nearly identical to that reported in biliary sludge. Given our previous observation that purified gallbladder mucin can bind bilirubin, it appears that the gallstone matrix originates from biliary sludge which is incorporated into gallstone structure during the nucleation and growth of stones. Biliary sludge identified by ultrasonography in humans may be the pathophysiologic equivalent of the tenacious mucus gel which accumulates in the gallbladder lumen of experimental animals during gallstone formation [14, 15]. In selected patients, prospective evaluation with serial ultrasonography has demonstrated the formation of gallstones within biliary sludge [16]. However, the only variable which has been consistently associated with the development of biliary sludge in humans is gallbladder stasis, particularly during periods of prolonged fasting. Physiologically, biliary sludge formation may be significantly different from the hypersecretion of gallbladder mucus which occurs in response to acute cholesterol feeding in experimental animals. However, the relationship between biliary sludge in humans and the risk of gallstone formation appears to be real. Direct extrapolation of the findings in experimental animals to human cholelithiasis cannot be supported at present, even though the aforementioned animal models appear to be the most satisfactory for the study of gallstone pathogenesis.

Mucin: Pronucleating Agent for Cholesterol Crystals

Because of the apparent importance of gallbladder mucus in cholesterol gallstone formation, our laboratory examined the ability of highly purified gallbladder mucin to accelerate the nucleation of cholesterol monohydrate crystals from supersaturated model bile in vitro [17]. Mucin was purified from human gallbladders and incubated in model bile which had a total lipid content of 10 g/dl and a cholesterol saturation index of 1.4. These values were chosen since they represent the average lipid composition of human lithogenic gallbladder bile. Mucin caused a concentration- and time-dependent increase in the nucleation of cholesterol monohydrate crystals from supersaturated model bile. Additional experiments revealed that mucin purified from gallbladders with and without stones accelerated the nucleation of cholesterol crystals as did mucin purified from bovine gallbladder and monkey cervix. These findings strongly suggest that human gallstone formation is not dependent on the secretion of an abnormal mucin, but rather that a quantitative defect in mucin secretion is responsible. Furthermore, our initial studies indicated that cholesterol monohydrate crystal nucleation in the presence of mucin was preceded by the appearance of cholesterol-lecithin liquid crystals in a fashion similar to that described by others in human and model biles. Mucin only promoted cholesterol crystal nucleation from supersaturated model biles with a total lipid content similar to gallbladder bile (10 g/dl) but not hepatic bile (3 g/dl). These studies indicate that mucin accelerates cholesterol crystal nucleation from supersaturated model bile in a manner which is relevant to what is known regarding the pathophysiology of cholesterol gallstone formation in humans.

We next examined whether the hydrophobic domains on the mucin peptide core contributes to the nucleation-promoting properties of mucin [4]. Multiple low-affinity binding sites for cholesterol and lecithin could be demonstrated on purified gallbladder mucin. Moreover, binding of cholesterol and lecithin to mucin increased as a function of increasing cholesterol saturation index of model bile. Proteolytic digestion of purified mucin disaggregated the native mucin polymer and eliminated the binding of small hydrophobic fluorescent probes to the mucin peptide core. In an analogous fashion, proteolysis of mucin decreased the binding of cholesterol and lecithin in model bile to mucin by 91% and 78%, respectively, indicating that these lipids bind to the hydrophobic domains on the mucin peptide core.

Proteolytic digestion of human and bovine gallbladder mucin abolished the ability of mucin to accelerate cholesterol crystal nucleation in model bile (Fig. 1). This finding indicates that structural integrity of the hyrophobic domains on the mucin peptide core is essential for the binding of biliary lipids to mucin as well as for the acceleration of cholesterol crystal nucleation by mucin. Furthermore, our data suggest that mucin does not simply facilitate cholesterol crystal growth but rather accelerates the initial nucleation of crystals.

Cholesterol is transported in supersaturated bile in mixed lipid micelles and in cholesterol-lecithin vesicles. In vivo nucleation of cholesterol monohydrate crystals appears to follow the fusion of unilamellar cholesterol-lecithin vesicles into multilamellar liposomes. Since mucin binds cholesterol and lecithin and accelerates cholesterol crystal nucleation, we sought to determine whether mucin preferentially interacts with either cholesterol-lecithin vesicles or mixed micelles [18]. Vesicles and micelles in supersaturated model bile were separated by Sephadex G-200 gel permeation chromatography. Vesicles which were recovered in the opalescent void volume of the column had a cholesterol-lecithin molar ratio of 1.00 while the smaller mixed micelles were recovered in the included volume of the column. Cholesterol crystal nucleated spontaneously from vesicles prepared by column chromatography but not from mixed micelles. Significant binding of cholesterol and lecithin to mucin occurred when these lipids were transported in vesicles, but not when they were in mixed micelles. In addition, mucin caused a concentration- and time-dependent acceleration of cholesterol crystal nucleation only from vesicles and not from mixed micelles. This study indicates that mucin binds and accelerates nucleation of cholesterol crystals from lipid particles in model bile with similar physical chemical properties to those particles which are responsible for cholesterol crystal nucleation in vivo.

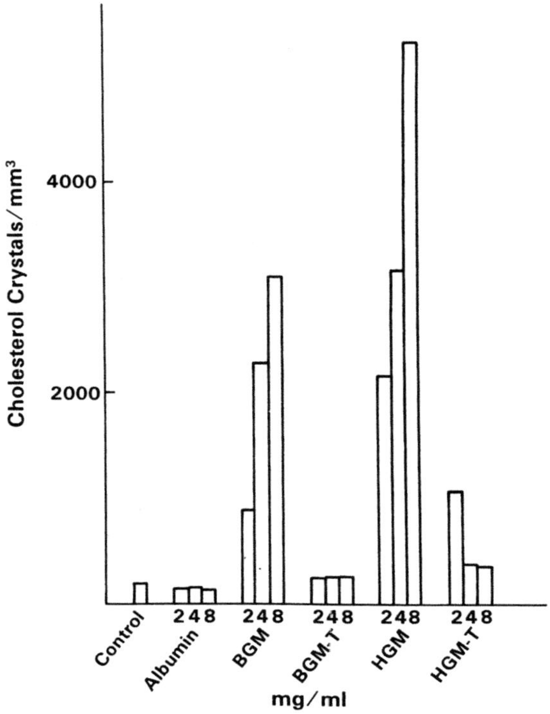

Fig. 1. Cholesterol crystal nucleation: effect of trypsin digestion of gallbladder mucin. Model bile was prepared with a cholesterol saturation index of 1.4 and a total lipid content of 10 g/dl. Aliquots of the same model bile were incubated at 37 °C under sterile conditions with either no protein addition (*control*, $n = 8$), bovine serum albumin (*albumin*), native bovine gallbladder mucin (*BGM*), trypsin-digested bovine gallbladder mucin (*BGM-T*), human gallbladder mucin (*HGM*), or trypsin-digested human gallbladder mucin (*HGM-T*). Protein incubations were performed in quadruplicate at concentrations of 2, 4, and 8 mg/ml. Cholesterol monohydrate crystals were quantitated by polarizing microscopy after 9 days of incubation and expressed as the number of cholesterol crystals/mm^3. HGM and BGM were significantly different from control, albumin-, and trypsin-digested mucin ($p < 0.0001$, for each)

Conclusion

This discussion has summarized the available lines of evidence which indicate that gallbladder mucin, the major organic constituent of gallbladder mucus, is a critical element in the pathogenesis of cholesterol gallstones. Mucin is the major secretory product of the gallbladder epithelium. In response to poorly defined stimuli, the gallbladder epithelium hypersecretes mucin, which results in the accumulation of a thick mucus gel on the mucosal surface of the gallbladder. Evidence obtained in experimental animals and in man indicates that mucus gel provides a nidus for the heterogeneous nucleation of cholesterol monohydrate crystals from supersaturated gallbladder bile, the initial event in the pathogenesis of cholesterol gallstones. Highly purified gallbladder mucin contains hydrophobic domains on its central peptide core which bind cholesterol and lecithin transported in vesicles in supersaturated model bile. Furthermore, mucin accelerates cholesterol crystal nucleation in a manner which appears to be pathophysiologically relevant to cholesterol gallstone formation in man. The ability to pharmacologically manipulate mucin synthesis and secretion promises to provide exciting and potentially useful therapies for the prevention of gallstones in selected patients in the future.

References

1. Makhlouf GM (1979) Transport and motor functions of the gallbladder. Viewpoints Dig Dis 11 (3):1
2. Smith BF, LaMont JT (1984) Hydrophobic binding properties of bovine gallbladder mucin. J Biol Chem 259:12170–12177
3. Smith BF, LaMont JT (1983) Bovine gallbladder mucin binds bilirubin in vitro. Gastroenterology 85:707–712
4. Smith BF (1987) Human gallbladder mucin binds biliary lipids and promotes cholesterol crystal nucleation in model bile. J Lipid Res 28:1088–1097
5. Smith BF, Peetermans JA, Tanaka T, Lamont JT (1989) Subunit interactions and physical properties of bovine gallbladder mucin. Gastroenterology 97:179–187
6. Lee SP, LaMont JT, Carey MC (1981) Role of gallbladder mucus hypersecretion in the evolution of cholesterol gallstones. Studies in the prairie dog. J Clin Invest 67:1712–1723
7. MacPerson BR, Pemsingh RS, Scott GW (1987) Experimental cholelithiasis in the ground squirrel. Lab Invest 56:138–142
8. Lee SP, Carey MC, LaMont JT (1981) Aspirin prevention of cholesterol gallstone formation in prairie dogs. Science 211:1429–1432
9. Womack N, Zeppa R, Irving G (1963) The anatomy of gallstones. Ann Surg 157:670–686
10. Maki T, Matsushiro T, Susuki N, Nakamura N (1974) Role of sulfated glycoproteins in gallstone formation. Surg Gnyecol Obstet 132:846–851
11. Been JM, Bills PM, Lewis DL (1979) Microstructure of gallstones. Gastroenterology 76:548–555
12. Bills PM, Lewis DL (1975) A structural study of gallstones. Gut 16:630–637
13. Smith BF, LaMont JT (1985) Identification of gallbladder mucin-bilirubin complex in human cholesterol gallstone matrix. Effects of reducing agents on in vitro dissolution of matrix and intact gallstones. J Clin Invest 76:439–445
14. Lee SP, Nichols JF (1986) Nature and composition of biliary sludge. Gastroenterology 90:677–686
15. Lee SP, Maher K, Nichols JF (1988) Origin and fate of biliary sludge. Gastroenterology 88:170–176
16. Messing B, Bories L, Kuntslinger F, Bernier J (1983) Does total parenteral nutrition induce gallbladder sludge formation and lithiasis? Gastroenterology 84:1012–1019
17. Levy PF, Smith BF, LaMont JT (1984) Human gallbladder mucin accelerates in vitro nucleation of cholesterol in artificial bile. Gastroenterology 87:270–275
18. Lee JT, Smith BF (1989) Bovine gallbladder mucin promotes cholesterol crystal nucleation from cholesterol transporting vesicles in supersaturated model bile. J Lipid Res 30:491–498

Biliary Proteins and Their Role as Nucleating Inhibitors/Promotors

P. R. C. Harvey and S. M. Strasberg

Department of Surgery and Research Institute, Mount Sinai Hospital, University of Toronto, 600 University Ave., Toronto, Ont. M5G 1X5, Canada

Introduction

The formation of cholesterol gallstones requires three major pathogenetic defects, namely supersaturation, nucleation, and crystal retention and cohesion. All three factors are necessary for the formation of cholesterol gallstones, and the presence of just one or two factors does not lead to stones. For example, many studies have shown not only that almost all patients with cholesterol gallstones have supersaturated bile, but that supersaturated bile is also very common in healthy individuals [1–3]. In other words, supersaturation is necessary but not sufficient for stone formation. Supersaturated gallbladder bile from normal persons is metastable; it nucleates cholesterol crystals before reaching equilibrium, but nucleation of crystals occurs slowly. Equally supersaturated bile from stone formers is labile, i.e., the nucleation is rapid [2, 3]. For instance the nucleation time (time of appearance of microscopic cholesterol crystals in a bile sample that has been initially cleared of all crystals) of bile obtained from cholesterol stone patients is rapid (1–2 days), whereas equally supersaturated bile from control patients nucleates slowly (up to 21 days) [2, 3]. But even the presence of defects in supersaturation and nucleation does not invariably lead to stones. Lee et al. have recently shown that most patients with cholesterol crystal-bearing sludge clear the crystals from bile over a period of time, and that only a few form stones [4]. We have recently identified a group of patients with cholesterol crystals in their bile but without stones [5]. It seems that a motility defect leading to crystal retention in the gallbladder is needed to turn crystals into stones. Stone formers may have an associated defect favoring adhesion of crystals as well as their retention. Although there are three defects necessary for gallstone production, much recent work including our own has focused on the second-stage defect – nucleation.

A possible role in the nucleation process has been suggested for several constituents of bile, including calcium salts [6–8], bilirubin [9], trace elements [10, 11], and proteins. All of these substances have been identified in the cholesterol stone itself [10–14]. This discussion focuses on the role of antinucleating and pronucleating proteins in human cholesterol gallstone formation.

Antinucleating Proteins

Apolipoproteins

The nucleation time of model bile is more rapid than that of equally supersaturated bile obtained from normal persons [15]. This observation suggested that normal bile contained stabilizing antinucleating factors. Holzbach et al. determined that these nucleation-inhibiting factors were bile proteins [15]; detergent-delipidated biliary proteins isolated from the bile of stone-free individuals prolonged the nucleation time when added to model bile [15]. Preincubation of these bile proteins with pronase destroyed the nucleation-inhibiting effect. This was the first study implicating biliary proteins as cholesterol crystal nucleation inhibitors. A preliminary attempt to isolate and identify the antinucleating protein by gel filtration showed that the major antinucleating activity eluted in the included volume of the column. Whether proteins which coeluted with the biliary lipids were associated with the lipids or eluted with lipids due to similar molecular size was not determined. The most likely explanation, however, as suggested by Holzbach et al., is that these proteins interact with bile lipids possibly forming complexes similar to the lipoproteins of serum.

Support for the role of apolipoproteins came from the work of Sewell et al. [16] and Ohisalo et al. [17], who demonstrated their presence in human gallbladder bile. Subsequently, purified serum apolipoproteins, namely apoproteins A-1, A-2, and C-3 were added to model biles to study their effect on nucleation time [18]. Apoproteins A-1 and A-2 inhibited the rate of formation of cholesterol crystals in supersaturated model bile systems; apoprotein C-3 had no effect. Furthermore, apoproteins A-1 and A-2 were identified in the included gel filtration fraction shown previously to contain the cholesterol nucleation-inhibiting factor [15]. These results strongly suggest that apoproteins A-1 and A-2 are proteins that inhibit cholesterol crystal nucleation in human supersaturated gallbladder bile. One might expect then that the concentration of these proteins would be higher in patients without gallstones. However, this was not found to be so. The concentration of apoprotein A-1 or A-2 is similar in patients with and without gallstones [16]. Possibly the presence of antinucleating proteins is the usual situation in persons with and without stones, and the presence of a nucleating protein(s) is the primary defect in patients with cholesterol gallstones.

Other Possible Nucleation-Inhibiting Proteins

Groen et al. [19] recently reported nucleation-inhibiting activity in human bile in the unbound protein fraction from a concanavalin A (ConA) Sepharose lectin column. The nucleation-inhibiting fraction was unstable; inhibiting activity was lost after 24 h at 37 °C. This nucleation-inhibiting protein may be apolipoprotein A-1, which does not contain carbohydrates [20] and would not bind to ConA. The activity of this factor is transient at 37 °C likely because it is denatured by endogenous proteolytic enzymes in gallbladder bile.

Holzbach's group [21] has used several lectins in order to isolate nucleating and antinucleating proteins from normal gallbladder bile. The protein fraction isolated by *Helix pomatia,* a lectin specific for *N*-acetyl-D-galactosamine [22] inhibited both nucleation and crystal growth. This protein fraction was reported to have greater potency than apolipoprotein A-1. The identity of this factor remains to be determined.

Nucleating Proteins

Mucous Glycoproteins

Mucous glycoproteins, a subgroup of glycoproteins, differ chemically and structurally from other classes of glycoproteins (serum glycoproteins and proteoglycans). Amino acid and carbohydrate content as well as the linkage of the sugars to the peptide backbone are characteristic and differ from those of other glycoproteins [23, 24]. The protein component is relatively rich in threonine, serine, and proline. Mucous glycoproteins characteristically have a high carbohydrate content (over 70% by weight) which contributes substantially to their high molecular weight (over 10^6 Da). The carbohydrate side chains consist of fucose, galactose, *N*-acetylgalactosamine, *N*-acetylglucosamine, and *N*-acetylneuraminic acid (sialic acid). Mucous glycoproteins are distinguished from serum glycoproteins by their low mannose content and from proteoglycans by lack of uronic acid. Linkage of the monosaccharides to the peptide in mucous glycoproteins occurs between *N*-acetylgalactosamine and the hydroxyl groups of threonine and serine (*O*-glycosidic linkage). This contrasts to the linkage in serum glycoproteins in which *N*-acetylglucosamine is attached to the nitrogen of asparagine (*N*-glycosidic linkage).

Mucous glycoproteins were implicated in stone formation by the observation that stones contained a mucopolysaccharide matrix [25–27]. Subsequently, it was found that some lithogenic diets caused hypersecretion of mucous glycoprotein in the gallbladder prior to stone formation in animals [28–31]. Aspirin inhibited the hypersecretion of mucous glycoprotein in the prairie dog model and prevented gallstone production without decreasing cholesterol saturation [32]. These studies suggested that mucous glycoprotein might be a pronucleator.

Lee et al. [31] directly examined the effect of mucous glycoprotein on nucleation. Human gallbladder mucin obtained from gallbladder mucosal scrapings accelerated the nucleation of cholesterol crystals when added to saturated prairie dog hepatic bile. Subsequently, it was shown that human gallbladder mucous glycoprotein accelerates the nucleation time of model bile systems [33] as well as that of control human gallbladder biles [34].

While there is no doubt that mucous glycoproteins are pronucleators, it is much less certain that either a quantitative or a qualitative abnormality of these compounds is the nucleation defect responsible for cholesterol gallstone formation. Lee et al. [35] found a significant increase in the gallbladder mucous glycoprotein concentration in patients with cholesterol gallstones compared to control patients, particularly if sludge was present. On the other hand, we found no significant difference in the gallbladder mucous glycoprotein concentration between the two patient groups, although there was a mild trend towards higher concentrations in patients with cholesterol gallstones [36]. There are at least two explanations for these discrepancies. Continuous feeding of the lithogenic diet is required to maintain hypersecretion of mucous glycoprotein in the prairie dog cholesterol gallstone model [31]. Perhaps, hypersecretion of mucous glycoprotein occurs in the human during stone formation but returns to normal after the stone is formed. This would be difficult to prove in the human. To clarify this issue we require studies comparing the mucous glycoprotein concentration in control patients that have cholesterol crystals in their bile (prestone formers) to those that do not have crystals. Secondly, it is well known that the gallbladder fills with mucous when the cystic duct is obstructed. Partial obstruction of the cystic duct by stone or inflammation secondary to the presence of stones might account for high mucous glycoprotein values. This artifact may be avoided by using the total lipid concentration of fasting gallbladder bile as a guide to cystic duct patency. Samples with total lipid concentration greater than 5 gm/dl probably indicate normal cystic duct patency [37].

In qualitative studies both the amino acid and carbohydrate content of mucous glycoproteins purified from patients with and without cholesterol gallstones were shown to be very similar [35, 36]. The only reported difference in mucous glycoprotein between groups is in the sulfate content. The bile of patients with cholesterol gallstones has been shown to contain a higher concentration of acidic mucous glycoprotein due to the increased sulfate [27, 35]. The significance of this finding is undetermined, but it seems unlikely that it can explain the difference in the in vitro nucleation time of the two patient groups. We have shown that the mucous glycoprotein purified from normal control bile was just as effective in accelerating the nucleation time as mucous glycoprotein obtained from stoneformer bile [34].

Proteins Other than Mucous Glycoproteins Acting as Nucleating Factors

Early investigations in our laboratory showed that patients with cholesterol gallstones contained a potent nucleating factor that was not removed by filtration through an Amicon XM-300 filter (mol. wt. cutoff approximately 300 kDa) [38]. Subsequent studies showing that filtration completely removed all mucous glycoproteins [34] suggested that another nucleating factor existed besides mucous glycoproteins. This led to the need for development of a method to purify biliary proteins from human bile. The method involved an adaptation of the method of Reuben et al. [39], used to separate rat bile proteins from bile lipids, and cesium chloride ultracentrifugation to separate mucous glycoproteins from other proteins of lower molecular weight. Although very tedious, the method provided a pure lipid-free mixture of biliary proteins other than mucous glycoproteins [40]. These purified proteins were used to perform an experiment very similar to the one described above for mucous glycoproteins. Purified gallbladder proteins obtained from patients with stones and controls without stones were added in identical amounts to control gallbladder bile. These results are shown in Fig. 1. We found that the proteins from patients with cholesterol gallstones were better pronucleators than the proteins of control patients. All protein samples from gallstone patients accelerated nucleation of control bile, but control patient proteins did so infrequently.

We also modified for use in bile the fluorescamine method for quantification of total protein concentration and validated the method by amino acid analysis. We found a small but significant difference in the mean total protein concentration between controls and cholesterol gallstone patients (1.76 ± 1.14 and 3.08 ± 2.32, respectively). A large number of patients had to be studied to detect this difference because of overlap in values between groups. Similar findings were subsequently reported by Antezana et al. [41]. Yamazaki et al. [42] were unable to substantiate these results in a small number of patients, but in more recent studies in a larger number of patients results similar to our own were reported [43]. Recently we have shown that control patients with crystals in their bile have higher total protein concentration than equally saturated controls without crystals [5]. Furthermore, the difference in protein concentration between control and

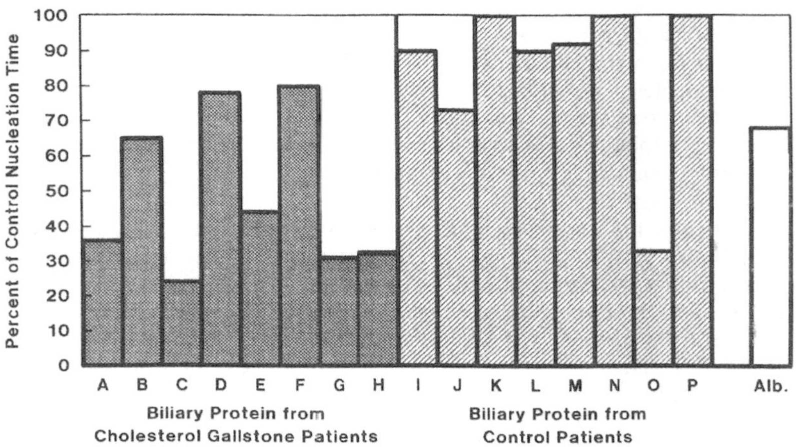

Fig. 1. Effect of addition of gallbladder proteins from patients with and without cholesterol gallstones on the nucleation time (NT) of control bile. Results are expressed as a percentage of control NT [(NT of protein mixture/NT of control) times 100]. *Letters A–P* represent results of proteins isolated from individual patients. Human serum albumin (Alb.) was used as a control protein

stone patients is much greater when only crystal-free supersaturated controls are compared to stone patients. We also found a correlation between protein concentration and nucleation time, i.e., patients with high protein concentrations had the most rapid nucleation time [40]. Furthermore, heating abnormal bile, which reduces the protein concentration by as much as 50%–60% results in prolongation of the nucleation time [34].

Further purification of the pronucleating protein has been achieved by using ConA affinity chromatography of hepatic bile samples [19]. Nucleation-promoting activity was also reported to be present in patients without cholesterol gallstones but was less potent. This ConA-binding glycoprotein has been shown to accelerate the nucleation time of model biles in a dose-response manner [44]. The number of crystals observed per day was also greater in models containing the higher concentration of ConA-binding glycoprotein. Since mucous glycoprotein does not bind to ConA, these results support the evidence that a nonmucous glycoprotein may have an important role in the formation of cholesterol gallstones. The glycoprotein must be rich in mannose and/or glucose since it binds to ConA. Subsequently Groen et al. [45] employing gel filtration chromatography with a Superose 12 column have found that nucleating promoting activity eluted in two peaks with molecular weights of 150 ± 30 kDa and below 5 kDa, respectively. The protein of below 5 kDa is believed to be a degraded product of the 150-kDa protein. The identity of the 150-kDa glycoprotein remains to be determined.

Proposed Mechanism of Action of Nucleating and Antinucleating Proteins

The concept that is emerging today is that both nucleating and antinucleating proteins exist in the same bile sample, and that cholesterol nucleation from a bile sample depends on the balance of these nucleating and antinucleating forces. This concept is analogous to the game of tug-of-war as depicted in Fig. 2. Patients with cholesterol gallstones have a greater propensity to nucleate cholesterol from their bile due to the overriding effect of the nucleating forces. It is likely that qualitative differences in proteins are much more important than the fact that stone patients have a slightly higher total protein concentration.

The question arises as to what the mechanism of action is of these pronucleating and antinucleating proteins. Do separate mechanisms exist or do the pronucleating and antinucleating proteins act by similar but opposite mechanisms? Clues to this question may be obtained if one looks at the form in which cholesterol is carried in the bile. Biliary cholesterol is transported in mixed bile salt-phospholipid-cholesterol micelles and in phospholipid-cholesterol vesicles [46–48]. Nucleation appears to be preceded by vesicle aggregation [49–52]. Vesicles and micelles can be separated from each other by gel filtration chromatography [48, 53]. Figure 3 shows the chromatographic results of a bile sample prelabeled with [^{3}H]-cholesterol and [^{14}C]-phospholipid. Two major peaks were observed: (a) cholesterol-phospholipid containing peak in the void volume, the vesicular peak, and (b) a cholesterol-phospholipid-bile salt peak in the included volume, the micellar peak. Figure 4 presents an electron micrograph of the vesicular peak separated by gel filtration.

Employing this technique, we have found that patients with cholesterol gallstones have a greater quantity of cholesterol carried in the vesicular state, that nucleation of cholesterol occurs from the vesicles and not the micelles, and that the chemistry of the vesicles, namely the cholesterol/phospholipid ratio of the vesicles from human bile, influences the nucleation of cholesterol [53, 54]. The critical importance of the vesicular cholesterol/phospholipid ratio in nucleation has also been described by Collins and Philips [55] and by Holzbach's group [50, 52] in model biles.

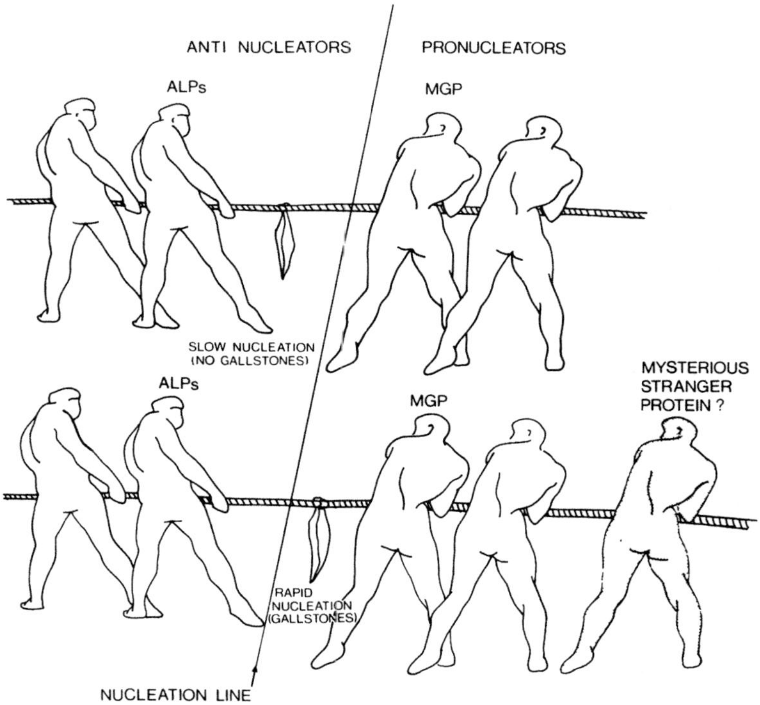

Fig. 2. The game of tug-of-war is analogous to the propensity of gallbladder bile to nucleate depending on the balance of nucleating and antinucleating forces. Patients with cholesterol gallstones have a greater propensity to nucleate cholesterol from their bile due to the overriding effect of the nucleating forces. ALPs, apolipoproteins; MGP, mucous glycoprotein

Vesicles may be classified as multilamellar or unilamellar. Multilamellar vesicles are larger, being several micrometers in size, and represent the thermodynamically most stable form [56]. Smaller unilamellar vesicles are a metastable form of higher free energy and revert to the more stable multilamellar form only when perturbed [57]. This process occurs by aggregation and fusion of the unilamellar vesicles. Fusion is a process in which one vesicle membrane is introduced into a second vesicle membrane with intermixing of their aqueous contents. Simultaneously as the vesicular bilayer structure opens up, bidirectional exchange of entrapped compounds with the external aqueous environment may occur. Such events may be operative in formation of cholesterol crystals from vesicles. When the concentration of cholesterol in phosphatidylcholine vesicles exceeds 30 mol%, cholesterol is asymmetrically distributed across the bilayer of vesicles, with a disproportionately larger amount of cholesterol present on the inner monolayer [58]. The possibility of cholesterol-to-cholesterol interaction is therefore greater on the inner monolayer as the relative decrease in phospholipid results in reduced solvation of each cholesterol molecule. Microcrystals may even form and be enclosed within these vesicles. Fusion of unilamellar vesicles with leakage of their contents to the external aqueous environment might then lead to the appearance of macroscopic cholesterol crystals.

The natural question to be answered is what is the relationship between vesicles from which nucleation occurs and pronucleating and antinucleating proteins. Figure 5 depicts the proposed mechanisms of cholesterol nucleation in gallstone disease. Several proteins

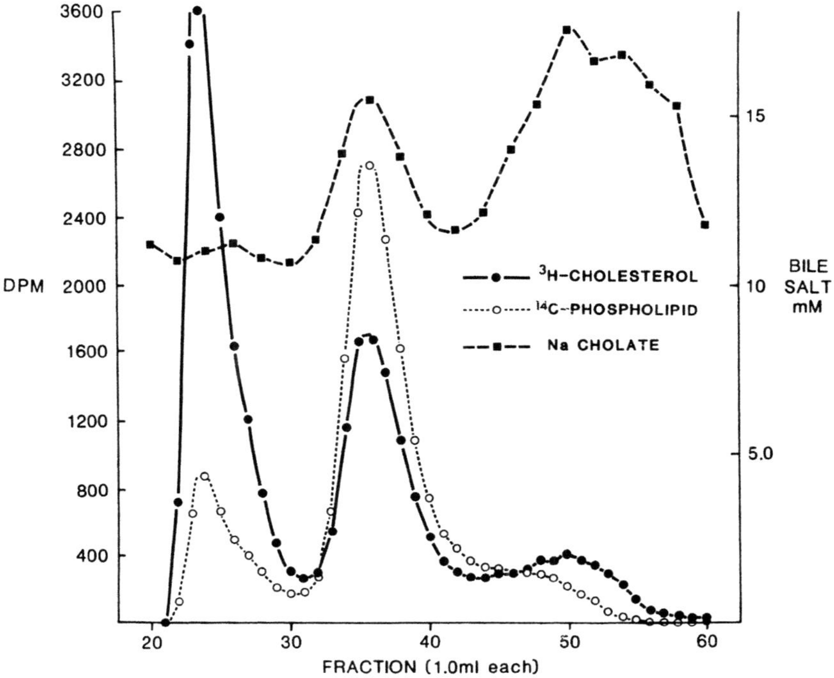

Fig. 3. Gel filtration of human gallbladder bile prelabeled with [^{3}H]-cholesterol and [^{14}C]-phospholipid to separate vesicles from micelles

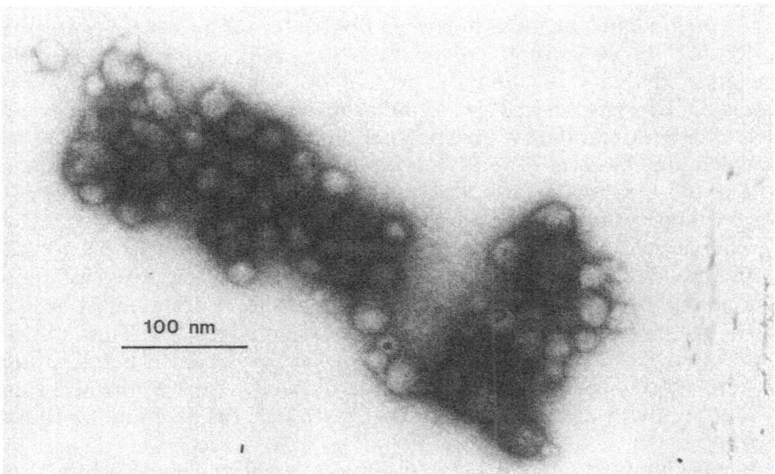

Fig. 4. Electron microscopy of the vesicular fraction isolated from human gallbladder bile by gel filtration

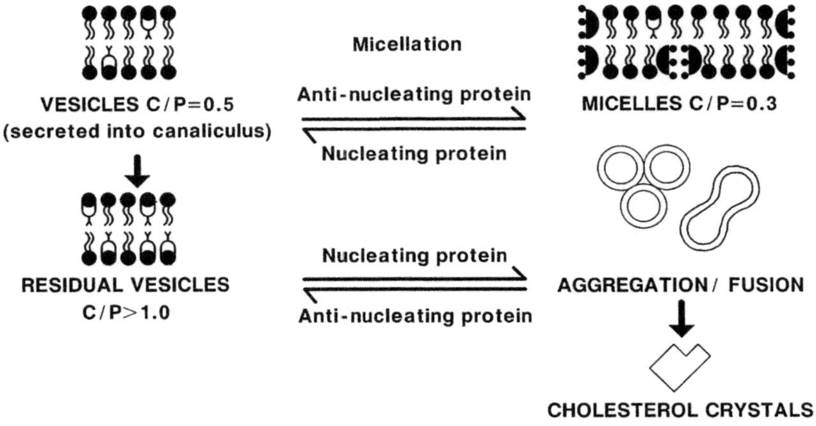

Fig. 5. Proposed mechanisms of action of nucleating and antinucleating proteins. Three major mechanisms may result in gallbladder bile becoming unstable with the consequence of favoring cholesterol nucleation. Lipid shifts may occur between micelles and vesicles resulting in more cholesterol being carried in the vesicular state. Micellation of vesicles with a low cholesterol/phospholipid (*C/P*) ratio could result in a residual vesicle with a higher C/P ratio due to the greater tendency of phospholipid to become micellarized in comparison to cholesterol. Aggregation or fusion of vesicles leads to cholesterol crystal formation. Biliary antinucleating proteins may delay, while nucleating proteins could accelerate these processes

have been shown to act as fusogenic agents. In early studies of protein–vesicle interactions of proteins, polylysine [59, 60] or polyhistidine [61], was used to fuse vesicles composed of acidic phospholipids. Such fusion is primarily due to interaction between positively charged peptide and negatively charged lipids promoting vesicle aggregration followed by fusion [62]. Other cationic polypeptides such as polymyxin B [63], melittin [64, 65], cytochrome C [59], and myelin basic protein [66] also interact with unilamellar vesicles containing acidic phospholipids by a similar mechanism. However the extent of fusion was noted to be greater if the cationic polypeptide contained hydrophobic residues [62]. Phosphatidylcholine vesicles have also been shown to fuse in the presence of a number of proteins [67–75] particularly at a low pH. It is believed that low pH causes a conformational change producing an amphipathic helix by exposure of hydrophobic domains [71, 75]. It should be noted that not all proteins require a low pH to induce fusion of phosphatidylcholine vesicles [64]. Therefore vesicles composed of the uncharged phospholipid phosphatidylcholine are hypothesized to be destabilized by hydrophobic residues of proteins in a fashion that results in fusion of vesicles. Thus a nucleating protein could interact with the phospholipid-cholesterol vesicles of bile resulting in their instability and subsequent fusion with cholesterol nucleation. On the other hand, a protein that interferes with this process and prevents vesicle fusion could be classified as an antinucleating protein.

Other possible mechanisms of action of nucleating and antinucleating proteins must be considered. These include interference with the equilibrium between vesicles and micelles [76, 77]. Indeed, Donovan et al. [76] have demonstrated that apolipoprotein A-1 can delay the micelle-to-vesicle transition and the growth of vesicle sizes for up to 48 h. Groen et al. [77], on the other hand, have shown that the nucleation-promoting ConA glycoprotein fraction induces a transfer of lipids from micelles to vesicles. It also appears that the nucleating protein interacts directly with vesicles rendering them less stable and resulting in cholesterol nucleation [77]. Whether an antinucleating protein stabilizes vesicles remains to be determined. It is also possible that a nucleating protein may act as a direct template for cholesterol nucleation, as suggested by Smith [78]. Future research will determine how and under what circumstances the nucleating and antinucleating protein interacts with vesicles or micelles to accelerate or delay nucleation.

References

1. Sedaghat A, Grundy SM (1980) Cholesterol crystals and the formation of cholesterol gallstones. N Eng J Med 302:1274–1277
2. Holan KR, Holzbach RT, Hermann RE, Cooperman AM, Claffey WJ (1979) Nucleation time: a key factor in the pathogenesis of cholesterol gallstone disease. Gastroenterology 77:611–617
3. Gollish SH, Burnstein MJ, Ilson RG, Petrunka CN, Strasberg SM (1983) Nucleation of cholesterol monohydrate crystals from hepatic and gall-bladder bile of patients with cholesterol gallstones. Gut 24:836–844
4. Lee SP, Maher K, Nicholls JF (1988) Origin and fate of biliary sludge. Gastroenterology 94:107–176
5. Strasberg SM, Toth JL, Harvey PRC (1988) High total protein and total lipid concentration are associated with reduced metastability in an early stage of cholesterol gallstones. Hepatology 8:1257
6. Moore EW, Celic L, Ostrow JD (1982) Interactions between ionized calcium and sodium taurocholate: bile salts are important buffers for prevention of calcium-containing gallstones. Gastroenterology 83:1079–1089
7. Moore EW (1984) The role of calcium in the pathogenesis of gallstones: Ca^{++} electrode studies of model bile salt solutions and other biologic systems. Hepatology 4:228s–243s
8. Williamson BWA, Anderson JL, Percy-Robb IW (1985) Cholesterol gallstones pathogenesis: morphology of cholesterol nucleation on calcium salt crystals. Gut 26:A561
9. Maki T (1966) Pathogenesis of calcium bilirubinate gallstones: role of E. coli beta-glucuronidase and coagulation by inorganic ions, polyelectrolytes and agitation. Ann Surg 164:90–100
10. Been JM, Bills PM, Lewis D (1977) Electron probe microanalysis in the study of gallstones. Gut 18:836–842
11. Been JM, Bills PM, Lewis D (1979) Microstructure of gallstones. Gastroenterology 76:548–555
12. Bogren H (1964) The composition and structure of human gallstones. Acta Radiol [Suppl] 226:7–47
13. Markkanen T, Aho AJ (1972) Metabolic aspects of trace metal content of gallstones and gallbladders. Acta Chir Scand 138:301–305
14. Al-Kinani AT, Watt DE, East BW, Harris IA (1984) Minor and trace element analysis of gallstones. Analyst 109:365–368
15. Holzbach TR, Kibe A, Thiel E, Howell JH, Marsh M, Hermann RE (1984) Biliary proteins: unique inhibitors of cholesterol crystal nucleation in human gallbladder bile. J Clin Invest 73:35–45
16. Sewell RB, Mao SJT, Kawamoto T, LaRusso NF (1983) Apolipoproteins of high, low, and very low density lipoproteins in human bile. J Lipid Res 24:391–401
17. Ohisalo JJ, Keso L, Ehnholm C (1983) Apolipoproteins AI and AII in human bile. Acta Physiol Scand 119:303–304
18. Kibe A, Holzbach RT, LaRusso NF, Mao SJT (1984) Inhibition of cholesterol crystal formation by apolipoproteins in supersaturated model bile. Science 225:514–516
19. Groen AK, Stout JPJ, Drapers JAG, Hoek FJ, Grijm R, Tytgat GNJ (1988) Cholesterol nucleation-influencing activity in t-tube bile. Hepatology 8:347–352
20. Mahley RW, Innerarity TL, Rall SC, Weisgraber KH (1984) Plasma lipoproteins: apolipoprotein structure and function. J Lipid Res 25:1277–1294
21. Busch N, Matiuck NV, Cottle A, Mancuso DJ, Tokumo H, Holzbach RT (1988) Inhibiting and promoting effects on cholesterol crystal nucleation and growth rate are found in protein fractions from normal human gallbladder bile. Hepatology 8:1224
22. Goldstein IJ, Hayes CE (1978) The lectins: carbohydrate-binding proteins of plants and animals. Adv Carbohydr Chem Biochem 35:127–340

23. Clamp JR (1977) Mucus in health and disease. In: Elstein M, Parke DV (eds) Mucus in health and disease. Plenum, New York, pp 1–15
24. Allen A (1983) Mucus – a protective secretion of complexity. Trends Biochem Sci 8:169–173
25. Womack NA, Zeppa R, Irvin GL (1963) The anatomy of gallstones. Ann Surg 157:670–686
26. Hulten O (1970) Contractions of the gallbladder and the formation of gallstones. Acta Chir Scand 136:53–56
27. Maki T, Matsushiro T, Suzuki N, Nakamura N (1971) Role of sulfated glycoprotein in gallstone formation. Surg Gynecol Obstet 132:846–854
28. Freston JW, Bouchier IAD, Newman J (1969) Biliary mucous substances in dihydrocholesterol-induced cholelithiasis. Gastroenterology 57:670–678
29. Womack NA (1971) The development of gallstones. Surg Gynecol Obstet 133:937–945
30. Lee SP (1981) Hypersecretion of mucus glycoprotein by the gallbladder epithelium in experimental cholelithiasis. J Pathology 134:199–207
31. Lee SP, LaMont JT, Carey MC (1981) Role of gallbladder mucus hypersecretion in the evolution of cholesterol gallstones. J Clin Invest 67:1712–1723
32. Lee SP, Carey MC, LaMont JT (1981) Aspirin prevention of cholesterol gallstone formation in prairie dogs. Science 211:1429–1431
33. Levy PF, Smith BF, LaMont JT (1984) Human gallbladder mucin accelerates nucleation of cholesterol in artificial bile. Gastroenterology 87:270–275
34. Gallinger S, Taylor RD, Harvey PRC, Petrunka CN, Strasberg SM (1985) Effect of mucous glycoprotein on nucleation time of human bile. Gastroenterology 89:648–658
35. Lee SP, Nicholls JF (1986) Nature and composition of biliary sludge. Gastroenterology 90:677–686
36. Harvey PRC, Rupar CA, Gallinger S, Petrunka CN, Strasberg SM (1986) Quantitative and qualitative comparison of gallbladder mucus glycoprotein from patients with and without gall stones. Gut 27:374–381
37. Tera H (1960) Stratification of human gallbladder bile in vivo. Acta Chir Scand [Suppl] 256:4–85
38. Burnstein MJ, Ilson RG, Petrunka CN, Taylor RD, Strasberg SM (1983) Evidence for a potent nucleating factor in the gallbladder bile of patients with cholesterol gallstones. Gastroenterology 85:801–807
39. Reuben A, Howell KE, Boyer JL (1982) Effects of taurocholate on the size of mixed lipid micelles and their associations with pigment and protein in rat bile. J Lipid Res 23:1039–1052
40. Gallinger S, Harvey PRC, Petrunka CN, Ilson RG, Strasberg SM (1987) Biliary proteins and the nucleation defect in cholesterol cholelithiasis. Gastroenterology 92:867–875
41. Antezana C, Covarrubias C, Severin C, Valdivieso V (1988) Cristalizacion del colesterol en la bilis vesicular. Rev Med Chil 116:858–862
42. Yamazaki K, Powers SP, LaRusso NF (1988) Biliary proteins: assessment of quantitative techniques and comparison in gallstone and nongallstone subjects. J Lipid Res 29:1055–1063
43. Perdigoto R, Yamazaki K, LaRusso NF (1988) Biliary glycoproteins: quantitative differences in subjects with and without gallstones. Hepatology 8:1257
44. Harvey PRC, Upadhya GA, Toth JL, Strasberg SM (1987) A concanavalin A binding glycoprotein accelerates the nucleation of cholesterol from model bile. Hepatology 7:1112
45. Groen AK, Stout JPJ, Noordam C, Korsen A, Hoek FJ, Jansen PLM, Tytgat GNJ (1987) Isolation and partial characterization of a cholesterol nucleation promoting factor from human bile. Hepatology 7:1023
46. Mazer NA, Schurtenberger P, Carey MC, Preisig R, Weigand K, Kanzig W (1984) Quasi-elastic light scattering studies of native hepatic bile from the dog: comparison with aggregative behaviour of model biliary lipid systems. Biochemistry 23:1994–2005
47. Sömjen GJ, Gilat T (1983) A non-micellar mode of cholesterol transport in human bile. FEBS Lett 156:265–268
48. Sömjen GJ, Gilat T (1985) Contribution of vesicular and micellar carriers to cholesterol transport in human bile. J Lipid Res 26:699–704
49. Kibe A, Dudley MA, Halpern Z, Lynn MP, Breuer AC, Holzbach RT (1985) Factors affecting cholesterol monohydrate crystal nucleation time in model systems of supersaturated bile. J Lipid Res 26:1102–1111
50. Halpern Z, Dudley MA, Lynn MP, Nader JM, Breuer AC, Holzbach RT (1986) Vesicle

aggregation in model systems of supersaturated bile: relation to crystal nucleation and lipid composition of the vesicular phase. J Lipid Res 27:295–306
51. Halpern Z, Dudley MA, Kibe A, Lynn MP, Breuer AC, Holzbach RT (1986) Rapid vesicle formation and aggregation in abnormal human biles. A time-lapse video-enhanced and polarizing light microscopy study. Gastroenterology 90:875–885
52. Holzbach RT, Halpern Z, Dudley MP, Lynn MP, Breuer AC (1987) Biliary vesicle aggregation and cholesterol crystal nucleation: evidence for a coupled relationship. In: Paumgartner G, Stiehl A, Gerok W (eds) Bile acids and the liver. Falk symposium 45, Oct 1986, Basel. MTP, Norwell, pp 301–316
53. Harvey PRC, Sömjen G, Lichtenberg MS, Petrunka CN, Gilat T, Strasberg SM (1987) Nucleation of cholesterol from vesicles isolated from bile of patients with and without cholesterol gallstones. Biochim Biophys Acta 921:198–204
54. Harvey PRC, Sömjen G, Gilat T, Gallinger S, Strasberg SM (1988) Vesicular cholesterol in bile. Relationship of protein concentration and nucleation time. Biochim Biophys Acta 958:10–18
55. Collins JJ, Phillips MC (1982) The stability and structure of cholesterol rich codispersions of cholesterol and phosphatidylcholine. J Lipid Res 23:291–298
56. Hauser H (1984) Some aspects of the phase behaviour of charged lipids. Biochim Biophys Acta 772:37–50
57. Strauss G, Schurtenberger P, Hauser H (1986) The interaction of saccharides with lipid bilayer vesicles: stabilization during freeze-thawing and freeze-drying. Biochim Biophys Acta 858:169–180
58. Dekruijff B, Cullis PR, Radda GK (1976) Outside-inside distribution and sizes of mixed phosphatidylcholine-cholesterol vesicles. Biochim Biophys Acta 436:729–740
59. Gad AE, Silver BL, Eytan GD (1982) Polycation-induced fusion of negatively-charged vesicles. Biochim Biophys Acta 690:124–132
60. Gad AE, Bental M, Elyashiv G, Weinberg H (1985) Promotion and inhibition of vesicle fusion by polylysine. Biochemistry 24:6277–6282
61. Wang CY, Huang L (1984) Polyhistidine mediates an acid dependent fusion of negatively charged liposomes. Biochemistry 23:4409–4416
62. Gad AE, Elyashiv G, Rosenberg N (1986) The induction of large unilamellar vesicle fusion by cationic polypeptides: the effects of mannitol, size, charge density, and hydrophobicity of cationic polypeptides. Biochim Biophys Acta 860:314–324
63. Gad AE, Eytan GD (1983) Chlorophylls as probes for membrane fusion. Polymyxin B-induced fusion of liposomes. Biochim Biophys Acta 727:170–176
64. Morgan CG, Williamson H, Fuller S, Hudson B (1983) Melittin induces fusion of unilamellar phospholipid vesicles. Biochim Biophys Acta 732:668–674
65. Batenburg AM, van Esch JH, Leunissen-Bijuelt J, Verkleij AJ, de Kruijff B (1987) Interaction of melittin with negatively charged phospholipids: consequences for lipid organization. FEBS Lett 223:148–154
66. Lampe PD, Wei GJ, Nelsestuen Gl (1983) Stopped-flow studies of myelin basic protein association with phospholipid vesicles and subsequent vesicle aggregation. Biochemistry 22:1594–1599
67. Subbarao NK, Parente RA, Szoka FC, Nadasdi L, Pongracz K (1987) pH-Dependent bilayer destabilization by an amphipathic peptide. Biochemistry 26:2964–2972
68. Parente RA, Nir S, Szoka FC (1988) pH-Dependent fusion of phosphatidylcholine small vesicles. Induction by a synthetic amphipathic peptide. J Biol Chem 263:4724–4730
69. Schenkman S, Soares de Araujo P, Dijkman R, Quina FH, Chaimovich H (1981) Effects of temperature and lipid composition on the serum albumin-induced aggregation and fusion of small unilamellar vesicles. Biochim Biophys Acta 649:633–641
70. Schenkman S, Soares de Araujo P, Sesso A, Quina FH, Chaimovich H (1981) A kinetic and structural study of two-step aggregation and fusion of neutral phospholipid vesicles promoted by serum albumin at low pH. Chem Phys Lipids 28:165–180
71. Garcia LAM, Soares de Araujo P, Chaimovich H (1984) Fusion of small unilamellar vesicles induced by a serum albumin fragment of molecular weight 9000. Biochim Biophys Acta 772:231–234
72. Blumenthal R, Henkart M, Steer CJ (1983) Clathrin-induced pH dependent fusion of phosphatidylcholine vesicles. J Biol Chem 258:3409–3415

73. Hung K, Yoshimura T, Papahadjopoulos D (1985) Interaction of clathrin with liposomes: pH dependent fusion of phospholipid membranes induced by clathrin. FEBS Lett 191:17–23
74. Farias RN, Vinals AL, Morero RD (1985) Insulin-mediated fusion of negatively charged phospholipid vesicles at low pH. Biochem Biophys Res Commun 128:68–74
75. Cabiaux V, Vandenbranden M, Falmagne P, Ruysschaert J-M (1984) Diphtheria toxin induces fusion of small unilamellar vesicles at low pH. Biochim Biophys Acta 775:31–36
76. Donovan JM, Benedek GB, Carey MC (1987) Formation of mixed micelles and vesicles of human apolipoproteins A-I and A-II with synthetic and natural lecithins and the bile salt sodium taurocholate: quasi-elastic light scattering studies. Biochemistry 26:8125–8133
77. Groen AK, Ottenhoff R, Jansen PLM, van Marle J, Tytgat GNJ (1989) Effect of cholesterol nucleation-promoting activity on cholesterol solubilization in model bile. J Lipid Res 30:51–58
78. Smith BF (1987) Human gallbladder mucin binds biliary lipids and promotes cholesterol crystal nucleation in model bile. J Lipid Res 28:1088–1097

Neurohormonal Aspects of Gallbladder Contractility in Gallstone Disease: The Role of Cholecystokinin

U. G. Klueppelberg *, X. Molero, H. Y. Gaisano, and L. J. Miller

Gastroenterology Research Unit, Mayo Clinic and Foundation, Rochester, MN 55905, USA

Introduction

In recent decades, studies examining the pathogenesis of gallstone disease have predominantly addressed changes in the physicochemical properties of bile. Disturbances of the equilibrium between biliary levels of bile acids, phospholipids, and cholesterol are well-established factors promoting gallstone disease [1, 7, 47, 51, 140]. Considerable progress has also been made in our understanding about biliary nucleation and antinucleation factors [11, 14, 50, 53, 75, 78–80, 147, 174]. The gallbladder mucosa plays an important role in the synthesis and secretion of nucleation factors as well as in modifying bile composition via epithelial absorption.

In this paper, we address the involvement of the gallbladder in the pathomechanisms of gallstone disease, focusing strictly on its contractile function as opposed to gallbladder secretion and absorption. In the first part, studies are reviewed which have uncovered the involvement of gallbladder motor function in the pathogenesis of gallstones. Further, recent studies are cited which have provided substantial progress in our understanding of the physiological regulation of gallbladder contraction. The cholecystokinin (CCK) system deserves special notice in this context, since for decades CCK has been considered the major hormonal stimulant of gallbladder smooth-muscle contraction. We then discuss studies which have identified factors affecting gallbladder function and speculate on potential mechanisms of their action. Finally, we discuss the role of the CCK system in gallstone disease with respect to hormone release and hormone–receptor interactions.

Role of Gallbladder Function in Gallstone Disease

The idea that disturbed gallbladder motor function, i.e., bile stasis, is involved in the pathogenesis of gallstones was proposed by von Helmsbach as early as 1856 [162]. For a review see LaMorte et al. [76]. Periodic gallbladder emptying during interdigestive cycles [94, 107, 137] as well as in response to meals [45] appears to play an important role in the enterohepatic circulation of the bile acid pool [63, 104, 141] as well as being a mechanism for clearance of nucleation factors, microcrystals, and even small stones [59].

Today, the availability of noninvasive methods for the examination of gallbladder dynamics, i.e., ultrasonography [8, 26] and cholescintigraphy [142, 150], permits detailed monitoring of gallbladder contraction and emptying, respectively. These methods have been employed to determine gallbladder function in selected groups of individuals known to be at increased risk to develop gallstone disease. Indeed, dramatically impaired gallbladder contractility has been shown in the second and third trimester of pregnancy [8, 27, 68] and may be one underlying mechanism responsible for the well-known correlation between pregnancy and increased occurrence of gallstones. Similarly, a decreased respon-

* Present address: Ludwig-Maximilians-University Munich, Internal Medicine II, Clinic Grosshadern, Marchioninistrasse 15, D-8000 Munich 70, FRG

siveness of the gallbladder has been reported in patients with diabetes mellitus [152] and obesity [93]. On the other hand, gallbladder emptying is also markedly impaired in patients with celiac disease [10, 90, 91]; however, this group has so far not been reported to have an increased risk for the development of gallstones. Whether the absence of biliary calculi in this particular group of patients is related to altered metabolic factors or to the juvenile age of these patients, this example clearly indicates that the cooperation of multiple lithogenic promoters is essential for the clinical manifestation of gallstones.

Animal studies have uncovered close relationships between physicochemical lithogenic factors and gallbladder contractility. In prairie dogs, a cholesterol-supplemented diet evoked not only biliary cholesterol supersaturation and changes in bile acids and phospholipids [9, 22, 52] but also increased gallbladder mucosal secretion of mucin glycoproteins [79]. Indeed, in the same species [34, 114] and in ground squirrels [34], a cholesterol-enriched diet also caused impaired gallbladder emptying in vivo [114] and decreased isometric tension of gallbladder strips in vitro [34]. Importantly, in both species impaired gallbladder contractility was detectable at an early stage, before gallstones had formed [34, 114].

The fact that dietary cholesterol provokes multiple potentially lithogenic factors in these animal models precludes an accurate estimation of the contribution of individual factors. Specifically, it was not clear whether sufficient gallbladder contraction could prevent the formation of gallstones in cholesterol-supersaturated bile containing nucleation factors. Therefore, the role of gallbladder kinetics in this model was addressed in studies performed by Hutton and coworkers [57, 58]. In prairie dogs, gallstone formation induced by a lithogenic diet could be prevented by sphincterotomy [57]. Since this prophylactic effect was reversible by cholinergic blockade [58], the authors concluded that a reduction of flow resistance by sphincterotomy facilitated more complete emptying of the gallbladder and consequently prevented the formation of calculi unless gallbladder contraction was inhibited by atropine [57, 58].

The absence of physiological stimuli mediating gallbladder contraction during parenteral nutrition may serve as a model for extreme gallbladder dysfunction in humans. Prolonged total parenteral nutrition is associated with the appearance of biliary sludge in about 50% of the patients after 4–6 weeks, reaching 100% after prolongation for more than 6 weeks [103]. Ultrasonographically detectable biliary sludge is likely to represent cholesterol monohydrate crystals and bilirubin [80, 81, 146] captured in biliary mucus and may provide the matrix for gallstone formation [75, 78–80, 147], especially in patients with additional lithogenic risk factors [124]. Prompt disappearance of gallbladder sludge upon oral refeeding [103] strongly suggests a pivotal role of periodic gallbladder contraction as its major clearance mechanism.

Several studies have investigated gallbladder function in gallstone patients in response to both endogenous stimuli (after standard meals) and/or exogenous stimulation with CCK. In these studies, controversial findings about gallbladder contractility (as assessed by ultrasonography) or emptying (as measured by cholescintigraphy) in gallstone patients as compared to healthy controls have been reported. In gallstone patients, investigators found increased gallbladder responses to meals [98] or CCK [108], decreased CCK-induced emptying [20, 142], or decreased responses to both standard meals and/or intravenous CCK [33]. In another report, gallbladder emptying in patients with cholelithiasis has been described as being decreased only after meals but normal after stimulation with CCK [31]. Others distinguish between "contractors" with normal response to a meal but increased gallbladder sensitivity to endogenous CCK versus "noncontractors" with diminished contractions after meals and decreased sensitivities to endogenous CCK [157, 159]. Finally, others distinguished two groups of patients, one with normal and the other one with decreased gallbladder emptying induced by exogenous CCK [117].

Table 1. Gallbladder motor function in gallstone patients

Reference	Patients *n*	Method	Gallbladder response to	
			Meal	CCK
Maudgal et al. [98]	34	Cystogr	+	
Northfield et al. [108]	18	Scinti		+
Shaffer et al. [142]	6	Scinti		−
Fisher et al. [31]	15	Scinti	−	±
Thompson et al. [157]	24	US	±, −	
Forgacs et al. [33]	39	Scinti + US	−	−
Pomeranz et al. [115]	26	Scinti		±, −
Upp et al. [159]	23	US	±, −	

Cystogr, Cholecystography; Scinti, cholescintigraphy; US, real-time ultrasonography; ±, no difference compared to controls; −, decreased compared to controls; +, increased compared to controls.

Indeed, taken together these results cover nearly all theoretically possible alterations in patients with gallstones (see Table 1). Differences in the methods employed in these studies (ultrasonography, cholecystography, and cholescintigraphy) are hardly the only variables to be blamed for the apparent disparity in the findings of these studies. Most likely we are dealing with a highly heterogeneous population of patients in whom various lithogenic factors contribute to their disease with different orders of dominance. Additionally, gallbladder contractility might be differently affected in various stages of the disease. Studies with prosthetic gallstones have shown that the maximum contractile response to CCK can be diminished by 20.5% when inert particles are present in the gallbladder, even when inflammatory infiltrations are absent [117]. For the identification of pathological mechanisms which might account for gallbladder dysfunction, it is essential to address the complicated hormonal and neural physiological regulation of gallbladder contraction.

Physiology of Gallbladder Contraction

Hormones

For decades CCK has been regarded as the major physiological stimulant of gallbladder contraction. However, multiple gastrointestinal hormones and neuronal substances have been demonstrated to be able to induce gallbladder contraction in vivo and/or in vitro. Postprandially, virtually every gastrointestinal hormone is detected in increased levels when compared to the fasting state [166]. Multiple hormones elicit contractile responses of the gallbladder in vivo or in vitro. Among these are bombesin [139] and substance P [19, 96, 101]. Receptors for both peptides have been functionally characterized on isolated gallbladder smooth-muscle cells [139]. Similarly, opioid receptor agonists cause smooth-muscle cells to contract via surface receptors [138]. On the other hand, in vivo morphine and an enkephalin analogue have been demonstrated to inhibit gallbladder emptying in humans [169]. Neurotensin mediates transient gallbladder contraction likely via cholinergic pathways in guinea pig gallbladder strips [172], but appears to mediate relaxation in vivo in humans [165]. An effect of motilin on the gallbladder could not be demonstrated in vitro [67, 116]; however, in vivo contractile responses have been described in dogs which were elicited only during the interdigestive period, and which are likely to be mediated by cholinergic neurons [155]. Substances such as glucagon or secretin appear to enhance gallbladder contractile responses to CCK in vivo [160] but have little [160] or even antagonistic effects in vitro [125].

Other hormones have been ascribed roles in the mediation of gallbladder relaxation. A relaxing effect on the prairie dog gallbladder has been shown in vivo for peptide YY [17]. This effect of peptide YY, however, could not be reproduced in the dog gallbladder in vivo and rabbit gallbladder strips in vitro [87]. Similarly, vasoactive intestinal peptide has been shown to induce gallbladder relaxation and antagonize CCK-mediated contraction in vitro in guinea pigs [128] and rabbits [88] and in vivo in the opossum [126], guinea pigs [160], and dogs [88], while these effects could not be reproduced in human gallbladders in vitro [30]. Pancreatic polypeptide has been reported to mediate gallbladder relaxation in vivo in prairie dogs [16], while human [116], rabbit [67, 88] and dog [88] gallbladders appear to be refractory to this hormone in vitro.

CCK release in response to a meal may also exert inhibitory effects on the gallbladder. CCK has been shown to mediate somatostatin release from pancreatic islet cells [2, 46, 122] as well as from fundic mucosa cells [149], and somatostatin has been recognized to inhibit gallbladder contraction in humans [18] and dogs [6].

Autonomic Nervous System

The multiplicity of hormonal actions and interactions is further complicated by the ability of hormones to mediate biological effects directly via receptors on target cells or indirectly via cholinergic or noncholinergic neurons. Peptides can reach their target either via blood (endocrine secretion) or by local release (neurocrine and paracrine secretion), thereby acting as hormone, neurotransmitter, or neuromodulator. For instance, bombesin may induce contraction of smooth muscle directly via surface receptors of smooth-muscle cells [138], indirectly via stimulation of intrinsic cholinergic nerves [99], or via stimulation of CCK release [24, 166].

Similarly, the final biological effect of CCK is not only an expression of hormonal interactions. In the feline biliary tract, CCK appears to interact (a) with excitatory receptors on smooth-muscle cells in the gallbladder and in the sphincter of Oddi, (b) with intramural, excitatory, postganglionic, cholinergic neurons in the gallbladder, and (c) with intramural, inhibitory, noncholinergic, nonadrenergic intrinsic neurons in the sphincter of Oddi [3, 4]. In contrast, in guinea pig [41], rabbit [67], and bovine gallbladder muscle strips [133], CCK-evoked contractions were affected neither by tetrodotoxin (TTX) nor by atropine, suggesting only direct interaction with smooth-muscle cells. Neurons are more susceptible to hypoxia than muscle cells, and consequently it has been suggested that in vitro studies could deal with almost pure muscle preparations [3]. However, TTX-sensitive acetylcholine release from guinea pig gallbladder strips could be evoked by field stimulation, demonstrating the presence of intact cholinergic neurons, while in the same preparation no acetylcholine release was detectable in response to CCK [173]. Others described scopolamine-sensitive release of acetylcholine in response to CCK in guinea pigs which could not be blocked by TTX or hexamethonium [170]. Future studies must show whether species differences or methodological factors are responsible for these controversial findings.

In vivo in dogs [153] and prairie dogs [113] atropine does not affect CCK-induced gallbladder contractions, however cholinergic blockade inhibited gallbladder emptying in response to the intraduodenal administration of oleate by 40% [153]. In a different in vivo study which was also performed in dogs, atropine did inhibit CCK-induced gallbladder contraction [155]. Indicating physiological relevance of cholinergic mechanisms in the regulation of gallbladder function in man, sham feeding has been reported to induce gallbladder contraction via an atropine-sensitive mechanism which is likely not mediated by CCK [55, 171]. Consistent with this is the partial contraction of the gallbladder following infusion of cholinergic agonists [32, 92]. Two lines of evidence suggest that cholinergic excitation of human gallbladder smooth muscle in response to a meal is primarily the result of peripheral neurohormonal interactions. First, after truncal vagotomy gallbladder contractility is unaltered in response to meals [113], and even augmented in response to CCK [32]. Second, cholinergic blockade with atropine inhibits both CCK-induced and meal-stimulated gallbladder contraction to a similar extent [32]. However, it is difficult to determine to what extent intrinsic cholinergic neurons contribute to gallbladder contraction in vivo since other groups have reported that gallbladder responses to CCK were merely abolished after premedication with atropine [42, 156].

Thus, the final biological effects mediated by hormones must be perceived as the net effect of their interactions with a variety of other hormones as well as cholinergic and noncholinergic neurons.

Eicosanoids and Histamine

Certain prostanoids and also histamine have been shown to elicit gallbladder contraction in vivo and in vitro. The physiological role of these substances is not well understood, however these substances may be relevant under pathological conditions particularly in inflamed gallbladders, and they are discussed below.

Cholecystokinin

Until recently, studies evaluating CCK as the major physiological stimulator of gallbladder contraction were indirect in nature depending on comparisons between the biological effects of endogenous postprandial levels of CCK and the response to similar serum levels after infusion of exogenous CCK [84]. Recently, the development of a potent and highly specific CCK antagonist, the benzodiazepine derivative L-364,718 [15, 89], has enabled us to further validate the physiological role of CCK in mediating gallbladder contraction. Indeed, gallbladder contraction in response to a meal is almost completely abolished after administration of L-364,718 [85]. Hence, considering the inhibitory effects of both atropine and L-364,718 (nearly 100% [85]), the data available at present strongly suggest that CCK is the dominant physiological stimulant of gallbladder contraction in humans, mediating this effect in part directly on smooth-muscle cells and in part indirectly via intrinsic cholinergic neurons.

The Cholecystokinin/Gastrin Family of Hormones

CCK was first described by Ivy and Oldberg in 1928 as a hormonal substance present in extracts from duodenal tissue which was able to induce gallbladder contraction [61]. In a similar approach, Harper and Raper discovered in 1943 a substance stimulating pancreatic enzyme release and called it pancreozymin [44]. Later, the identity of CCK and pancreozymin was disclosed when Mutt and Jorpes isolated and partially characterized the structure of CCK-33 as a single-chain polypeptide that possessed both cholecystokinetic and pancreozymic activity [105].

Subsequently, multiple biologically active CCK forms have been identified in tissue extracts and plasma varying in length between 4 and 58 amino acid residues [28, 29, 36, 119, 120]. Homology between gastrin and CCK is evident in the carboxyl-terminal parts of the molecules with the last five amino acids being identical. In addition to their known gastrointestinal effects, CCK and gastrin interact with targets in the central nervous system mediating a large variety of biological effects [23, 48, 49, 100, 129, 148]. This family of hormones exhibits differential principality in that in different tissues different CCK/gastrin forms predominate and interact with receptors which have different affinities for CCK/gastrin peptides depending on their length (macroheterogeneity), differential amino acid sequences or derivatization of single residues localized within the biologically active domain (microheterogeneity) [121]. We distinguish subtypes of CCK receptors according to their ability to bind different CCK forms with different affinities.

Extensive structure-activity studies have identified the carboxyl-terminal heptapeptide as the fully biologically active segment of CCK [64, 65] with sulfation of the tyrosine residue in position 27 being crucial for the cholecystokinetic [13, 133, 143, 151] and pancreozymic activity [64, 65, 161].

Pathophysiology of Gallbladder Function

In the previous section we have reviewed extensive work that substantiates the role of CCK as the predominant physiological hormonal stimulant of gallbladder contraction. In order to detect potential pathophysiological dysfunctions, investigators have studied the release of this hormone, numbers of CCK receptors, and biochemical characteristics of gallbladder CCK receptors in gallstone patients.

Cholecystokinin Release

To date, studies examining fasting levels of CCK and the meal-stimulated release of this hormone in gallstone patients are rare. In two of these studies [157, 159], patients were assigned to groups of "contractors" and "noncontractors" depending on their gallbladder response to a meal. Simultaneously with the ultrasonographic assessment of gallbladder contraction, the postprandial output of CCK was measured by radioimmunoassay employing the same antibody (UT 132) which cross-reacts with only CCK-33/39 and has negligible cross-reactivity with CCK-8 and gastrin [157, 159]. Although comparable numbers of patients were studied with similar distributions of age and sex, and the same radioimmunoassay was employed, the CCK output in response to the same standard meal given in the same dose was different in "noncontractors." While in one study the mean postprandial output of CCK was similar in "noncontractors" and in healthy controls [157], „noncontractors" had a more than twofold higher mean CCK output in the other study (Table 2) [159]. In both studies, "contractors" had a lower postprandial output of CCK than healthy controls [157, 159]. Partly corroborating these findings, Masclee and coworkers [95] assigned gallstone patients to three different subgroups depending on their meal-stimulated CCK release and gallbladder emptying. In first group CCK release and gallbladder emptying were within the normal range, a second group was characterized by reduced CCK release but normal gallbladder emptying, and a third group had reduced CCK release and diminished gallbladder emptying (Table 3) [95].

The fact that only few studies have addressed the important question of CCK release in gallstone patients [95, 157, 159] may be partly related to the problems encountered in attempts to determine the levels of bioactive CCK in plasma. Determinations of CCK serum levels by radioimmunological methods are particularly difficult due to the immunovariability of various biologically active CCK forms and the cross-reactivity with gastrin. Antibodies directed against the biologically active domain of CCK, the carboxyl-terminal heptapeptide, often cross-react with gastrin, whereas antibodies directed against

Table 2. CCK release and gallbladder response after a meal in controls and in gallstone patients defined as "contractors" and "noncontractors". (From Upp et al. [159])

Group	*n*	CCK output [a] (ng min/ml)	Gallbladder response [b]
Controls	10	5.5 ± 1.2	Normal
"Contractors"	13	1.6 ± 0.2	Normal
"Noncontractors"	10	11.1 ± 2.1	Decreased

[a] CCK output in response to standard meal (mean ± SEM).
[b] Gallbladder response assessed by real-time ultrasonography

Table 3. CCK release and gallbladder emptying in controls and three subgroups of patients with gallstones. (From Masclee et al. [95])

Group	*n*	CCK output [a] (pmol l^{-1} h^{-1}	Emptied [b] (%)
Control	20	191 ± 11	60 ± 4
Group 1	7	181 ± 22	57 ± 10
Group 2	6	58 ± 11	70 ± 8
Group 3	6	45 ± 10	8 ± 5

[a] CCK output in response to a standard meal (mean ± SEM).
[b] Gallbladder emptying assessed by cholescintigraphy (mean ± SEM)

other parts of the molecule may interact with biologically inactive degradation products and fail to react with major biologically active forms. Thus, either at least two antibodies must be used, or chromatographic purification of the samples is required prior to the incubation with antibodies to eliminate the interference of the assay with gastrin [28, 120].

These problems have been approached with the use of antisera which specifically bind to the sulfated tyrosine residue of CCK in position 27 [12, 62, 69, 131] or the in vitro bioassay of CCK bioactivity in plasma via the determination of stimulation of amylase release from dispersed pancreatic acini [84]. Fasting and postprandial CCK serum levels determined by these radioimmunoassays [54, 69] and this bioassay [84] are very similar, indicating the usefulness of these assays for reliable measurements of CCK in human plasma. Future studies employing these techniques are likely to give us more information about fasting and postprandial CCK serum levels in gallstone patients.

Nevertheless, a subgroup of gallstone patients has been identified in which inadequate release of CCK may be responsible for diminished gallbladder emptying [95]. Differently, in another group of patients the gallbladder fails to respond adequately to normal [157] or increased [159] CCK levels. Similar observations have been reported in patients with celiac disease [10, 91]. These findings clearly suggest that in these patients the mediation of gallbladder contraction is disturbed at a more distal step in the stimulus-contraction cascade following hormone release. Theoretically, this may be due to pathologically increased levels of inhibitory substances. These may affect the stimulus-contraction cascade via different mechanisms, including desensitization of CCK or other stimulatory receptors and/or interactions with intracellular pathways mediating smooth-muscle cell contraction.

Role of Inhibitory Substances in Gallbladder Contraction

Peptide Hormones

A pathophysiological mechanism can be proposed in which the gallbladder response to adequate stimulation is impaired due to excessive levels of inhibitory substances which may be elevated acutely or chronically. This model may be valid in various subgroups of patients. For instance, gallstones are frequently diagnosed in patients with somatostatinomas [35, 38, 74, 158], and somatostatin has been demonstrated to inhibit CCK-mediated gallbladder contraction [6, 18, 43]. The increasing use of somatostatin as a therapeutic agent may provide further evidence for the clinical relevance of the inhibitory action of this hormone on gallbladder function. Also consistent with this pathophysiological model is the report that neurotensin induces gallbladder relaxation in vivo in humans and was found in increased postprandial serum levels in gallstone patients [165].

Steroid Hormones

Similarly, the markedly impaired gallbladder contraction found in pregnant women [8, 68] is likely due to elevated progesterone serum levels. Indeed, preincubation with progesterone reduces stimulated isometric tension of guinea pig gallbladder strips in vitro [21, 127]. It has been speculated that this action may be mediated by specific interactions of progesterone with intracellular receptors [145]. This hypothesis is supported by the finding that the presence of progesterone receptors in guinea pig gallbladder tissue is inversely related to the contractile response to CCK [56]. Similar findings have also been described in humans [20] in that gallstone patients with receptor-positive gallbladder tissue had a lower contractility than normal volunteers. This observation is still preliminary, since (a) for obvious reasons the progesterone receptor status of the control group was unknown, and (b) differences in gallbladder function between receptor-negative and -positive gallstone patients failed to reach statistical significance [20]. This may either be due to the number of patients studied, or be related to the fact that progesterone receptors in this study were assayed in the cytosolic fraction while these receptors are primarily localized in the cell nucleus [40].

Very little is known about the "cross talk" between receptors localized in the plasma membrane, i.e., the CCK receptor, and steroid receptors which are localized intracellularly and regulate DNA transcription. Similarly, the mechanism by which progesterone receptors inhibit the contractile response of smooth-muscle cells is unknown. This mechanism is likely directed against postreceptor steps in excitation-contraction coupling since after progesterone pretreatment (a) the ED_{50} of acetylcholine and CCK remained unaltered [21], and (b) gallbladder contractions were diminished similarly after stimulation via potassium depolarization [21] and after stimulation with CCK or acetylcholine [21, 127].

Cholesterol

Similarly, suggesting dysfunctions of the excitation-contraction cascade on an intracellular, postreceptor level in the prairie dog model, are the observations that after feeding a high-cholesterol diet (a) the response to multiple stimuli is impaired [34], and (b) permeabilized muscle strips appear also to be partly refractory to calcium stimulation [83]. Consequently, it has been speculated that disturbed interactions between calmodulin and myosin light-chain kinase may play an important role in this pathomechanism [14, 83].

Multiple substances are candidates to interfere with this interaction, including leukotrienes and prostanoids [14] (see "Eicosanoids and Histamine," below).

The underlying mechanism by which cholesterol inhibits gallbladder contractility in this model is the matter of numerous speculations. Cholesterol has multiple biological effects, including influences on fluidity and stability of plasmalemmal membranes, variables which may have important implications for receptor function [130]. Cholesterol effects may even be mediated transcriptionally, similar to those of steroid hormones. Structural similarities between steroids and cholesterol have given rise to speculation about the existence of intracellular cholesterol receptors as members of this class of receptors [25].

Bile Acids

Discussing alterations of gallbladder contractility in gallstone patients, it is important to note the apparent inhibitory effects of bile acids on gallbladder contraction and emptying. Both chenodeoxycholic acid (CDCA) and ursodeoxycholic acid (UDCA) are commonly used alone or in combination for dissolution treatment of cholesterol gallstones. Shaffer and coworkers [142] first described the adverse effect of chronic CDCA administration on gallbladder filling and particularly emptying in a single patient. Since then the effects of chronic administration of UDCA [33, 154] and CDCA [154] have been evaluated in larger series of patients. In these studies gallbladder function was already impaired before therapy [33, 154] and further deteriorated with respect to gallbladder emptying [33, 154] or contraction [33] in response to CCK. Additionally, disturbed gallbladder filling was detected and was found to be decreased to a higher degree in patients in whom the gallstones could not be dissolved [154].

So far, the mechanism of these inhibitory effects of bile acids on gallbladder contractility has not been unequivocally characterized. Adverse effects may in part be related to the solubilizing properties of bile acids on plasmalemmal proteins [123]. In addition, bile acids appear to exert inhibition of CCK release in dogs and humans [39]. On the other hand, significantly increased levels of β-endorphinlike immunoreactivity have been measured after acute administration of both UDCA and CDCA [97]. Although the effect of chronic bile acid intake on β-endorphins remains to be elucidated, it is intriguing to speculate that the inhibitory effect of endogenous opioids on CCK-stimulated gallbladder contraction in vivo [169] may in part be responsible for contractile gallbladder dysfunction seen after chronic administration of UDCA and CDCA.

Eicosanoids and Histamine

The role of prostaglandins and thromboxanes as members of the class of eicosanoids in mediating gallbladder contraction is not well understood. These hormonelike substances may mediate their biological effects via cell surface receptors or as intracellular messengers [5]. Wood and coworkers [168] reported isolated guinea pig gallbladders and human gallbladder strips to be relatively insensitive to various prostanoids, responding only weakly or not at all to high concentrations of various members of this class. Nakano et al. [106] reported that the effect of prostaglandins in vivo in dogs was dependent on the initial intraluminal gallbladder pressure. In their studies [106], PGE_1 and PGE_2 lowered the gallbladder pressure when the initial pressure exceeded 5 mmHg but had no effect when the initial prssure was below 3 mmHg. In contrast, when the cystic duct was clamped, PGE_1 and PGE_2 increased the gallbladder pressure. PGF_2 elicited increases in gallbladder pressure regardless of the initial pressure or clamping of the cystic duct. In other studies [73], chronically inflamed human gallbladder strips responded with concentration-dependent contractions to PGF_2, PGB_2, and PGD_2. In these studies, the effects of PGE_1 and PGE_2 were variable, however, after pretreatment with indomethacin contractions could be recorded [73]. In contrast, acutely inflamed muscle strips were unresponsive to all prostaglandins tested even after pretreatment with indomethacin [73]. Disparities in studies examining the biological effects of prostaglandins on gallbladder muscle may be related to the biphasic dose-response curves produced by these hormone-like substances [73]. Jivegård and Svanvik [66] were able to show inhibition of secretory and contractile effects of PGE_2 by morphine and loperamide. Thus effects of prostanoids on the gallbladder may be regulated by endogenous opioids.

Generally, a physiological role of prostanoids in mediating gallbladder contraction is questionable since the contractile forces elicited by these substances are weak compared to muscle tensions induced by acetylcholine [73] and CCK. On the other hand, dramatic alterations of these substances in inflamed tissues may be relevant under pathological conditions. Increased levels of prostaglandins under the metabolic conditions present in the prairie dog model have been recognized to be crucial for the increased glycoprotein synthesis [77, 78]. Indeed, arachidonic acid as the fatty acid precursor in the synthesis of eicosanoids (prostaglandins, thromboxanes, and leukotrienes) may be an important factor in receptor signaling (a) as part of inositol phospholipid pathways or (b) as intracellular messenger and precursor of other messengers [5].

Stimulatory (H_1) histamine receptors mediating gallbladder contraction and inhibitory (H_2) receptors mediating relaxation of gallbladder smooth muscle have been shown to be present in the gallbladder [60]. In vitro, the sensitivity of human gallbladder strips to contract in response to histamine correlated positively with the severity of inflammation [82]. Preincubation of gallbladder muscle strips with an H_2 antagonist led to increased CCK-induced contractions with a significant leftward shift in the CCK dose-response curve [164]. These data suggest that excitation of H_2 receptors may induce heterologous desensitization of gallbladder CCK receptors. The role of histamine-mediated gallbladder contraction under physiological conditions is not well characterized. However, desensitization of CCK receptors via excitation of H_2 receptors may be relevant in gallstone patients especially when the disease is associated with inflammatory reactions of gallbladder tissue.

Gallbladder CCK Receptors

In recent years, the gallbladder CCK receptor has been studied morphologically [133], functionally [134, 143, 151], and biochemically [134, 143] in various species. Using a large variety of CCK receptor probes, the bovine gallbladder [143], human gallbladder [134], and rat pancreatic CCK receptors [70, 110, 112, 118] have been biochemically characterized in affinity labeling studies. These studies disclosed molecular heterogeneity of these receptors from different species identifying glycoproteins of apparent $M_r = 85\,000$–$95\,000$ in the human gallbladder, $M_r = 70\,000$–$80\,000$ in the bovine gallbladder, and $M_r = 85\,000$–$95\,000$ in the rat pancreas [70, 110, 112, 118, 134, 143]. These differences appear to be due primarily to differential glycosylation since the core proteins of these glycoproteins have similar molecular masses of $M_r = 42\,000$ (in rat pancreas) [72, 111, 118] and $M_r = 43\,000$ (in human and bovine gallbladder) [132], and similarities were also found in the pattern of fragments generated by protease peptide mapping [71, 132]. Pancreatic and gallbladder CCK receptors from the same species have additionally been compared in functional studies and were found to be similar in their selectivity to bind various CCK receptor agonists and antagonists [163].

Little is known about potential pathological alterations of gallbladder CCK receptors in gallstone disease. Studies have so far addressed questions about changes in receptor density [159] as well as functional and biochemical characteristics [134] of these receptors in gallstone patients. In one report [159], the number of receptors in 23 gallbladders obtained at cholecystectomy was found to be inversely related to their preoperative contractility. The authors concluded that the differences in gallbladder contractility between contractors versus noncontractors resulted from a decrease in the population of CCK receptors. Subsequently, this paper has been criticized with the question being raised as to whether the methodological strategies employed in this work were appropriate to draw this attractive conclusion [109].

In a recent study performed in our laboratory, we focused strictly on functional and biochemical comparisons of CCK receptors in the muscularis layer from 50 diseased and seven healthy gallbladders (obtained at time of resection of liver metastases). Indeed, employing binding studies and affinity-labeling techniques, we were unable to demonstrate any differences in CCK receptors in healthy versus diseased gallbladders (Table 4) [134]. The number of CCK receptors per milligram protein found in these tissues varied over a wide range with the mean value in diseased gallbladders being even higher than in normal gallbladders (Table 4) [134]. However, due to variable amounts of fibrous

Table 4. CCK binding to normal and healthy gallbladder plasma membranes. (From Schjoldager et al. [134])

Group	*n*	Binding affinity K_d (nM)	Number of sites[a] (fmol/mg protein)
Healthy	7	1.1 ± 0.1[b]	230 ± 47[b]
Diseased	50	0.9 ± 0.1[b]	366 ± 47[b]

[a] Number of CCK binding sites as determined by Scatchard analysis. Data presented as means ± SEM
[b] $p > 0.05$

tissue and inflammatory infiltrates in the diseased gallbladders, the protein content of these tissues had to be expected to vary significantly, thereby affecting the calculations of receptor density to a significant degree. Consequently, we were careful not to draw any conclusions from the binding capacities assessed in these organs [134].

Obviously, we cannot exclude that in a subgroup of patients biochemical defects of CCK receptors account for impaired gallbladder function. However, our studies indicate that in the majority of gallstone patients the CCK receptor is biochemically intact and not affected in its ability to bind CCK [134]. On the other hand, we speculate that the signaling of CCK receptors is subject to important functional regulations.

The intracellular events mediating the biological response stimulated by CCK occupancy of cell-surface receptors have been difficult to characterize because of the complex binding and biological response characteristics of this hormone. In pancreatic acinar cells, the present model for intracellular CCK signaling following agonist binding to its receptor includes association and activation of a guanine nucleotide binding protein (G-protein) [102, 167], which activates phospholipase C to catalyze cleavage of phosphatidylinositol bisphosphate to generate diacylglycerol and inositol phosphates [102, 135, 136]. However, recently it has become evident that CCK receptor signaling in pancreatic acinar cells may additionally involve an important alternate pathway which is yet to be defined [37, 86]. At present it cannot be decided whether this pathway is also relevant in smooth-muscle cells.

Nevertheless, striking similarities have been found to exist among receptors coupled to G-proteins. These include their biochemical structure and functional aspects, such as the regulation of their transmembrane signaling by receptor phosphorylation [144]. So far, phosphorylation of the CCK receptor has not been demonstrated. However, considering the complex dose-response characteristics of CCK, it is logical to predict that phosphorylation events may play a pivotal role in the regulation of CCK receptor signaling. Therefore, it is intriguing to speculate that the inhibitory action of some substances on gallbladder contraction may be mediated by heterologous desensitization of CCK receptors. In the future, the purification of the CCK receptor will hopefully enable us to develop the techniques necessary to answer these exciting questions.

Conclusions

Disturbed gallbladder motor function may play a critical role for the development of gallstones in certain groups of patients. The observation that during bile acid therapy gallbladder motor function can deteriorate, but that gallstones can still be dissolved under these conditions [33, 154] may serve as an important hint that pathological alterations in the physicochemical properties of bile are essential factors for gallstone growth in man. Thus, gallbladder contractile dysfunction must be considered as not more than a pathogenic *co*factor in the development of gallstone disease. On the other hand, disturbed gallbladder contractility is closely linked to other lithogenic factors in that it could cause alterations in the enterohepatic circulation of bile acids and/or account for retention of factors promoting cholesterol nucleation in the gallbladder. Finally, alterations in bile composition have been identified to cause contractile gallbladder dysfunction, thus identifying the gallbladder as part of a vicious circle in which gallstone formation occurs.

The complex neurohormonal regulation of gallbladder motor function offers a variety of pathomechanisms which may be present in yet unidentified distinct subgroups of patients to cause impaired gallbladder motor function. Potential defects may occur in cholinergic and noncholinergic innervation, release of antagonistic and agonistic hormones, interactions with their receptors, functional coupling of receptors to their effectors, intracellular signaling via messengers, and function of intracellular contractile proteins. Future studies may elucidate these potential pathomechanisms and may enable us to develop new therapeutic approaches in the clinical management of gallstone disease.

Summary

Already in the last century investigators suggested that defective gallbladder contractility with bile stasis in the gallbladder may play an important role in the pathogenesis of gallstone disease. Meanwhile, the availability of noninvasive methods for monitoring gallbladder motility (i.e., ultrasonography and cholescintigraphy) provide important means to assess potential abnormalities in gallbladder function. Employing these methods, impaired kinetics of gallbladder contraction have been demonstrated in selected groups of individuals known to be at increased risk to develop gallstone disease. Other studies in gallstone patients investigating gallbladder contraction in response to both endogenous or exogenous stimuli have generated apparently contradictory results with increased or decreased gallbladder contractile responses. These findings may reflect a wide range of physiological or pathophysiological variations in gallbladder sensitivity and/or pronounced heterogeneity within the population of gallstone patients. Studies conducted in animal models have uncovered close relationships between major lithogenic factors. Cholesterol-supplemented diets induce (a) biliary cholesterol supersaturation,

(b) increased secretion of glycoproteins from the gallbladder mucosa, and (c) depression of gallbladder contractility. Periodic gallbladder emptying appears to be the major mechanism for clearance of biliary mucus which has been shown to provide a matrix for cholesterol nucleation. The complicated system of hormonal and neuronal stimuli involved in the regulation of gallbladder motility offers multiple possibilities for defects within the cascade mediating the contractile response of the gallbladder. This system might be affected within different axes and levels in distinct subgroups of gallstone patients. Potential defects may include cholinergic and noncholinergic innervation, release of antagonistic and agonistic hormones, interactions with receptors, functional coupling of receptors to their effectors, intracellular signaling via messengers, and function of intracellular contractile proteins. Studies conducted to reveal such defects have investigated in vitro gallbladder responses to various stimuli. Since CCK is the predominant physiological hormonal stimulant of gallbladder contraction, investigators have examined release of this hormone, numbers of CCK receptors, as well as functional and biochemical characteristics of gallbladder CCK receptors. These studies await careful reevaluation in order to outline future directions aimed at the elucidation of a possible role of CCK in the pathogenesis of gallstone disease.

References

1. Admirand WH, Small DM (1968) The physicochemical basis of cholesterol gallstone formation in man. J Clin Invest 47:1043–1052
2. Ahrén B, Mårtensson H, Nobin A (1988) Cholecystokinin (CCK)-4 and CCK-8 stimulate islet hormone secretion in the pig. Pancreas 3:279–284
3. Behar J, Biancani P (1980) Effect of cholecystokinin and the octapeptide of cholecystokinin on the feline sphincter of Oddi and gallbladder: mechanisms of action. J Clin Invest 66:1231–1239
4. Behar J, Biancani P (1987) Pharmacologic characterization of excitatory and inhibitory cholecystokinin receptors of the cat gallbladder and sphincter of Oddi. Gastroenterology 92:764–770
5. Berridge MJ (1987) Inositol triphosphate and diacylglycerol: two interacting second messengers. Ann Rev Biochem 56:159–193
6. Bloom SR, Joffe SH, Polak JM (1975) Effect of somatostatin on pancreatic and biliary function. Gut 16:836–837
7. Bouchier IAD (1984) Debits and credits: a current account of cholesterol gall stone disease. Gut 25:1021–1028
8. Braverman DZ, Johnson ML, Kern F Jr (1980) Effects of pregnancy and contraceptive steroids on gallbladder function. N Engl J Med 302:362–364
9. Brenneman DE, Connor WE, Forker EL, DenBesten L (1972) The formation of abnormal bile and cholesterol gallstones from dietary cholesterol in the prairie dog. J Clin Invest 51:1495–1503
10. Brown AM, Bradshaw MJ, Richardson R, Wheeler JG, Harvey RF (1987) Pathogenesis of impaired gall bladder contraction of coeliac disease. Gut 28:1426–1432
11. Burnstein MJ, Ilson RG, Petrunka CN, Taylor RD, Strasberg SM (1983) Evidence for a potent nucleating factor in the gallbladder bile of patients with cholesterol gallstones. Gastroenterology 85:801–807
12. Cantor P (1986) Evaluation of a radioimmunoassay for cholecystokinin in human plasma. Scand J Clin Lab Invest 46:213–221
13. Cantor P, Petronijevic L, Pedersen JF, Worning H (1986) Cholecystokinetic and pancreozymic effect of O-sulfated gastrin compared with nonsulfated gastrin and cholecystokinin. Gastroenterology 91:1154–1163
14. Carey MC, Cahalane MJ (1988) Whither biliary sludge? Gastroenterology 95:508–523
15. Chang RSL, Lotti VJ (1986) Biochemical and pharmacological characterization of an extremely potent and selective nonpeptide cholecystokinin antagonist. Proc Natl Acad Sci USA 83:4923–4926

16. Conter RL, Roslyn JJ, DenBesten L, Taylor IL (1987) Pancreatic polypeptide enhances post-contractile gallbladder filling in the prairie dog. Gastroenterology 92:771–776
17. Conter RL, Roslyn JJ, Taylor IL (1987) Effects of peptide YY on gallbladder motility. Am J Physiol 252 (Gastrointest Liver Physiol 15):G736–G741
18. Creutzfeld W, Lankisch PG, Fölsch UR (1975) Hemmung der Sekretin- und Cholezystokinin-Pankreozymin-induzierten Saft- und Enzymsekretion des Pankreas und der Gallenblasenkontraktion beim Menschen durch Somatostatin. Dtsch Med Wochenschr 100:1135–1138
19. Dahlstrand C, Björck S, Edin R, Dahlström A, Ahlman H (1988) Substance P in the control of extrahepatic biliary motility in the cat. Regul Pept 20:11–24
20. Daignault PG, Fazekas AG, Rosenthall L, Fried GM (1988) Relationship between gallbladder contraction and progesterone receptors in patients with gallstones. Am J Surg 155:147–151
21. Davis M, Ryan JP (1986) Influence of progesterone on guinea pig gallbladder motility in vitro. Dig Dis Sci 31:513–518
22. DenBesten L, Safaie-Shirazi S, Connor WE, Bell S (1974) Early changes in bile composition and gallstone formation induced by a high cholesterol diet in prairie dogs. Gastroenterology 66:1036–1045
23. Dockray GJ (1982) The physiology of cholecystokinin in brain and gut. Br Med Bull 38:253–258
24. Erspamer V, Improta G, Melchiorri P, Sopranzi N (1974) Evidence of cholecystokinin release by bombesin in the dog. Br J Pharmacol 52:227–232
25. Evans RM (1988) The steroid and thyroid hormone receptor superfamily. Science 240:889–895
26. Everson GT, Braverman DZ, Johnson ML, Kern F Jr (1980) A critical evaluation of real-time ultrasonography for the study of gallbladder volume and contraction. Gastroenterology 79:40–46
27. Everson GT, McKinley C, Lawson M, Johnson M, Kern F Jr (1982) Gallbladder function in the human female: effect of the ovulatory cycle, pregnancy, and contraceptive steroids. Gastroenterology 82:711–719
28. Eysselein VE, Deveney CW, Sankaran H, Reeve JR, Walsh JH (1983) Biological activity of canine intestinal cholecystokinin-58. Am J Physiol 245 (Gastrointest Liver Physiol 8):G313–320
29. Eysselein VE, Eberlein GA, Hesse WH, Singer MV, Goebell H, Reeve JR (1987) Cholecystokinin-58 is the major circulating form of cholecystokinin in canine blood. J Biol Chem 262:214–217
30. Feeley TM, Clanachan AS, Scott GW (1984) The effects of vasoactive intestinal polypeptide on the motility of human and guinea pig gallbladder. Can J Physiol Pharmacol 62:356–359
31. Fisher RS, Stelzer F, Rock E, Malmud LS (1982) Abnormal gallbladder emptying in patients with gallstones. Dig Dis Sci 27:1019–1024
32. Fisher RS, Rock E, Malmud LS (1985) Cholinergic effects on gallbladder emptying in humans. Gastroenterology 89:716–722
33. Forgacs IC, Maisey MN, Murphy GM, Dowling RH (1984) Influence of gallstones and ursodeoxycholic acid therapy on gallbladder emptying. Gastroenterology 87:299–307
34. Fridhandler TM, Davison JS, Shaffer EA (1983) Defective gallbladder contractility in the ground squirrel and prairie dog during the early stages of cholesterol gallstone formation. Gastroenterology 85:830–836
35. Friesen SR (1982) Tumors of the endocrine pancreas. N Engl J Med 306:580–590
36. Gaisano HY, Reilly W, Go VLW, Olivero D, Miller LJ (1986) Large molecular forms of cholecystokinin circulating in humans. Pancreas 1:148–153
37. Gaisano HY, Klueppelberg UG, Pinon DI, Pfenning MA, Powers SP, Miller LJ (1989) Novel tool for the study of cholecystokinin-stimulated pancreatic enzyme secretion. J Clin Invest 83:321–325
38. Ganda OP, Weir GC, Soeldner JS, Legg MA, Chick WL, Patel YC, Ebeid AM, Gabbay KH, Reichlin S (1977) "Somatostatinoma": a somatostatin-containing tumor of the exocrine pancreas. N Engl J Med 296:963–967
39. Gomez G, Upp JR Jr, Lluis F, Alexander RW, Poston GJ, Greeley GH, Thompson JC (1988) Regulation of the release of cholecystokinin by bile salts in dogs and humans. Gastroenterology 94:1036–1046

40. Green S, Chambon P (1986) A superfamily of potentially oncogenic hormone receptors. Nature 324:615–617
41. Grider JR, Makhlouf GM (1987) Regional and cellular heterogeneity of cholecystokinin receptors mediating muscle contraction in the gut. Gastroenterology 92:175–180
42. Gullo L, Bolondi L, Priori P, Casanova P, Labò G (1984) Inhibitory effect of atropine on cholecystokinin-induced gallbladder contraction in man. Digestion 29:209–213
43. Gullo L, Bolondi L, Scarpignato C, Priori P, Casanova P, Labò G (1986) Effect of somatostatin and thyrotropin-releasing hormone on cholecystokinin-induced gallbladder emptying. Dig Dis Sci 31:1345–1350
44. Harper HA, Raper HS (1943) Pancreozymin, a stimulant of the secretion of pancreatic enzymes in extracts of small intestine. J Physiol 102:115–125
45. Hepner GW (1975) Effect of decreased gallbladder stimulation on enterohepatic cycling and kinetics of bile acids. Gastroenterology 68:1574–1581
46. Hermansen K (1984) Effects of cholecystokinin (CCK)-4, nonsulfated CCK-8, and sulfated CCK-8 on pancreatic somatostatin, insulin, and glucagon secretion in the dog: studies in vitro. Endocrinology 114:1770–1775
47. Hofmann AF, Grundy SM, Lachin JM, Lan SP, Baum RA, Hanson RF, Hersh T, Hightower NC Jr, Marks JW, Mekhjian H, Shaefer RA, Soloway RD, Thistle JL, Thomas FP, Tyor MP, group a NCGS (1982) Pretreatment biliary lipid composition in white patients with radiolucent gallstones in the National Cooperative Gallstone Study. Gastroenterology 83:738–752
48. Hokfelt T, Rehfeld JF, Skirboll L, Ivemark B, Goldstein M, Markey K (1980) Evidence for coexistence of dopamine and CCK in mesolimbic neurons. Nature 285:476–478
49. Hokfelt T, Johansson O, Goldstein M (1984) Chemical anatomy of the brain. Science 225:1326–1334
50. Holan KR, Holzbach RT, Herman RE et al. (1979) Nucleation time: a key factor in the pathogenesis of cholesterol gallstone disease. Gastroenterology 77:611–617
51. Holzbach, RT, Marsh M, Olszewski M, Holan K (1973) Cholesterol solubility in bile: evidence that supersaturated bile is frequent in man. J Clin Invest 52:1467–1479
52. Holzbach RT, Corbusier C, Marsh M, Naito HK (1976) The process of cholesterol cholelithiasis induced by diet in the prairie dog: a physicochemical characterization. J Lab Clin Med 87:987–998
53. Holzbach RT, Kibe A, Thiel E, Howell JH, Marsh M, Hermann RE (1984) Biliary proteins: unique inhibitors of cholesterol crystal nucleation in human gallbladder bile. J Clin Invest 73:35–45
54. Hopman WPM, Rosenbusch G, Jansen JBMJ, de Jong AJL, Lamers CBHW (1985) Gallbladder contraction: effects of fatty meals and cholecystokinin. Radiology 157:37–39
55. Hopman WPM, Jansen JBMJ, Rosenbusch G, Lamers CBHW (1987) Cephalic stimulation of gallbladder contraction in humans: role of cholecystokinin and the cholinergic system. Digestion 38:197–203
56. Hould FS, Fried GM, Fazekas AG, Tremplay S, Mersereau WA (1988) Progesterone receptors regulate gallbladder motility. J Surg Res 45:505–512
57. Hutton SW, Sievert CE Jr, Vennes JA, Duane WC (1981) The effect of sphincterotomy on gallstone formation in the prairie dog. Gastroenterology 81:663–667
58. Hutton SW, Sievert CE Jr, Vennes JA, Duane WC (1982) Inhibition of gallstone formation by sphincterotomy in the prairie dog: reversal by atropine. Gastroenterology 82:1308–1313
59. Hutton SW, Sievert CE Jr, Vennes JA, Shaffer RB, Duane WC (1988) Spontaneous passage of glass beads from the canine gallbladder: facilitation by sphincterotomy. Gastroenterology 94:1031–1035
60. Impicciatorre M (1978) Occurrence of H_1 and H_2 histamine receptors in the guinea pig gallbladder in situ. Br J Pharmacol 64:219–222
61. Ivy AC, Oldberg E (1928) A hormone mechanism for gallbladder contraction and evacuation. Am J Physiol 86:599–613
62. Jansen JBMJ, Lamers CBHW (1983) Radioimmunoassay of cholecystokinin in human tissue and plasma. Clin Chim Acta 131:305–316
63. Jazrawi RP, Northfield TC (1986) Effects of a pharmacological dose of cholecystokinin on bile salt kinetics and biliary cholesterol saturation in man. Gut 27:355–362
64. Jensen RT, Lemp GF, Gardner JD (1980) Interaction of cholecystokinin with specific membrane receptors on pancreatic acinar cells. Proc Natl Acad Sci USA 77:2079–2083

65. Jensen RT, Lemp GF, Gardner JD (1982) Interactions of the COOH-terminal fragments of cholecystokinin with receptors on dispersed acini from guinea pig pancreas. J Biol Chem 257:5554–5559
66. Jivegård L, Svanvik J (1986) The influence of morphine, loperamide and naloxone on gallbladder response to prostaglandin E_2 in the anaesthetized cat. Acta Physiol Scand 127:275–279
67. Johnson AG, Marshall CE, Wilson IAI (1982) Effects of some drugs and peptide hormones on the responsiveness of the rabbit isolated gall-bladder to cholecystokinin. J Physiol 332:415–425
68. Kern F Jr, Everson GT, DeMark B, McKinley C, Showalter R, Erfling W, Braverman DZ, Szczepanik-van Leeuwen P, Klein PD (1981) Biliary lipids, bile acids, and gallbladder function in the human female: effects of pregnancy and the ovulatory cycle. J Clin Invest 68:1229–1242
69. Kerstens PJSM, Lamers CBHW, Jansen JBMJ, de Jong AJL, Hessels M, Hafkenscheid JCM (1985) Physiological plasma concentrations of cholecystokinin stimulate pancreatic enzyme secretion and gallbladder contraction in man. Life Sci 36:565–569
70. Klueppelberg UG, Powers SP, Miller LJ (1988) Biochemical characterization of the CCK-receptor and its active site: efficiency of covalent labeling using a battery of probes. Biomed Res [Suppl] 1:54
71. Klueppelberg UG, Powers SP, Miller LJ (1989) Protease peptide mapping of affinity labeled rat pancreatic cholecystokinin-binding proteins. Biochemistry 28:7124–7129
72. Klueppelberg UG, Gaisano HY, Powers SP, Miller LJ (1989) Use of a nitro-tryptophancontaining peptide for photoaffinity labeling the active site of the pancreatic cholecystokinin receptor. Biochemistry 28:3463–3468
73. Kotwall CA, Clanachan AS, Baer HP, Scott GW (1984) Effects of prostaglandins on motility of gallbladders removed from patients with gallstones. Arch Surg 119:709–712
74. Krejs GJ, Orci L, Conlon JM, Ravazzola M, Davis GR, Raskin P, Collins SM, McCarthy DM, Baetens D, Rubenstein A, Aldor TAM, Unger RH (1979) Somatostatinoma syndrome – biochemical, morphologic and clinical features. N Engl J Med 301:285–292
75. LaMont JT, Smith BF, Moore JRL (1984) Role of gallbladder mucin in the pathophysiology of gallstones. Hepatology 4:51S–56S
76. LaMorte WW, Schoetz DJ Jr, Desmond HB, Williams LF Jr (1979) The role of the gallbladder in the pathogenesis of gallstones. Gastroenterology 77:580–592
77. LaMorte WW, Booker ML, Scott TE, Williams LF (1985) Increases in gallbladder prostaglandin synthesis before the formation of cholesterol gallstones. Surgery 98:445–451
78. Lee SP, Carey MC, LaMont JT (1981) Aspirin prevention of cholesterol gallstone formation in prairie dogs. Science 211:1429–1431
79. Lee SP, LaMont T, Carey M (1981) Role of gallbladder mucus hypersecretion in the evolution of cholesterol gallstones: studies in the prairie dog. J Clin Invest 67:1712–1723
80. Lee SP, Maher K, Nicholls JF (1988) Origin and fate of biliary sludge. Gastroenterology 94:170–176
81. Lee SP, Nicholls JF (1986) Nature and composition of biliary sludge. Gastroenterology 90:677–686
82. Lennon F, Feeley TM, Clanachan AS, Scott GW (1984) Effects of histamine receptor stimulation on diseased gallbladder and cystic duct. Gastroenterology 87:257–262
83. Li YF, Weisbrodt NW, Moody FG, Coelho JC, Gouma DJ (1987) Calcium-induced contraction and contractile protein content of gallbladder smooth muscle after high-cholesterol feeding of prairie dogs. Gastroenterology 92:746–750
84. Liddle RA, Goldfine ID, Rosen MS, Taplitz RA, Williams JA (1985) Cholecystokinin bioactivity in human plasma – molecular forms, responses to feeding, and relationship to gallbladder contraction. J Clin Invest 75:75
85. Liddle RA, Kanayama S, Beccaria L (1988) The ability of a new cholecystokinin receptor antagonist, L-364,718, to inhibit CCK- and meal-stimulated gallbladder contraction in humans. Biomed Res [Suppl] (abstr) 1:59
86. Lignon M, Galas M, Rodriquez M, Gaillon G, Martinez J (1987) A CCK-analogue that exhibits part of the CCK reponse on rat pancreatic acini: relationships among amylase release, receptor affinity and phosphoinositide breakdown. In: Bali J, Martinez J (eds) Gastrin and cholecystokinin. Chemistry, physiology, pharmacology. Elsevier, New York, pp 57–60
87. Lluis F, Fujimura M, Lonovics J, Guo Y, Gomez G, Greeley GH Jr, Townsend CM Jr,

Thompson JC (1988) Peptide YY and gallbladder contraction: studies in vivo and in vitro. Gastroenterology 94:1441–1446
88. Lonovics J, Devitt P, Rayford PL, Thompson JC (1979) Actions of VIP, somatostatin, and pancreatic polypeptide on gallbladder tension and CCK-stimulated gallbladder contraction in vitro. Surg Forum 30:407–409
89. Lotti VJ, Pendleton RG, Gould RJ, Hanson HM, Chang RSL, Clineschmidt BV (1987) In vivo pharmacology of L-364,718, a potent nonpeptide peripheral cholecystokinin antagonist. J Pharmacol Exp Ther 241:103–109
90. Low-Beer TS, Heaton KW, Heaton ST, Read AE (1971) Gallbladder inertia and sluggish enterohepatic circulation of bile-salts in cœliac disease. Lancet ii:991–994
91. Low-Beer TS, Harvey RF, Davies ER, Read AE (1975) Abnormalities of serum cholecystokinin and gallbladder emptying in celiac disease. N Engl J Med 292:961–963
92. Marzio L, Capone F, Neri M, di Felice F, Celiberti V, Mezzetti A, Giorgi D, Cuccurullo F (1987) Effect of cholinergic agonists and antagonists on gallbladder volume in fasting man. Eur J Clin Pharmacol 33:151–153
93. Marzio L, Capone F, Neri M, Mezzetti A, De Angelis C, Cuccurullo F (1988) Gallbladder kinetics in obese patients: effect of a regular meal and low-calorie meal. Dig Dis Sci 33:4–9
94. Marzio L, Neri M, Capone F, Di Felice F, De Angelis C, Mezzetti A, Cuccurullo F (1988) Gallbladder contraction and its relationship to interdigestive duodenal motor activity in normal human subjects. Dig Dis Sci 33:540–544
95. Masclee AAM, Geuskens LM, Driessen WMM, Jansen JBMJ, Lamers CBHW (1988) Impaired plasma cholecystokinin and gallbladder responses to fat in gallstone patients. Hepatology 8:1256 (abstr)
96. Mate L, Sakamoto T, Greeley GH, Thompson JC (1986) Effect of substance P on contractions of the gallbladder. Surg Gynecol Obstet 163:163–166
97. Matsumura M, Shimizu I, Ohura M, Mori H, Saito S (1988) Effects of bile salts on plasma concentration of β-endorphin-like immunoreactivity in men. Dig Dis Sci 33:692–696
98. Maudgal DP, Kupfer RM, Zentler-Munro PL, Northfield TC (1980) Postprandial gallbladder emptying in patients with gallstones. Br Med J 280:141–143
99. Mayer EA, Elashoff J, Walsh JH (1982) Characterization of bombesin effects on canine gastric muscle. Am J Physiol 243:G141–G147
100. McCulloch J (1983) Peptides and the microregulation of blood flow in the brain. Nature 304:120
101. Meldrum LA, Bojarski JC, Calam J (1987) Effects of substance P and other neuropeptides on guinea pig gall-bladder muscle. Digestion 37:193–199
102. Merritt JE, Taylor CW, Rubin RP, Putney VW Jr (1986) Evidence suggesting that a novel guanine nucleotide regulatory protein couples receptors to phospholipase C in exocrine pancreas. Biochem J 236:337–343
103. Messing B, Bories C, Kunstlinger F, Bernier J (1983) Does total parenteral nutrition induce gallbladder sludge formation and lithiasis? Gastroenterology 84:1012–1019
104. Mok HYI, von Bergmann K, Grundy SM (1977) Regulation of pool size of bile acids in man. Gastroenterology 73:684–690
105. Mutt V, Jorpes JE (1968) Structure of porcine cholecystokinin-pancreozymin. I. Cleavage with thrombin and trypsin. Eur J Biochem 6:156–162
106. Nakano J, McCloy RE, Gin AC, Nakano SK (1975) Effect of prostaglandin E_1, E_2 and F, and pentagastrin on the gall bladder pressure in dogs. Eur J Pharmacol 30:107–112
107. Nally CV, McMullin LJ, Clanachan AS, Scott GW (1987) Periodic gallbladder contraction maintains bile acid circulation during the fasting period: a canine study. Br J Surg 74:1134–1138
108. Northfield TC, Kupfer TM, Maudgal DP, Zentler-Munro PL, Meller ST, Garvie NW, McCready R (1980) Gall-bladder sensitivity to cholecystokinin in patients with gallstones. Br Med J 280:143–144
109. Ouyang A (1988) Cholecystokinin receptor and gallbladder contractility. Gastroenterology 94:241–242
110. Pearson RK, Miller LJ (1987) Affinity labeling of a novel cholecystokinin-binding protein in rat pancreatic plasmalemma using new short probes for the receptor. J Biol Chem 262:869–876

111. Pearson RK, Miller LJ, Hadac EM, Powers SP (1987) Analysis of the carbohydrate composition of the pancreatic plasmalemmal glycoprotein affinity labeled by short probes for the cholecystokinin receptor. J Biol Chem 262:13850–13856
112. Pearson RK, Miller LJ, Powers SP, Hadac EM (1987) Biochemical characterization of the pancreatic cholecystokinin receptor using monofunctional photoactivatable probes. Pancreas 2:79–84
113. Pellegrini CA, Lewin M, Patti MG, Thomas MJ, Ryan T, Way LW (1985) Gallbladder filling and response to cholecystokinin are not affected by vagotomy. Surgery 98:452–458
114. Pellegrini CA, Ryan T, Broderick W, Way LW (1986) Gallbladder filling and emptying during cholesterol gallstone formation in the prairie dog. Gastroenterology 90:143–149
115. Pomeranz IS, Shaffer EA (1985) Abnormal gallbladder emptying in a subgroup of patients with gallstones. Gastroenterology 88:787–791
116. Pomeranz IS, Davison JS, Shaffer EA (1983) In vitro effects of pancreatic polypeptide and motilin on contractility of human gallbladder. Dig Dis Sci 28:539–544
117. Pomeranz IS, Davison IS, Shaffer EA (1986) The effects of prosthetic gallstones on gallbladder function and bile composition. J Surg Res 41:47–52
118. Powers SP, Fourmy D, Gaisano H, Miller LJ (1988) Intrinsic photoaffinity labeling probes for cholecystokinin (CCK)-gastrin family receptors. J Biol Chem 263:5295–5300
119. Reeve JR Jr, Eysselein V, Walsh JH, Ben-Avram CM, Shively JE (1986) New molecular forms of cholecystokinin: microsequence analysis of forms previously characterized by chromatographic methods. J Biol Chem 261:16392–16397
120. Rehfeld JF (1978) Immunohistochemical studies on cholecystokinin. II. Distribution and molecular heterogeneity in the central nervous system and intestine of man and hog. J Biol Chem 253:4022–4030
121. Rehfeld JF (1981) Four basic characteristics of the gastrin-cholecystokinin system. Am J Physiol 240 (Gastrointest Liver Physiol 3):G255–G266
122. Rehfeld JF, Larsson LI, Goltermann NR, Schwartz TW, Holst JJ, Jensen SL, Morley JS (1980) Neural regulation of pancreatic hormone secretion by the C-terminal tetrapeptide of CCK. Nature 284:33–38
123. Reuben A (1984) Biliary proteins. Hepatology 4:46S–50S
124. Roslyn JJ, Pitt HA, Mann LL, Ament ME, DenBesten L (1983) Gallbladder disease in patients on long-term parenteral nutrition. Gastroenterology 84:148–154
125. Ryan J, Cohen S (1976) Interaction of gastrin I, secretin, and cholecystokinin on gallbladder smooth muscle. Am J Physiol 230:553–556
126. Ryan J, Cohen S (1977) Effect of vasoactive intestinal peptide on basal and cholecystokinin-induced gallbladder pressure. Gastroenterology 73:870–872
127. Ryan JP, Pellecchia D (1982) Effect of progesterone pretreatment on guinea pig gallbladder motility in vitro. Gastroenterology 83:81–83
128. Ryan JP, Ryave S (1978) Effect of vasoactive intestinal peptide on gallbladder smooth muscle in vitro. Am J Physiol 234 (Endocrinol Metab Gastrointest Physiol 3):E44–E46
129. Saito A, Sankaran H, Goldfine ID, Williams JA (1980) Cholecystokinin receptors in the brain: characterization and distribution. Science 208:1155–1156
130. Sargent DF, Schwyzer R (1986) Membrane lipid phase as catalyst for peptide–receptor interactions. Proc Natl Acad Sci USA 83:5774–5778
131. Schafmayer A, Werner M, Becker HD (1982) Radioimmunological determination of cholecystokinin in tissue extracts. Digestion 24:146–154
132. Schjoldager B, Klueppelberg UG, Powers SP, Miller LJ (1988) Biochemical characterization of the CCK-binding subunit of the bovine gallbladder receptor using an intrinsic photoaffinity labeling probe. Gastroenterology 94:A408
133. Schjoldager B, Shaw MJ, Powers SP, Schmalz PP, Szurszewski J, Miller LJ (1988) Bovine gallbladder muscularis: source of a myogenic receptor for cholecystokinin. Am J Physiol 254 (Gastrointest Liver Physiol 17):G294–G299
134. Schjoldager B, Molero X, Miller LJ (1989) Functional biochemical characterization of the human gallbladder muscularis cholecystokinin receptor. Gastroenterology 96:1119–1125
135. Schnefel S, Banfic H, Eckhardt L, Schultz G, Schulz I (1988) Acetylcholine and cholecystokinin receptors functionally couple by different G-proteins to phospholipase C in pancreatic acinar cells. FEBS Lett 230:125–130

136. Schulz I, Streb H, Bayerdörffer E, Imamura J (1986) Intracellular messengers in stimuli-secretion coupling of pancreatic acinar cells. Cardiovasc Pharmacol 8 [Suppl 8]:S91–S96
137. Scott RB, Eidt PB, Shaffer EA (1985) Regulation of fasting canine duodenal bile acid delivery by sphincter of Oddi and gallbladder. Am J Physiol (Gastrointest Liver Physiol 12) 249:G622–G633
138. Severi C, Grider JR, Makhlouf GM (1988) Characterization of opioid receptors on isolated canine gallbladder smooth muscle cells. Life Sci 42:2373–2380
139. Severi C, Grider JR, Makhlouf GM (1988) Identification of separate bombesin and substance P receptors on isolated muscle cells from canine gallbladder. J Pharmacol Exp Ther 245:195–198
140. Shaffer EA, Small DM (1976) Gallstone disease: pathogenesis and management. Curr Probl Surg 13:1–72
141. Shaffer EA, Small DM (1977) Biliary lipid secretion in cholesterol gallstone disease: the effect of cholecystectomy and obesity. J Clin Invest 59:828–840
142. Shaffer EA, McOrmond P, Duggan H (1980) Quantitative assessment of gallbladder filling and emptying and duodenogastric reflux. Gastroenterology 79:899–906
143. Shaw MJ, Hadac EM, Miller LJ (1987) Preparation of enriched plasma membranes from bovine gallbladder muscularis for characterization of cholecystokinin receptors. J Biol Chem 262:14313–14318
144. Sibley DR, Benovic JL, Caron MG, Lefkowitz RJ (1987) Regulation of transmembrane signaling by receptor phosphorylation. Cell 48:913–922
145. Singletary BK, Van Thiel DH, Eagon P (1986) Estrogen and progesterone receptors in human gallbladder. Hepatology 6:574–578
146. Smith BF (1987) Human gallbladder mucin binds biliary lipids and promotes cholesterol crystal nucleation in model bile. J Lipid Res 28:1088–1097
147. Smith BF, LaMonte JT (1984) Hydrophobic binding properties of bovine gallbladder mucin. J Biol Chem 259:12170–12177
148. Smith GP, Jerome C, Cusnin BJ, Eterno R, Simansky KJ (1981) Abdominal vagotomy blocks the satiety effect of cholecystokinin in the rat. Science 213:1036–1037
149. Soll AH, Amirian DA, Park J, Elashoff JD, Yamada T (1985) Cholecystokinin potently releases somatostatin from canine fundic mucosa cells in short-term culture. Am J Physiol 248 (Gastrointest Liver Physiol 11):G569–G573
150. Spellman SJ, Shaffer EA, Rosenthall L (1979) Gallbladder emptying in response to cholecystokinin. Gastroenterology 77:115–120
151. Steigerwalt RW, Goldfine ID, Williams JA (1984) Characterization of cholecystokinin receptors on bovine gallbladder membranes. Am J Physiol 247 (Gastrointest Liver Physiol 10):G709–G714
152. Stone BG, Gavaler JS, Belle SH, Shreiner DP, Peleman RR, Sarva RP, Yingvorapant N, van Thiel DH (1988) Impairment of gallbladder emptying in diabetes mellitus. Gastroenterology 95:170–176
153. Strah KM, Pappas TN, Melendez RL, Debas HT (1986) Contrasting cholinergic dependence of pancreatic and gallbladder responses to cholecystokinin. Am J Physiol 250 (Gastrointest Liver Physiol 13):G665–G669
154. Sylwestrowicz TA, Shaffer EA (1988) Gallbladder function during gallstone dissolution. Gastroenterology 95:740–748
155. Takahashi I, Suzuki T, Aizawa I, Itoh Z (1982) Comparison of gallbladder contractions induced by motilin and cholecystokinin in dogs. Gastroenterology 82:419–424
156. Takahashi T, Yamamura T, Ishikawa Y, Kantoh M, Utsunomiya J (1986) Effects of cholecystokinin-octapeptide on the human gallbladder both in vivo and in vitro. Gastroenterol Jpn 21:49–54
157. Thompson JC, Fried GM, Ogden WD, Fagan CJ, Inoue K, Wiener I, Watson LC (1982) Correlation between release of cholecystokinin and contraction of the gallbladder in patients with gallstones. Ann Surg 195:670–676
158. Unger RH (1977) Somatostatinoma. N Engl J Med 296:998–1000
159. Upp JR, Nealon WH, Singh P, Fagan CJ, Jonas AS, Greeley GH, Thompson JC (1987) Correlation of cholecystokinin receptors with gallbladder contractility in patients with gallstones. Ann Surg 205:641–648

160. Vagne M, Troitskaja V (1976) Effect of secretin, glucagon and VIP on gallbladder contraction. Digestion 14:62–67
161. Villanueva ML, Collins SM, Jensen RT, Gardner JD (1982) Structural requirements for action of cholecystokinin on enzyme secretion from pancreatic acini. Am J Physiol 242 (Gastrointest Liver Physiol 5):G416–G422
162. von Helmsbach M (1856) Mikrogeologie. Reimer, Berlin
163. von Schrenck T, Moran TH, Heinz-Erian P, Gardner JD, Jensen RT (1988) Cholecystokinin receptors on gallbladder muscle and pancreatic acinar cells – a comparative study. Am J Physiol 255 (Gastrointest Liver Physiol 18):G512–G521
164. Waldman DB, Zfas AM, Makhlouf GM (1977) Stimulatory (H_1) and inhibitory (H_2) histamine receptors in gallbladder muscle. Gastroenterology 22:932–936
165. Walker JP, Khalil T, Wiener I, Fagan CJ, Townsend CM, Greeley GH, Thompson JC (1985) The role of neurotensin in human gallbladder motility. Ann Surg 201:678–683
166. Walsh JH (1981) Gastrointestinal hormones and peptides. In: Johnson LR (ed) Physiology of the gastrointestinal tract. Raven, New York, pp 59–144
167. Williams JA, McChesney DJ (1987) Cholecystokinin induces the interaction of its receptor with a guanine nucleotide binding protein. Regul Pept 18:109–117
168. Wood JR, Saverymuttu SH, Ashbrooke AB, Stamford IF (1980) Effects of various prostanoids on gallbladder muscle. Adv Prostaglandin Thromboxane Res 8:1569–1571
169. Worobetz LJ, Baker RJ, McCallum JA, Wells G, Sullivan SN (1982) The effect of naloxone, morphine, and an enkephalin analogue on cholecystokinin octapeptide-stimulated gallbladder emptying. Am J Gastroenterol 77:509–511
170. Yamamura T, Takahashi T, Kusunoki M, Kantoh M, Ishikawa Y, Utsunomiya J (1986) Cholecystokinin octapeptide-evoked [^{3}H]acetylcholine release from guinea pig gallbladder. Neurosci Lett 65:167–170
171. Yamamura T, Takahashi T, Kusunoki M, Kantoh M, Seino Y, Utsunomiya J (1988) Gallbladder dynamics and plasma cholecystokinin responses after meals, oral water, or sham feeding in healthy subjects. Am J Med Sci 295:102–107
172. Yamasato T, Nakayama S (1988) Effects of neurotensin on the motility of the isolated gallbladder, bile duct and ampulla in guinea-pigs. Eur J Pharmacol 148:101–106
173. Yau WM, Youther ML (1984) Modulation of gallbladder motility by intrinsic cholinergic neurons. Am J Physiol 247 (Gastrointest Liver Physiol 10):G662–G666
174. Zak RA, Frenkiel PG, Marks JW, Bonorris GG, Allen A, Schoenfield LJ (1984) Cyclic nucleotides and glycoproteins during formation of cholesterol gallstones in prairie dogs. Gastroenterology 87:263–269

Environmental Factors and Gallstones

J. G. Wechsler

University Clinic of Ulm, Department of Internal Medicine II, Robert-Koch-Str. 8, D-7900 Ulm, FRG

Most gallstones are symptomless and therefore often remain undiagnosed. Exact data for national incidence rates could theoretically be obtained by an ultrasonographic screening of defined samples of the population. Epidemiologic data are available from autopsy surveys, cholecystographies, and ultrasound examinations [1]. These data show well-known cultural and geographic differences. In North America, in Europe, especially the northern parts, and in other industrialized countries gallstones are much more common than in most parts of Asia and Africa. Frequency rates for gallstones of between 40% and 60% can be found in Sweden and Finland, for example. In the United Kingdom, Federal Republic of Germany, and Greece an incidence between 20% and 40% has been described.

Most published studies relating to gallstone disesae show a strong correlation between dietary intake and nutritional status. These interactions can be seen clearly in Japan, where people moving from a region with low incidence to a region with high incidence develop gallstones at the higher rate.

The recurrence rate of gallstones after successful medical dissolution is about 50%. Under these circumstances dietary and nutritional factors may be important not only during dissolution but also for the postdissolution prevention of gallstone recurrence [2].

Age

Advanced age is a risk factor for gallstone formation. Statistical significance was found by Einarsson et al. [3] for the relationship between age and cholesterol secretion. Cholesterol saturation of bile increases with age as a consequence of an increased rate of hepatic secretion of cholesterol. A negative correlation between age and the rate of bile acid synthesis ($r = -0.60$) was observed both in patients with gallstones and in gallstone-free subjects with supersaturated bile. Both mechanisms, the increased secretion of cholesterol and the decreased synthesis of bile acid, can be explained by the activities of the rate-determining enzymes β-hydroxy-β-methylglutaryl coenzyme A reductase and 7α-hydroxylase, respectively.

Sex

Gallstones are more common in women than in men. The prevalence of gallstones is the same in both sexes until puberty, however during the fertility period and after menopause gallstones are more frequent in women. In a cross-sectional study reported by Jorgenson et al. [4] on women, gallstone disease was significantly associated with young age at menarche, with abortions, and with multiple child births. Use of oral contraceptives was significantly associated with gallstone disease in univariate analysis but not in multivariate analysis. Breast feading, age at menopause, and menopausal hormone therapy were not associated with gallstones. The formation of gallstones often can be observed during pregnancy in the mother. Fetal gallstones are considered extremely rare. Some cases of fetal gallstones with spontaneous resolution in the neonatal period were diagnosed by ultrasound examination [5]. The exact factors promoting the formation of gallstones during pregnancy are unknown. The hormonal changes in pregnancy may alter the composition of bile. Gallbladder motility is diminished. Weight gain during pregnancy may increase hepatic cholesterol secretion and increase the saturation of bile with cholesterol.

And finally, progestin and not estrogen may be responsible for gallstone formation.

Genetics

Gallstone disease seems to cluster in some families. Genetic influences may be at work, independent of other environmental risk factors for gallstone formation.

Race

In some races gallstones are more common than in others. American Indians have one of the highest incidence rates of cholesterol gallstones. The prevalence found in Central and South America is relatively high. Bile acid deficiency caused by diminished bile acid synthesis seems to induce supersaturation of bile. Furthermore, obesity is very common in Indians [6]. Black populations in America reveal a low incidence of gallstone disease. No studies on lipid metabolism or nucleating factors are available to explain the varying rates of gallstone formation in blacks, whites, and Indians.

Obesity

In obese persons the frequency of cholesterol gallstones is two to four times that found than in the general population. The Framingham study [7] showed a twofold increased risk for gallstones in persons whose weight was 20% above the median. The link between obesity and gallstones involves supersaturated bile. Obese individuals have a higher energy intake and eat more dietary fat and cholesterol than lean persons. Plasma concentrations of low-density and very low density lipoproteins are elevated in overweight individuals. The overproduction of total body cholesterol leads to an increased biliary cholesterol secretion into the bile and therefore to cholesterol supersaturation relative to the concentrations of bile acids and lecithin.

Rapid weight loss may be associated with increased risk for gallstones. L. J. Schoenfield (1987, personal communication) placed superobese patients (160% of ideal body weight) on a 520 calorie per day diet. Four of 13 patients developed gallstones by the 16th week of weight reduction. Decrease in synthesis and pool size in bile acids, mobilization of cholesterol from adipose tissue stores, and decreased gallbladder motility may be the factors responsible for supersaturation of bile during weight reduction.

Cholesterol saturation of bile has been studied in our clinic in ten patients after successful weight reduction with a very low calorie diet (modified fasting) providing 450 calories per day over 4 weeks. The mean weight loss was 12.6 kg (from 110.4 ± 4.9 kg to 97.8 ± 4.6 kg). The bile was obtained endoscopically through prepapillary suction after stimulation of the gallbladder with 5 μg ceruletide. The procedure was carried out before and after weight reduction during isocaloric energy intake over 3 days for equilibration.

The cholesterol saturation index decreased from 1.34 ± 0.08 to 1.08 ± 0.06 (statistically significant). However, in most cases of the still overweight persons no normalization of cholesterol saturation could be achieved. Nevertheless, we are convinced that treatment and avoidance of obesity are of importance in the prevention of cholesterol gallstone formation.

Fiber

It is well known from epidemiologic and experimental studies that fiber-depleted foods cause cholesterol-rich gallstones. Many studies, on the other hand, show that dietary fiber in the form of wheat bran reduces the risk of gallstones. A reduced amount of fiber is often associated with high energy intake and high refined carbohydrate intake. When bran was given to subjects with unsaturated bile, it had no effect; in individuals with supersaturated bile, however, the bile became less saturated and in some cases unsaturated [8].

We have studied the influence of dietary fiber (30 g wheat bran per day) on lithogenicity of the bile in ten healthy persons. Mean body weight was 76.8 ± 2.3 kg, mean height was 189.9 ± 2.1 cm, and mean age was 25.5 ± 0.26 years. Twice daily 15 g wheat bran was given additional to the normal diet over 6 weeks. Bile was obtained by prepapillary suction endoscopically following stimulation of the gallbladder with ceruletide. Gallbladder contraction was controlled sonographically. Increased dietary fiber intake resulted in significant lowering of cholesterol concentration in the bile from 3.27 ± 0.89 to 2.50 ± 0.67 mmol/l. The lithogenic index decreased from 1.01 ± 0.14 to 0.67 ± 0.11 (statistically significant) [9]. The mechanism of this effect is not clearly understood. Diminished absorption of dietary cholesterol and alteration in the gut bacterial flora that would favor decreased formation of deoxycholic acid might be consequences of increased fiber intake. Furthermore deoxycholic acid could displace chenodeoxycholic acid from the bile.

It is likely that a diet rich in fiber helps to prevent the formation and recurrence of gallstones.

Alcohol

The study of Scragg et al. [10] demonstrated that consumption of alcoholic beverages was associated with a decreased risk for gallstone formation. Thornton et al. [11] found that in individuals with moderate alcohol intake bile cholesterol saturation decreased and the plasma level of high-density lipoprotein cholesterol increased. The Rome Group for the Epidemiology and Prevention of Cholelithiasis [12] reported a tendency toward an increased incidence of gallstones with increased wine consumption. Increasing the frequency of consumption of high-alcohol drinks, however, decreased incidence of gallstones. Schwesinger et al. [13] observed in ethanol- and cholesterol-fed prairie dogs a lower incidence of gallstones than in cholesterol-fed controls; the cholesterol saturation index was reduced from 1.22 to 0.81 in the ethanol group. The mechanism of ethanol on cholelithiasis is still incompletely understood.

The activity of HMG coenzyme A reductase, the enzyme responsible for hepatic cholesterol synthesis, has been found both to be increased [14] and to be decreased in rats fed with ethanol [15]. The other major rate-limiting enzyme, 7α-hydroxylase, is also discussed controversially. Furthermore, qualitative changes in the bile acid composition, modulation of cholesterol solubility, and crystal nucleation in ethanol-fed animals may contribute to a lower incidence of gallstone formation.

Cholesterol

No relationship exists between serum cholesterol and gallstone disease. However, cholesterol feeding induces cholesterol hypersecretion in bile. DenBesten et al. [16] observed in some persons after cholesterol feeding increases biliary cholesterol concentration; other authors could not confirm this effect, however. Le et al. [17] studied the effect on biliary cholesterol secretion of giving diets containing 500, 750, or 1000 mg cholesterol/day. The percentage of cholesterol in bile and the cholesterol saturation index increased significantly in gallstone patients (9.2% to 12.4% and 1.25 to 1.53, respectively; $p<0.01$).

In conclusion, excess dietary intake of cholesterol may lead to supersaturation of gallbladder bile in some patients. In these patients a low-cholesterol diet should be recommended.

Hyperlipidemia (Hypertriglyceridemia)

Patients with hypertriglyceridemia have an increased probability of developing cholesterol gallstones. Concentrations of low-density and very low density lipoproteins in patients with hypertriglyceridemia are elevated, followed by an increased secretion of cholesterol in bile. Hypertriglyceridemia and obesity often are associated.

Lipid-lowering drugs such as clofibrate enhance the cholesterol saturation of bile. The Clofibrate Study of the World Health Organization [18] demonstrated an increased risk for development of cholesterol gallstones during treatment with fibric acid. The bile acid sequestrants cholestyramine and colestipol do not influence biliary cholesterol concentrations. Nicotinic acid, however, increases the cholesterol saturation of bile. Potent plasma cholesterol lowering drugs such as probucol, compactin, mevinolin, and synvinolin seem to have beneficial effects not only on plasma cholesterol concentrations but also on biliary cholesterol saturation.

Considering long-term treatment of hyperlipidemias, supersaturation of bile may occur only over a limited period of time. Nevertheless, the development of silent gallstones ought to be considered during lipid-lowering regimens.

Fatty Acid Composition

Polyunsaturated fatty acids can lower elevated plasma cholesterol levels. The mechanisms for this effect have not been elucidated completely. Evidence of increased risk for development of gallstones after long-term treatment with large amounts of polyunsaturated fatty acids was gained from the Los Angeles sutdy of Sturdevant et al. [19]. Other groups could not confirm this effect. It is likely that a decrease in plasma cholesterol is followed by an increase in biliary cholesterol secretion for a limited period. Results of studies on the effects of ω-3 fatty acids on biliary lipid concentrations are still contradictory and are under investigation [20].

Refined Carbohydrate Intake

The term refined carbohydrates refers to white or brown sugar, syrups, and white flour. Thornton et al. [21] found that excess intake of refined carbohydrates is followed by an elevated cholesterol saturation index. A high-fiber, low-sugar diet lowered biliary cholesterol concentration and the mean cholesterol saturation index from 1.5 to 1.2 in a 6-week cross-over study in 13 patients with asymptomatic gallstones. Further studies giving diets either high or low in refined sucrose did not lead to supersaturated bile [22]. A high energy intake with high amounts of refined carbohydrates and a reduced fiber intake could alter the gut bacterial flora. Increased formation of deoxycholic acid might increase biliary cholesterol secretion.

Conclusion

Environmental factors are the principle cause for the high prevalence of gallstones in various populations. Factors such as age, sex, genetics, and race may predispose to gallstone formation and should be compensated by dietary or other preventive measures. The most important risk factors for cholelithiasis are obesity, hypertriglyceridemia, and a diet high in cholesterol and low in fiber intake. Patients with gallstone disease and individuals after successful gallstone dissolution should be encouraged to reduce body weight and to take a low-calorie, low-cholesterol, and fiber-rich diet.

References

1. Barbara L (1984) Epidemiology of gallstone disease: The "Sirmione Study". In: Capocaccia L, Ricci G, Angelico F, Angelico M, Attili AF (eds) Epidemiology and prevention of gallstone disease. MTP Press, Lancaster, pp 23–250
2. Grundy SM, Kalser SC (1987) Highlights of the meeting on prevention of gallstones. Hepatology 7:946–951
3. Einarsson K, Nilsell K, Leijd B, Angelin B (1985) Influence of age on secretion of cholesterol and synthesis of bile acids by the liver. N Engl J Med 313:277–282
4. Jorgensen T (1988) Gallstones in a Danish population: fertility period, pregnancies, and exogenous female sex hormones. Gut 29:433–439
5. Klingensmith WC, Cioffi-Ragan DT (1988) Fetal gallstones. Radiology 167:143–144
6. Grundy SM, Metzger AL, Adler RD (1972) Mechanisms of lithogenic bile formation in American Indian women with cholesterol gallstones. J Clin Invest 51:3026–3043
7. Friedman G, Kannel W, Dawber T (1966) The epidemiology of gallbladder disease: observations in the Framingham study. J Chronic Dis 19:273–292
8. Heaton KW (1987) Effect of dietary fiber on biliary lipids. In: Barbara L et al. (eds) Nutrition in gastrointestinal disease. Raven, New York
9. Wechsler JG, Wenzel H, Swobodnik W, Ditschuneit H (1987) Influence of increased fibre intake on biliary lipids. Scand J Gastroenterol 22 [Suppl 129]:185–191
10. Scragg R, McMichael A, Baghurst P (1984) Diet, alcohol, and relative weight in gallstone disease: a case-control study. Br Med J 288:1113–1119
11. Thornton J, Symes C, Heaton K (1983) Moderate alcohol intake reduces bile cholesterol saturation and raises HDL cholesterol. Lancet 2:819–822
12. Attili AF, the Rome Group for the Epidemiology and Prevention of Cholelithiasis (GREPCO): (1987) Diet and gallstones: results of an epidemiologic study performed in male civil servants. In: Barbara L et al. (eds) Nutrition in gastrointestinal disease. Raven, New York
13. Schwesinger WH, Kurtin WE, Johnson R (1988) Alcohol protects against cholesterol gallstone formation. Ann Surg 207:641–647
14. Lakshmanan M, Veech R (1977) Short- and long-term effects of ethanol administration in vivo on rat liver HMG-CoA reductase and cholesterol 7 alpha-hydroxylase activities. J Lipid Res 18:325–330
15. Maruyama S, Murawaki Y, Hirayama C (1986) Effect of chronic ethanol administration on hepatic cholesterol and bile acid synthesis in relation to serum high density lipoprotein cholesterol in rats. Res Commun Chem Pathol Pharmacol 53:3–21
16. DenBesten L, Connor WE, Bell S (1973) The effect of dietary cholesterol on the composition of human bile. Surgery 73:266–273

17. Lee DWT, Gilmore CJ, Vonorris G, Cohen H, Marks JW et al. (1985) Effect of dietary cholesterol on biliary lipids in patients with gallstones and normal subjects. Am J Clin Nutr 42:414–420
18. Einarsson K, Angelin B (1986) Hyperlipoproteinemia, hypolipidemic treatment, and gallstone disease. In: Grundy SM (ed) Bile acids and atherosclerosis, vol 15. Raven, New York, pp 67–97
19. Sturdevant RAL, Pearce ML, Dayton S (1973) Increased prevalence of cholelithiasis in men ingesting a serum-cholesterol lowering diet. N Engl J Med 288:24–27
20. Wechsler JG, Swobodnik W, Wenzel H, Saal D, Janowitz P, Ditschuneit H (1989) Veränderungen der Plasmalipide, Lipoproteine und biliären Lipide nach Omega-3-Fettsäurenzufuhr bei Normalpersonen. Aktuelle Ernährungsmedizin 14:12–15
21. Thornton JR, Emmett PM, Heaton KW (1983) Diet and gallstones: effects of refined and unrefined carbohydrate diets on bile cholesterol saturation and bile acid metabolism. Gut 24:2–6
22. Werner D, Emmett PM, Heaton KW (1984) Effects of dietary sucrose on factors influencing cholesterol gallstone formation. Gut 25:269–274

Different Therapeutic Approaches to Gallstone Disease

Is Therapeutic Intervention Necessary in Gallstone Disease: The Surgeon's Point of View

B. S. Ashby

Southend Hospital, Southend, Essex SS0 0RY, UK

Introduction

Is therapeutic intervention necessary in gallstone disease? That is, if we find gallstones, should we do anything about them? As a surgeon expressing a view on this question, I shall consider the incidence of gallstones in the general population and describe the natural history of untreated gallstone disease, particularly the influence of advancing age. I shall then assess the results of gall-bladder surgery in the elderly compared with younger, fitter patients, in terms of the morbidity and mortality associated with increasing age. I shall also comment on an alternative to cholecystectomy commonly used in the treatment of elderly and medically unfit gallstone patients.

Incidence of Gallstones in the General Population

A number of studies have been published which attempt to establish the incidence of gallstones; these have generally been based on large series of routine post-mortem examinations [1–4]. The figures are roughly similar for Western Europe, the United States and Australia, and stones are generally more common in white persons than in coloured. Some of these series are quite large. Lieber, for instance, reviewed nearly 30000 post-mortem examinations in persons over 20 years old, with gallstones occurring in 11.6% [1], and Bouchier included nearly 5000 cases, with an incidence of 15.5% [4]. Most pathologists would agree that at autopsy they may find gallstones in up to 20% of cases, and presumably these are largely asymptomatic gallstones.

There is a marked difference between the sexes, with gallstones more than twice as common in women than in men. Lieber reported 21.7% of women having stones compared with 9.7% of men [1], and Bouchier reported 19.2% and 9.5%, respectively [4]. Also, the incidence increases with each decade of age; the same authors showed that between 20 and 30 years of age about 2.5% of the population have gallstones, that between 50 and 60 years the incidence rises to around 11%, and that over 80 years an average of 27% have stones. The increase in incidence with age is also greater in women than men. This increasing incidence reaches a peak in women between the ages of 50 and 60 years and in men between 60 and 70 years. In patients with gall-bladder stones who come to operation the incidence of stones in the common bile duct varies from 10% to 24% depending on the age of the patients, the extent of use of operative cholangiography, and the degree of aggression of the surgeon towards the common bile duct [5–9]. It is general experience that the common bile duct is explored in approximately 20% of patients undergoing cholecystectomy, and stones are actually found in about 15%.

Thus the incidence of gall-bladder stones in the general population is between 10% and 20%, greater in women, and increasing with age to reach nearly 30% in those aged over 80. The incidence of common bile duct stones also increases with age, and up to one-third of patients aged over 80 with gall-bladder stones also have common bile duct stones [10, 11]. As I shall show below, it is the elderly patients with gallstone disease, particularly those with common bile duct stones, who are also more likely to develop complications either from the disease or the operation.

Natural History of Untreated Gallstones

What happens to the patient in whom gallstones are diagnosed but not treated? Predictably, there are not many such series published on this. That of Wenckert and Robertson [6] is a large recent series of 781 patients with gall-bladder stones diagnosed but untreated and followed up for 10 years. Half the patients remained asymptomatic, 16% developed symptoms that were not serious, but 35% developed disease serious enough to require eventual surgery. Also, the risks of developing severe complications or jaundice were much higher in the elderly; 29% of those over the age of 60 had complications compared with 14% under 60 [6]. In another series 137 patients with gallstones were left untreated and followed up for up to 15 years [12]. Of these, 24% eventually came to operation because of severe symptoms or complications. The mortality amongst these cases was 48%, because, of course, they included the most medically unfit patients, which is the reason that they had remained surgically untreated in the first place.

Gall Bladder Surgery in the Elderly

There are many published series of younger patients with uncomplicated gall-bladder and common bile duct disease who undergo elective surgery. The morbidity rate is close to 0%, and mortality is less than 1%. A number of studies of biliary surgery in the elderly, on the other hand, show a rather different picture [7, 8, 10, 13]. Unfortunately, these studies present data that are not exactly comparable due to the variable age groups reported. Nevertheless, there is clearly general agreement regarding the greater mortality associated with advancing age. Ganey et al. [8], for example, showed no mortality with cholecystectomy for those below the age of 65 and a 3.2% mortality for those over 75 years. Similarly, Irvin and Arnstein [10] reported no mortality in the younger patients but 2% in those aged over 80.

In most series the mortality rate is very similar regardless of whether a simple cholecystectomy is performed or an exploration of the common bile duct. Complications are related more to age and emergency status than to the operation performed, as is, indeed, the mortality rate. In patients over the age of 65 the mean mortality reported for elective cholecystectomy is 0.75% and that for urgent or emergency cholecystectomy 10.4% [7, 13–15]. Also the need for emergency surgery increases with age. Houghton et al. [13] found that 10% of his patients aged over 60 needed urgent or emergency surgery, but that the figure rose to 20% in those over the age of 70. Addison and Finan [15] recorded 16% of those over 60 and 35% of those over 70 requiring urgent or emergency cholecystectomy. Thus, patients over 70 years of age required urgent or emergency surgical intervention more than twice as often as those aged between 60 and 70. The former also showed an appreciably higher mortality rate.

The effect of advanced age is seen particularly well in the study by Irvin and Arnstein [10]. In a series of 544 patients with symptomatic gall-bladder stones the difference between those under 70 and those over 70 years of age was marked. In those over 70 more than twice as many required emergency admission, needed common bile duct exploration, required permanent internal drainage of the bile duct, and developed postoperative complications. In addition, the mortality was confined entirely to those over 70.

The outcome of surgery for gallstones in younger patients (those aged under 65) with no complications is good regardless of the type of operation that is performed. Morbidity and mortality rates are almost nil. It is with advancing age and the need for urgent or emergency surgery that results deteriorate. Furthermore, it is the elderly who are more likely to develop the complications associated with gallstones such as jaundice, gangrene or perforation of the gall-bladder which require urgent surgical intervention. And it is the elderly who have the highest morbidity and mortality rates. Thus, once acute symptoms and pathology have been allowed to develop in elderly patients, they enter a vortex of surgical and medical complications from which it is increasingly difficult to extricate them alive.

We often have difficulty persuading our physician colleagues that an elective operation to remove a gall-bladder that is full of stones is the wise course in a patient who has few or no symptoms. However, the surgeon's response is that this is the very best and safest time to perform such an operation.

Cholecystectomy in Combination with Other Operations

Simple cholecystectomy for gallstones has also been shown to be safe when combined with other intra-abdominal operations. Incidental appendicectomy was performed during cholecystectomy in a controlled series of 108 cases [16]. There was no difference in postoperative course, including wound infection rate, between those who had a cholecystectomy alone and those whose cholecystectomy was combined with appendicectomy. Similarly, cholecystectomy performed during the course of colonic surgery makes no difference to the outcome [17]. Most of the cases were those of right hemicolectomy, with a few cases of left hemicolectomy and total colectomy. Other abdominal operations described in conjunction with cholecystectomy include hernia repair, hysterectomy, vagotomy and gastrectomy [8].

A word of caution should be added regarding pregnant women; these patients do not respond well to biliary surgery, particularly urgent surgery for acute biliary disease, and particularly in the first 3 months of pregnancy. Loss of the fetus is a common result. If at all possible, these women should be allowed to settle down conservatively, and operation be delayed until after pregnancy [18].

Endoscopic Papillotomy

Therapeutic intervention in the case of gallstones does not necessarily mean surgery. A number of other possible modalities are to be discussed in this symposium. Endoscopic papillotomy is one technique for removing gallstones from the common bile duct without resorting to surgery. This has become widely used as the primary treatment for choledocholithiasis in the elderly and in medically unfit patients with obstructive biliary disease (jaundice, cholangitis, etc.), but without symptoms attributable to their gall-bladder stones. Common bile duct stones are removed endoscopically, but the gall-bladder is left in situ, and many of these patients do not require any further surgery. However, in a study recently conducted in Australia [19], on an admittedly small series of 18 cases, the patency of the cystic duct was assessed at ERCP. A papillotomy was then performed, and the patients were sent home with intact gall-bladders. There were ten patients with a patent cystic duct and eight with an obstructed cystic duct. Those with a patent cystic duct required no further surgery. Of those discharged from hospital with an obstructed cystic duct 75% eventually required operation; there were four deaths in this group, three of which were directly related to the surgery.

Endoscopic papillotomy is a very useful technique in the management of common bile duct stones in the elderly and unfit, however those with an obstructed cystic duct should perhaps not be discharged with an intact gall-bladder but offered rather an early cholecystectomy.

Conclusion

The results of surgical intervention for gallstone disease in the younger, fitter patient are very good. However, with advancing age the patient is more likely to need emergency surgery or common bile duct surgery and is more likely to develop complications from the disease or the surgery. Thus in most patients it is reasonable to offer active treatment for gallstones at diagnosis regardless of whether they are symptomatic or not. What form this treatment should take, however, is open to discussion, whether it should be surgery or some other modality.

Is therapeutic intervention necessary in gallstone disease? This surgeon's view is: yes – but in what form?

References

1. Lieber MM (1952) The incidence of gallstones and their correlation with other diseases. Ann Surg 135:394–405
2. Torvick A, Hoivik B (1960) Gallstones in an autopsy series. Acta Chir Scand 120:168–174
3. Friedman GD, Kannel WB, Dawber TR (1966) The epidemiology of gall bladder disease. J Chronic Dis 19:273–292
4. Bouchier IAD (1969) Post mortem study of the frequency of gallstones in patients with cirrhosis of the liver. Gut 10:705–710
5. Crump C (1931) The incidence of gallstones and gall bladder disease. Surg Gynecol Obstet 53:447–455
6. Wenckert A, Robertson B (1966) The natural course of gallstone disease. Gastroenterol 50:376–381
7. Crumplin MKH, Jenkinson LR, Kassab JY, Whittaker CM, Al Boutiahi FH (1985) Management of gallstones in a District General Hospital. Br J Surg 72:428–432
8. Ganey JB, Johnson PA, Prillaman PE, McSwain GR (1986) Cholecystectomy: clinical experience with a large series. Am J Surg 151:352–357
9. Johnson AG, Hosking SW (1987) Appraisal of the management of bile duct stones. Br J Surg 74:555–560
10. Irvin TT, Arnstein PM (1988) Management of symptomatic gall stones in the elderly. Br J Surg 75:1163–1165
11. Glenn F, McSherry CK (1975) Calculous biliary tract disease. In: Ravitch MM (ed) Current problems in surgery. Year Book, Chicago, pp 1–38
12. Maroske D, Stroh M, Roher HD (1985) Early operation for acute cholecystitis as a therapeutic principle. (in German) Dtsch Med Wochenschr 110:1108–1114
13. Houghton PWJ, Jenkinson LR, Donaldson LA (1985) Cholecystectomy in the elderly: a prospective study. Br J Surg 72:220–222
14. Harness JK, Strodel WE, Talsma SE (1986) Symptomatic biliary disease in the elderly patient. Am Surg 52:442–445
15. Addison NV, Finan PJ (1988) Urgent and early cholecystectomy for acute gall bladder disease. Br J Surg 75:141–143
16. O'Malley VP, Finch DRA, Powley PH (1986) Wound sepsis after cholecystectomy. Influence of incidental appendicectomy. J Clin Gastroenterol 8:435–437
17. Shennib H, Fried GM, Hampson LG (1986) Does simultaneous cholecystectomy increase the risk of colonic surgery? Am J Surg 151:266–268
18. Hiatt JR, Hiatt JCG, Williams RA, Klein SR (1986) Biliary disease in pregnancy: strategy for surgical management. Am J Surg 151:263–265
19. Worthley CS, Toouli J (1988) Gall bladder non-filling: an indication for cholecystectomy after endoscopic sphincterotomy. Br J Surg 75:796–798

Surgical Therapy for Acute Gallstone Complications

W. Oettinger, K. Orth, and B. Leibl

Department of General Surgery, University of Ulm, Steinhoevelstraße 9, D-7900 Ulm, FRG

Gallstone complications are one of the last few unquestioned domains of surgical interventions since elective surgery faces the challenge of alternative therapeutical approaches by means of litholysis and/or lithotripsy.

Patients

Between May 1982 and December 1988 we operated on a total of 1245 patients for gallstone disease. Of these patients, 237 (19%) presented with gallstone complications that needed urgent or even emergency surgery. In addition, 48 patients underwent necrosectomy of the pancreas for necrotizing biliary pancreatitis. Gallstone complications are listed in Fig. 1; this list is headed in terms of frequency by acute cholecystitis, followed by necrotizing pancreatitis, biliary edematous pancreatitis, and intestinal gallstone obstruction. Since the latter disease occurs particularly in elderly patients, pancreatitis assumed a substantial role in this series, while residual stones either after a common bile duct exploration or endoscopy played a minor role.

Surgical Procedures

The surgical procedures performed in our patients (Table 1) included cholecystectomy, simple drainage, and pancreatic necrosectomy. A total of 187 patients with cholecystitis required local or even general lavage because of diffuse peritonitis; of these, three patients died, presenting the only mortality after surgery of gallstone complications in this series. In 26 patients common bile duct exploration and T-tube drainage was indicated. A comparatively rare event favoring the endoscopic approach was transduodenal papillo-

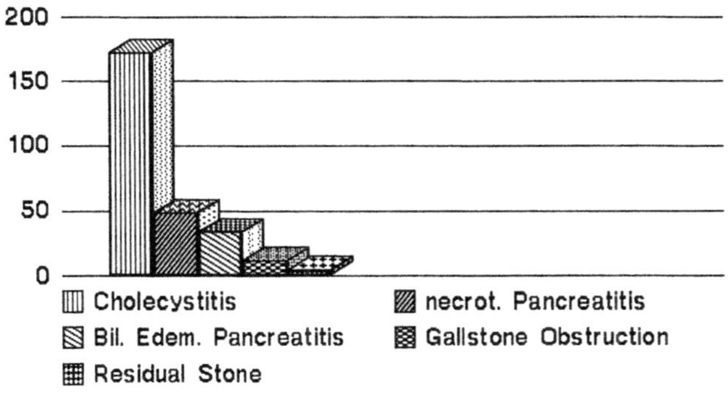

Fig. 1. Frequency of gallstone complications in 1293 patients undergoing surgery for gallstone disease

Table 1. Surgical procedures for complicated gallstones

	n	Deaths
CCE and simple drainage	95	0
CCE and local lavage	77	0
CCE and general lavage	15	3
Choledochotomy and T-type	26	0
Transduodenal papillotomy	5	0
Choledochoduodenostomy	8	0
Enterotomy alone	2	0
Enterotomy + simultaneous biliary tract repair	9	0
Pancreatic necrosectomy	48	0

CCE, Cholecystectomy

Table 2. Complications leading to reoperations

	n	%
Residual stones in CBD	5	0.4
Wound infection	2	0.16
Peritonitis	2	0.16
Bleeding	2	0.16
Adhesions	1	0.08
Bile fistula	1	0.08
Necrosis of CBD	1	0.08

CBD, Common bile duct

tomy. Also rare was choledochoduodenostomy, performed in eight elderly patients with impacted stones. Our experience is generally good with simultaneous biliary tract repair in patients with intestinal gallstone obstruction (see Table 1).

Complications

The therapeutic effect of dealing with gallstone complications should be measured against the complications generated by performing surgery itself. Table 2 presents the types of surgical complications which led to reoperations; these included residual or recurrent stones in the common bile duct, wound infection, peritonitis, bleeding, adhesions, bile fistulas, and necroses of the common bile duct. We found these complications in a lower frequency than 1 or 0.1%. The mortality rate in patients undergoing reoperation was 0%. The rate of overall hospital mortality among the total 1293 patients was 0.5% and was accounted for by two patients undergoing elective cholecystectomy, two with preoperatively known carcinomas, and three with severe cholecystitis and subsequent sepsis.

Unexpected Carcinoma

Among patients being operated for gallstone disease 20 presented with unexpected carcinoma of the biliary tract – 15 patients in the gallbladder and 5 in the common bile duct. This represents an incidence of 1.6% in the total series.

Conclusion

As can be seen in these data and in the relevant literature [1, 2], the incidence of complicated gallstones requiring urgent surgery varies among various institutions between 8% and 46%. In almost unanimous experience, the leading indication is acute cholecystitis, followed by biliary pancreatitis, residual stones in the common bile duct, and intestinal gallstone obstruction. While mortality rates after elective surgery in patients under 70 years of age range from 0% to 0.9% [3, 4], the above-mentioned complications and age over 70 years [5] can increase the mortality rate to 53%, e.g., in cases of biliary pancreatitis [6]. Mortality after elective surgery in our series was 0.56% and that after urgent surgery 1.26%. Average age of the patients accounting for the mortality was 76.85 years. The incidence of biliary tract carcinoma was 1.6%, involving 20 patients aged 25–84 years.

These data confirm that even emergency surgery for gallstone complications is a safe and effective procedure yielding little morbidity and no mortality in patients younger than 70 years. Moreover, up to now surgery remains the only tool to detect and remove preoperatively unknown carcinomas of the biliary tract. Hidden carcinoma might thus not be a complication of gallstones, but it can evolve to a complication of modern nonsurgical gallstone therapy, with well only 1.6% in the overall statistics, however, with 100% for the patient involved.

References

1. Haertisch A, Hartman G (1988) Ergebnisse bei der Frühoperation der akuten Galle. Zentralbl Chir 113(5):952–958
2. Crumplin MKH, Jenkinson LR, Kassab JY, Whitaker CM, Al-Boutiahi FH (1985) Management of gallstones in a district general hospital. Br J Surg 72:428–432
3. DenBesten L, Berci G (1986) The current status of biliary tract surgery: an international study of 1072 consecutive patients. World J Surg 10:116–122
4. Roukema JA, Carol EJ, Liem F, Jakimowicz JJ (1986) A retrospective study of surgical common bile duct exploration: ten years experience. Neth J Surg 38(1):11–14
5. Huber DF, Martin EW, Cooperman M (1983) Cholecystectomy in elderly patients. Am J Surg 146(6):719–722
6. Cave-Bigley DJ, Aukland P, Kane JF, Hardy EG (1984) Transduodenal exploration of the common bile duct in a district general hospital. Ann R Coll Surg Engl 66(3):187–189

Therapeutic Interventions in Patients with Gallbladder Stones: The Internist's View

G. Paumgartner

Department of Medicine II, University of Munich, Klinikum Großhadern, Marchioninistraße 15, D-8000 Munich 70, FRG

The past two decades have witnessed not only the advance of a number of nonsurgical treatments of gallstone disease but also a considerable increase in our knowledge about the natural history of gallstone disease. As a result, we must now ask the following questions: (a) for which patients with gallbladder stones are therapeutic interventions necessary, and (b) which therapeutic modalities can be recommended?

Indications for Therapeutic Interventions

Most of my conclusions are based on a Working Team Report on the nonsurgical therapeutic approach to biliary stones which was presented at the International Congress of Gastroenterology in Rome in 1988 [1].

Prior to a decision as to the appropriate therapeutic approach, the following stages of gallstone disease must be defined. We must distinguish between asymptomatic gallbladder stones, i.e., those that do not cause specific biliary symptoms [2], and symptomatic gallbladder stones. For the diagnosis of symptomatic gallbladder stones, specific biliary symptoms are required. These are characterized by one or more episodes of acute biliary pain, commonly called biliary colic, which is the most frequent and specific symptom of gallstones. This is defined arbitarily as a steady pain lasting more than 15 min but less than 5 h [1]. This pain is usually located in the epigastrium and/or upper right quadrant and often radiates to the back. Episodes of pain occur irregularly, separated by symptom-free intervals of weeks or even years. The pain is often accompanied by nausea. Pain lasting more than 5 h raises the suspicion that other processes, such as acute inflammation of the gallbladder, may be involved.

To decide in which stage of gallstone disease a therapeutic intervention is indicated, we must know the natural history of asymptomatic and symptomatic gallstone disease.

Table 1 summarizes four follow-up studies [3–6] of patients with asymptomatic gallbladder stones. These have been selected because the follow-up period was specified, and because biliary pain, complications, and deaths due to gallstone disease during the follow-up period were reported. A total of 279 patients were studied for up to 24 years; of these, 52 (19%) developed biliary pain or complications. Only three patients died from gallstone disease. The largest and most important of these studies are those of Comfort et al. [4] and of Gracie and Ransohoff [6], who followed 112 patients for a period of 10–20 years and 123 patients for 11–24 years, respectively. The results of these two studies are in good agreement with one another. They found that 13%–19% of the patients with symptomatic gallstones developed biliary pain or complications within a follow-up period of about 20 years. Gracie and Ransohoff [6] also analyzed their data by life-table analysis. The cumulative probability to develop biliary pain or complications was 10% after 5 years, 15% after 10 years, and 18% after 15 years; it did not increase thereafter. Thus, the yearly risk to develop biliary pain decreased with the

Table 1. Natural history of asymptomatic gallstone disease

Reference	Number of patients	Follow-up period (years)	Biliary pain or complications	Deaths from gallstone disease
Truesdell 1944 [3]	30	1–20	11	0
Comfort et al. 1948 [4]	112	10–20	21	3
Ralston and Smith 1965 [5]	14	15–30	4	0
Gracie and Ransohoff 1982 [6]	123	11–24	16	0
Total	279		52 (19%)	3

passage of time. These studies indicate that the natural history of asymptomatic gallstones is generally benign. About 20% of patients with asymptomatic gallstones develop biliary pain or complications within 20 years.

The issue of natural history is only one of several that must be considered in making the decision about therapy. Another important consideration is the mortality rate with prophylactic cholecystectomy. In addition, we must ask about the risks with respect to morbidity, the costs, and the inconvenience of therapy. Ransohoff et al. [7] used decision analysis to determine the outcome of asymptomatic gallstone disease in hypothetical cohorts of 30-year-old and 50-year-old persons using the data on the natural history of asymptomatic gallstone disease and data on age-specific operative mortality rates. It was assumed that an operation is performed soon after the occurrence of the initial episode of biliary pain or complications. This analysis revealed that for a cohort of 100000 30-year-old men the number of operative deaths after prophylactic cholecystectomy would be 107. With expectant management, 292 deaths must be expected, but these deaths occur at a much higher age. For a cohort of 100000 50-year-old men the number of operative deaths after prophylactic cholecystectomy would be 540. There would only be 383 deaths with expectant management, again occurring in later years as the subjects grow older, develop pain or complications, and have a cholecystectomy.

Another way to compare prophylactic cholecystectomy with expectant management is to look at life expectancy. Direct evidence from follow-up studies is not available. Therefore, such comparisons must again be made by decision analysis. Provided that an operation is performed soon after the initial biliary problem occurs, the life expectancy of a patient with asymptomatic gallstone disease managed expectantly is only about 1 week less than that of a person in the general population [7, 8]. For a 30-year-old man with asymptomatic gallstones who chooses prophylactic cholecystectomy instead of expectant management, life expectancy is decreased on average by about 4 days. With a perfect prophylactic therapy, with no morbidity and no mortality, there would be only a small gain in life expectancy, namely about 6 days of life. One can conclude from these data that asymptomatic cholelithiasis should be managed expectantly.

The situation is quite different if the patient has had a biliary colic. At least four studies [5, 9–11] on the natural history of symptomatic gallstone disease show that the percentage of patients who develop biliary pain or complications is high (Table 2). A total of 378 patients were followed in these studies for up to 30 years; 222 patients (59%) developed biliary pain or complications. If we look at complications only, the percentage is also high, namely 28%. These data indicate that symptomatic gallstones have a less benign natural history. The majority of patients who have had symptoms will in the following years develop symptoms again and will have a risk of acute cholecystitis of about 3% per year.

Table 2. Natural history of symptomatic gallstone disease

Reference	Number of patients	Follow-up period (years)	Biliary pain or complications	Complications only
Ehnmark 1939 [9]	6	4–15	28	20
Lund 1960 [10]	201	5–20	117	54
Ralston and Smith 1965 [5]	71	15–30	48	ND
Gomand et al. 1966 [11]	40	8–17	29	11
Total	378		222 (59%)	85 (28%)[a]

[a] Data of Ralston and Smith not included

These results have been substantiated more recently by the Natural Cooperative Gallstone Study in the United States [12]. This study distinguished two groups of patients, one of 112 patients who reported biliary pain in the year before study entry and one of 193 patients who did not. Within a follow-up period of 24 months, 69% of the patients with prior biliary pain but only 31% of patients without prior biliary pain developed specific biliary symptoms. These data justify therapeutic intervention in the patient with symptomatic gallbladder stones.

Choice of Therapeutic Modality

Having answered the first question, we must now answer the second question: which therapeutic modalities can be recommended for the patient with symptomatic gallbladder stones?

Cholecystectomy was first performed by Carl Langenbuch about 100 years ago [13], and this must still be regarded as the gold standard against which all other therapeutic modalities must compete.

During the past two decades, several nonsurgical therapies for gallbladder stones have been developed, such as dissolution of radiolucent gallbladder stones by bile acids [14] or by solvents [15]. Since dissolution of gallbladder stones by oral bile acid treatment has been limited by stone size and by the time required for complete dissolution [16–19], and since direct solvent dissolution by methyl *tert*-butyl ether [20] is an invasive procedure, extracorporeal shock-wave lithotripsy has been introduced for the treatment of gallstones [21, 22]. These various therapeutic modalities are discussed in other chapters of this volume.

For the decision as to whether a nonsurgical approach may be considered for a patient with symptomatic gallbladder stones, we must ask whether the patient has uncomplicated symptomatic gallbladder stones. Patients with uncomplicated gallstone disease have episodes of biliary colic which last only less than 5 h. Patients with complicated symptomatic gallstone disease are characterized by prolonged biliary pain, signs or symptoms of acute cholecystitis, biliary obstruction, acute cholangitis, or acute biliary pancreatitis. Nonsurgical treatments of gallbladder stones appear justified only in patients with uncomplicated symptomatic gallbladder stones [1].

On the basis of these considerations, what do we tell a patient with gallbladder stones who opts for a nonsurgical treatment of his gallstones, and who prefers the least invasive modality that can be justified from a medical point of view? My answer is summarized in a grossly simplified algorithim in Fig. 1 [23].

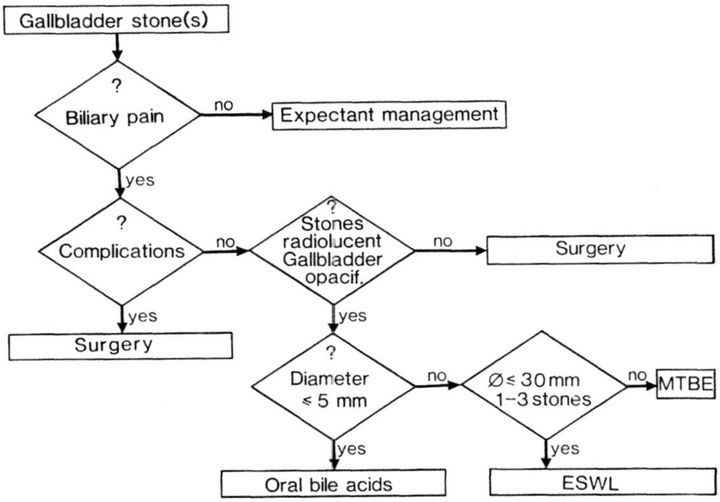

Fig. 1. Algorithm for the therapy of gallbladder stones, if the least invasive method is to be chosen. Methyl *tert*-butyl ether (*MTBE*) is still an investigational drug. *ESWL*, Extracorporeal shock wave lithotripsy. (From Paumgartner [23])

References

1. Paumgartner G, Carr-Locke DL, Roda E, Thistle JL (1988) Biliary stones: non-surgical therapeutic approach. Gastroenterol Int 1:17–24
2. Schoenfield LJ, Carulli N, Dowling RH, Ransohoff D, Sama C, Wolpers C (1989) Asymptomatic gallstones: definition and treatment. Gastroenterol Int 2:25–29
3. Truesdell ED (1944) The frequency and future of gallstones believed to be quiescent or symptomless. Ann Surg 119:232
4. Comfort MW, Gray HK, Wilson JM (1948) The silent gallstone: a ten to twenty year follow-up study of 112 cases. Ann Surg 128:931–937
5. Ralston DE, Smith LA (1965) The natural history of cholelithiasis: a 15 to 30-year follow-up study of 112 cases. Minn Med 48:327–332
6. Gracie WA, Ransohoff DF (1982) The natural history of silent gallstones: the innocent gallstone is not a myth. N Engl J Med 307:798–800
7. Ransohoff DF, Gracie WA, Wolfenson LB, Neuhauser D (1983) Prophylactic cholecystectomy or expectant management for persons with silent gallstones: a decision analysis to assess survival. Ann Intern Med 99:199–204
8. Gracie WA, Ransohoff DF (1985) Natural history and expectant management of gallstone disease. In: Cohen S, Soloway R (eds) Gallstones. Churchill Livingstone, New York, pp 27–43
9. Ehnmark E (1939) The gallstone disease: a clinical-statistical study. Acta Chir Scand [Suppl] 57:1–238
10. Lund J (1960) Surgical indications in cholelithiasis: prophylactic cholecystectomy elucidated on the basis of long-term follow up on 526 nonoperated cases. Ann Surg 151:153–162
11. Gomand L, Vandenbroucke J, DeGroote J (1966) De naturlijke evolutie van colelithiase. Tijdschr Gastroenterol 9:594
12. Thistle JL, Cleary PA, Lachin JM, et al. (1984) The natural history of cholelithiasis: the national cooperative gallstone disease. Ann Intern Med 101:171–175
13. Langenbuch C (1882) Ein Fall von Exstirpation der Gallenblase wegen chronischer Cholelithiasis. Berl Klin Wochenschr 18:725–727
14. Danzinger RG, Hofmann AF, Schoenfield LS, Thistle JL (1972) Dissolution of cholesterol gallstones by chenodeoxycholic acid. N Engl J Med 286:1–8

15. Allen MJ, Borody TJ, Bugliosi TF, May GR, LaRusso NF, Thistle JL (1985) Rapid dissolution of gallstones by methyl *tert*-butyl ether: preliminary observations. N Engl J Med 312:217–220
16. Hofmann AF, Paumgartner G (1985) Chenodeoxycholic acid therapy of gallstones. Progress report 1975. Schattauer, Stuttgart
17. Erlinger S, Le Go A, Husson JM, Fevery J (1984) Franco-Belgian cooperative study of ursodeoxycholic acid in the medical dissolution of gallstones: a double-blind, randomized, dose-response study, and comparison with chenodeoxycholic acid. Hepatology 4:308–314
18. Bachrach WH, Hofmann AF (1982) Ursodeoxycholic acid in the treatment of cholesterol cholelithiasis. Dig Dis Sci 27:833–856, 737–761
19. Podda M, Zuin M, Battezzati PM, Ghezzi C, de Fazio C, Dioguardi ML (1989) Efficacy and safety of a combination of chenodeoxycholic acid and ursodeoxycholic acid for gallstone dissolution: a comparison with ursodeoxycholic acid alone. Gastroenterology 96:222–229
20. Thistle JL, May GR, Bender CE, et al. (1989) Dissolution of cholesterol gallbladder stones by methyl tert-butyl ether administered by percutaneous transhepatic catheter. N Engl J Med 320:633–639
21. Sauerbruch T, Delius M, Paumgartner G, et al. (1986) Fragmentation of gallstones by extracorporeal shock waves. N Engl J Med 314:818–822
22. Sackmann M, Delius M, Sauerbruch T, et al. (1988) Shock-wave lithotripsy of gallbladder stones: the first 175 patients. N Engl J Med 318:393–397
23. Paumgartner G (1989) Shock-wave lithotripsy of gallstones. AJR 153:235–242

Acute Biliary Pancreatitis

P. Malfertheiner

Department of Internal Medicine II, University of Ulm, Robert-Koch-Str. 8, D-7900 Ulm, FRG

Introduction

Gallstones are a well established pathogenetic factor in acute pancreatitis and recognized as one of its two major causes. While alcohol has a higher prevalence among cases with acute pancreatitis reported in series from North America [1] and Germany [2], gallstones are the commonest etiological factor of acute pancreatitis in the United Kingdom, where they account for more than 50% of cases [3]. No definite explanation is available for these geographic discrepancies.

The high incidence of gallstones, with 10% in the general population, compared with the low incidence of gallstone-associated acute pancreatitis, opens two questions:

1. What is the relative risk of pancreatitis in patients with gallstones?
2. What factors predispose patients with gallstones to develop acute pancreatitis?

A recent attempt to answer the first question by Moreau et al. [4] led to the conclusion that gallstone patients' relative risk of developing acute pancreatitis is considerably increased, being 12 to 35 times higher than in the general population.

The definition of factors that predispose patients with gallstones to acute pancreatitis and other factors that prevent from it is far from complete. The current hypotheses on pathophysiology and the available information on predisposing factors is summarized in the following sections.

Pathogenesis of Gallstone-Induced Pancreatitis

Since Opie's original observation in 1901 of a gallstone impacted at the ampulla of Vater in a patient who had died from severe acute pancreatitis [5], obstruction of the common channel has been widely accepted as the initial pathogenic event in biliary pancreatitis. Further support for and progress concerning this theory was provided by several groups of clinical researchers, who have stressed that just a transient migration of one or more stones would be sufficient for initiating acute pancreatitis [6–8]. These conclusions were based on the recovery of gallstones in the feces, following an episode of acute pancreatitis, which were similar in their chemical composition to the ones removed at biliary surgery from the gallbladder [6–8].

It is not clear if, in addition to the transient or persisting obstruction caused by gallstones, obstruction of the outflow from the pancreatic ductal system alone suffices to induce the acute event, or if both pancreatic and biliary outflow need to be obstructed together. It is also uncertain if biliary reflux into the pancreatic duct system has to occur, or if increased pressure in the pancreatic duct system alone is sufficient. Recent experimental studies showed that bile salts alter the pancreatic ductal barrier, and this could favor the diffusion of activated pancreatic enzymes into the parenchyma [9].

Important objections, as proposed by Steer in a recent review article [10], call into question the pathogenetic role of biliary reflux:

1. The common channel present in most subjects is so short that obstruction would involve the biliary as well as the pancreatic duct, thus making bile reflux into the pancreatic duct impossible.
2. Bile duct pressure is lower than pancreatic duct pressure, which would favor a reflux in the other direction, from the pancreatic ductal system into the biliary system.

The alternative hypothesis, that hypertension in the pancreatic ductal system may be the essential event in the development of acute pancreatitis, assumes that either (a) ductal hypertension leads to rupture of pancreatic ductules, with extravasation of activated pancreatic juice into the pancreatic parenchyma and subsequent inflammation, or (b) ductal hypertension prevents acinar cell secretion of digestive enzymes and stimulates intracellular events (activation of intracellular enzymes) that result in pancreatitis [11].

On the basis of the proposed data and assumptions, the events of gallstone-associated pancreatitis are summarized in Table 1.

Predisposing Factors

According to the proposed concepts of pathophysiological events in acute biliary pancreatitis, relevant mechanical and anatomic factors have been established that predispose patients with gallstones to develop acute pancreatitis.

Several different investigators have found that the frequency of acute pancreatitis is inversely proportional to the size of gallstones [12–14]; patients with stones less than 3 mm in diameter appear at highest risk. Other features of gallstones which affect the risk for acute pancreatitis are their number and irregularity of shape. Besides the observation, using cholangiography, that pancreatic duct reflux occurs more frequently in patients who had a previous episode of gallstone pancreatitis [15], some other specific anatomic features were found to be more frequent in these patients [12, 15]: (a) a wider angle of entry between the common bile duct and pancreatic duct, (b) a longer functioning common channel, greater than 5 mm, and (c) a large-caliber cystic duct.

Table 1. Pathogenesis (hypothetic model) of gallstone-associated pancreatitis

Cholecystolithiasis
▼
Gallstone migration in common bile duct
▼
Transient obstruction or impaction of the ampulla Vateri
▼
Pancreatic ductal hypertension with or without bile reflux
▼
Damage to pancreatic ductular barrier
▼
Extravasation of "activated" pancreatic juice into the pancreatic parenchyma
or
Activation of intracellular enzymes (crinophagy)
▼
Acute pancreatitis

Epidemiological surveys showed that women have gallstone pancreatitis more often than men, and that obesity is a common feature in these patients [16]. Patients with gallstone pancreatitis are frequently older than those with alcoholic pancreatitis [17].

Diagnosis and Prognosis of Gallstone Pancreatitis

Acute pancreatitis is diagnosed when a patient has acute abdominal pain together with raised serum concentrations of pancreatic-specific enzymes, among pancreatic amylase, lipase, trypsin, and elastase. There are clinical tools specific enough to help in identifying the etiology as biliary rather than any of the other various possible causes [18].

An accurate clinical history helps in distinguishing patients with alcohol-related acute pancreatitis from those with gallstone pancreatitis. Nevertheless, in a carefully performed prospective study by McMahon and Mayer in 1984, as many as 20% of apparently alcohol-related attacks of pancreatitis could also have been attributed to gallstones [19]. This indicates the necessity for routine investigation of the biliary tract in all patients with acute pancreatitis, irrespective of the suspected etiology, except those with recurrent attacks due to established chronic pancreatitis [18–20].

In search for gallstones an erect abdominal X-ray, often performed at admission, can reveal the presence of stones in up to 15% of patients [17]. The first mandatory investigation to search for gallstones is ultrasound. Ultrasonography is hampered by the fact that initially the gallbladder may not be visualized in over 30% of patients [21], but results are substantially improved if serial examinations are performed [17]. Absence of stones in the gallbladder does not rule out the possibility that one or more stones may have been evacuated and passed the papilla; the only positive proof for gallstones in these cases is their recovery from feces.

Another pitfall of ultrasonography to be borne in mind is that a dilated common bile duct may also be observed in cases where the etiology is other than biliary and is than simply due to swelling of the inflamed pancreas [18].

Among several biochemical parameters, a transient elevation of aspartatate amino transferase in serum (>60 U/l) has proven more helpful than parameters indicating cholestasis (bilirubin, alkaline phosphatase) [22].

The gold standard for detection of gallstones during an attack of acute pancreatitis is endoscopic retrograde cholangiopancreaticography (ERCP). Fear and reluctance to use this technique in acute pancreatitis has been overcome since its safety – when properly performed – has been proven. ERCP makes possible the detection of gallstones in cases where all other techniques have failed; moreover, when stones are impacted in the ampullary region or in the common bile duct, this technique allows instantaneous treatment by endoscopic sphincterotomy. The detection rate of stones in the common bile duct obviously depends on timing, since stones pass through the papilla spontaneously in the majority of cases within 48 h [6].

The prognosis of the clinical outcome in acute biliary pancreatitis is no different from that of other etiologies [23]. As for the other etiologies, the prognosis in biliary pancreatitis depends on whether parenchymal necrosis is present, and it is further aggravated if the necrosis becomes infected [24]. Several staging systems as well as determination of individual biochemical parameters are available for assessing the severity of acute pancreatitis [18, 25].

Therapeutic Management

At present, two different approaches are recommended for causal treatment of acute gallstone-associated pancreatitis: biliary surgery and endoscopic sphincterotomy. These treatments have their specific indications and are competitive in some circumstances and complementary in others.

Biliary Surgery

Cholecystectomy is the standard procedure in treatment of acute biliary pancreatitis when stones are detected in the gallbladder during or following an acute episode. The risk of recurrent episodes of pancreatitis is reduced to a miniumum when cholecystectomy can be performed and all stones removed from the biliary tree [26, 27]. While general agreement has been achieved that cholecystectomy has to be performed during the initial admission of the patient with acute pancreatitis, the exact timing remains controversial. This controversy arises from the observation that common bile duct stones are detected in 63%–78% of patients undergoing surgery during the acute phase, but only in 5%–15% when surgery is delayed [28, 29]. The latter observation indicates that the majority of stones pass spontaneously through the ampulla of Vater soon after the onset of pancreatitis.

An important contribution to the discussion about timing of surgery in gallstone pancreatitis has recently been made by Kelly and Wagner [30]. These authors found that, irrespective of the severity of acute pancreatitis at admission, early operation (within 48 h after hospital admission) is never of any benefit; indeed, they found that patients presenting with more than three Ranson's signs had higher morbidity and mortality with early surgery. Frei et al. came to similar conclusions and did not find any benefit from emergency operations compared to medical management followed by delayed operation during the same hospitalization [31].

From this surgical experience we have learned that gallstones initiate the pathologic event of acute pancreatitis, but appear not to be responsible for progression of the disease, and early removal of a "migrated stone" seems not to ameliorate progression. Conflicts about the timing of surgery may still go on, but the tendency is swinging to delayed surgical intervention during the initial hospitalization [30, 31].

Endoscopic Sphincterotomy

The current concept of endoscopic sphincterotomy (ES) in acute pancreatitis is based on the assumption that rapid disimpaction of the obstructed ampulla would favorably influence the course of the disease. This assumption was supported by the study of Acosta et al. [28], which reported 75% of stones to be present in the ampulla within 48 h after the onset of symptoms, and only 25% at day 4.

In the study of Acosta et al., rapid clinical remission was obtained in patients in whom patency of the ampulla was restored within 48 h, and similar results were obtained in another study [29]. More prolonged ampullary obstruction led to irreversible lesions. Following earlier encouraging results with ES [32, 33], Neoptolemos et al. [34] conducted the first and so far only prospective randomized study to prove the value of ES in acute gallstone pancreatitis. In this study, patients with suspected gallstone-induced pancreatitis were treated either by conventional management or received "urgent" ERCP within 72 h of admission. Additional ES was performed only when stones were detected in the common bile duct. The findings from this study showed that morbidity was lower and hospital stay shorter among patients with severe pancreatitis and stones in the common bile duct who underwent ERCP and additional ES. ERCP and ES were confirmed to be safe procedures during acute pancreatitis.

This study awaits further confirmation from other centers before several criticisms to this approach are rebutted and a general recommendation may be stated for this strategy.

Conclusions

Gallstones are the most or second most important cause of acute pancreatitis depending on regional differences. The pathogenesis is still based on a hypothetical model, for which transient ampullary obstruction, pancreatic ductal hypertension, and possibly bile reflux are the cornerstones. Predisposing factors for the development of acute pancreatitis in patients with gallstones include inherent factors such as female sex, old age, and obesity, and anatomical characteristics of the biliary tree, and size and number of gallstones. Differential diagnosis of gallstone-associated pancreatitis relies on biochemical parameters, ultrasound, and ERCP.

The standard therapeutic management to prevent recurrent attacks is still cholecystectomy, but operation is preferably performed with some delay during the initial admission of the patient. ERCP with ES is a valid alternative in patients with common bile duct stones and in those considered at risk for operation. ES and cholecystectomy may be combined in selected cases. The role of urgent ERCP and ES is still under debate and awaits confirmation of usefulness from further clinical studies.

References

1. Ranson JHC (1982) Etiological and prognostic factors in human acute pancreatitis: a review. Am J Gastroenterol 77:633–638
2. Goebell H, Hotz J (1976) Die Ätiologie der akuten Pankreatitis. In: Forell MM (ed) Handbuch der Inneren Medizin, vol 6: Pankreas. Springer, Berlin Heidelberg New York, pp 615–675
3. Corfield AP, Cooper MJ, Williamson RCN (1985) Acute pancreatitis: a lethal disease of increasing incidence. Gut 26:724–729
4. Moreau JA, Zinsmeister AR, Melton LJ, DiMagno EP (1988) Gallstone pancreatitis and the effect of cholecystectomy: a population-based cohort study. Mayo Clin Proc 63:466–473
5. Opie EL (1901) The etiology of acute hemorrhagic pancreatitis. Bull Johns Hopkins Hosp 12:182–188
6. Acosta JM, Ledesma CL (1974) Gallstone migration as a cause of acute pancreatitis. N Engl J Med 290:484–488
7. Kelly TR (1976) Gallstone pancreatitis: pathophysiology. Surgery 80:488–492
8. Mayer AD, McMahon MJ, Benson EA, Axon ATR (1984) Operations upon the biliary tract in patients with acute pancreatitis: aims, indications and timing. Ann R Coll Surg Eng 66:179–183
9. Reber HA, Farmer RC, Maslin SC (1982) Effects of bile on the permeability of the pancreatic duct to macromolecules. Gastroenterology 82:1156
10. Steer ML (1986) Etiology and pathophysiology of acute pancreatitis. In: Go VLW (ed) The exocrine pancreas: biology, pathobiology, and diseases. Raven, New York, pp 465–474
11. Steer ML, Meldolesi J, Figarella C (1984) Pancreatitis. The role of lysosomes. Dig Dis Sci 29:934–938
12. McMahon MJ, Shetta JR (1980) Physical characteristics of gallstones and the calibre of the cystic duct in patients with acute pancreatitis. Br J Surg 67:6–9
13. Armstrong CP, Tylor TV, Jeacock J, Lucas S (1985) The biliary tract in patients with acute gallstone pancreatitis. Br J Surg 72:551–555
14. Houssin D, Castaing D, Lemoine J, Bismuth H (1983) Microlithiasis of the gallbladder. Surg Gynecol Obstet 157:20–24
15. Armstrong CP, Taylor TV (1986) Pancreatic-duct reflux and acute gallstone pancreatitis. Ann Surg 204:59–64
16. Creutzfeldt W, Lankisch PG (1985) Acute pancreatitis: etiology and pathogenesis. In: Berk JE (ed) Bockus Gastroenterology, vol. 6, 4th edn. Saunders, Philadelphia, pp 3971–3992
17. Imrie CW (1987) Gallstone-associated acute pancreatitis. In: Beger HG, Büchler M (eds) Acute pancreatitis. Springer, Berlin Heidelberg New York, pp 227–232

18. Malfertheiner P, Büchler M (1987) Clinical symptoms and signs and diagnostic requirements in acute pancreatitis. In: Beger HG, Büchler M (eds) Acute pancreatitis. Springer, Berlin Heidelberg New York, pp 103–109
19. McMahon MJ, Mayer AD (1984) Comparison of the clinical features of acute pancreatitis due to gallstones and alcohol. In: Gyr KE, Singer MV, Sarles H (eds) Pancreatitis – concepts and classification. Elsevier, Amsterdam, pp 379–388
20. Lankisch PG (1988) Aetiology of acute pancreatitis. In: Glazer G, Ranson JHC (eds) Acute pancreatitis: experimental and clinical aspects of pathogenesis and management. Baillière Tindall, Eastbourne, pp 167–181
21. Blamey SL, Osborne DH, Gilmour WH, O'Neill J, Carter DC, Imrie CW (1983) The early identification of patients with gallstone-associated pancreatitis using clinical and biochemical factors only. Ann Surg 198:514–518
22. Mayer AD, McMahon MJ (1985) Biochemical identification of patients with gallstones associated acute pancreatitis on the day of admission to hospital. Ann Surg 201:68–75
23. Uhl W, Büchler M, Malfertheiner P, Beger HG (1988) Severity of acute pancreatitis is unrelated to the etiology. Digestion XX Meeting of the European Pancreatic Club 6:120
24. Beger HG, Block S, Bittner R (1987) The significance of bacterial infection in acute pancreatitis. In: Beger HG, Büchler M (eds) Acute pancreatitis. Springer, Berlin Heidelberg New York, pp 79–86
25. Büchler M, Uhl W, Malfertheiner P (1987) Biochemical staging of acute pancreatitis. In: Beger HG, Büchler M (eds) Acute pancreatitis. Springer, Berlin Heidelberg New York, pp 143–153
26. Kelly TR (1980) Gallstone pancreatitis: the timing of surgery. Surgery 38:345–350
27. Kelly TR, Swaney PE (1982) Gallstone pancreatitis: second time around. Surgery 92:571–574
28. Acosta JM, Rossi R, Galli DM (1978) Early surgery for acute gallstone pancreatitis: evaluation of a systemic approach. Surgery 83:367–371
29. Stone HH, Fabian TC, Dunlop EW (1981) Gallstone pancreatitis, biliary tract pathology in relation to time of operation. Ann Surg 194:305–312
30. Kelly TR, Wagner DS (1988) Gallstone pancreatitis: a prospective randomized trial of the timing of surgery. Surgery 104:600–605
31. Frei GJ, Frei VT, Thirlby RC, McClelland RN (1986) Biliary pancreatitis: clinical presentation and surgical management. Am J Surg 151:170–175
32. Van Spuy DS (1981) Endoscopic sphincterotomy in the managment of gallstone pancreatitis. Endoscopy 13:25–26
33. Safrany L (1982) Controversies in acute pancreatitis. Springer, Berlin Heidelberg New York, pp 214–218
34. Neoptolemos JP, Carr-Locke DL, London NJ, Bailey IA, James D, Fossard DP (1988) Controlled trial of urgent endoscopic retrograde cholangiopancreatography and endoscopic sphincterotomy versus conservative treatment for acute pancreatitis due to gallstones. Lancet ii:979–983

Systemic Litholysis with Bile Acids

Principles of Gallstone Dissolution with Chenodeoxycholic Acid, Ursodeoxycholic Acid, and the Combination of both Bile Acids

A. Stiehl

Medizinische Universitätsklinik, Klinikum der Universität Heidelberg, Bergheimerstr. 58, D-6900 Heidelberg, FRG

Composition of Gallstones

Gallstones in man consist of cholesterol or pigment or a combintion of both and contain variable amounts of calcium salts. Approximately 80% of the gallstones reported in European patients are cholesterol stones (Table 1). Stones in the common bile duct removed during cholecystectomy mainly contain cholesterol [25], however those removed from the bile ducts years after cholecystectomy generally consist of pigment [23]. Only cholesterol gallstones may be dissolved with bile acids by oral treatment.

Table 1. Composition of gallstones in the gallbladder and the common duct ($n=45$). (From Sieg et al. [25])

Stone type	Gall-bladder	Common duct
Cholesterol	33	36
Mixed	8	5
Brown pigment	3	3
Black pigment	1	1

Patient Selection

The ideal patient for gallstone dissolution has only minor symptoms and no complications of gallbladder disease. The asymptomatic patient, in general, should not be treated since follow-up studies have shown that the probability of developing biliary problems is only 20%–25% after more than 20 years [9]. Severe and frequent biliary colic is a relative contraindication to bile acid therapy since this takes too long to dissolve the stones; such patients preferably should have surgical treatment. Several studies have shown that dyspepsia and colic decrease during bile acid therapy, and this is probably the reason that this therapy is well accepted by patients. With respect to stone composition the ideal patient for bile acid therapy has small radiolucent gallstones floating in the gallbladder. Calcified and pigment stones do not dissolve during bile acid treatment. Another important prerequisite for litholysis is that the gallbladder opacifies on oral cholecystography. Failure of the contrast medium to enter the gallbladder indicates that bile which is unsaturated during bile acid therapy may not enter the gallbladder, and that therefore the stones will not be dissolved.

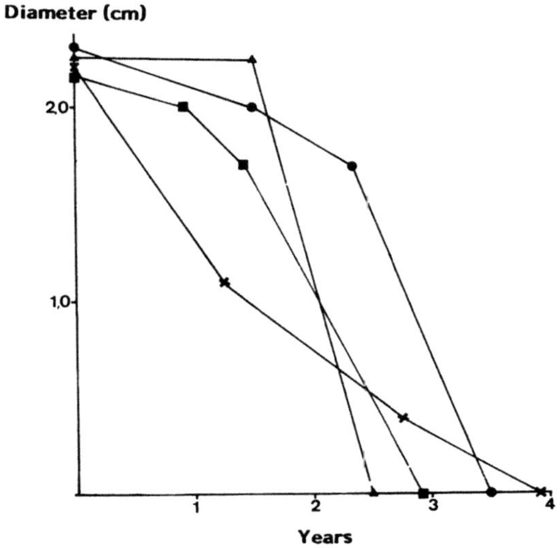

Fig. 1. Dissolution of large gallstone by oral treatment with bile acids. The largest diameter measured on oral cholecystograms is indicated. Dissolution of such large stones is rather slow, and therefore prior fragmentation should be performed

Radiolucency by standard X ray indicates a 80%–85% probability that the stones are composed predominantly of cholesterol. More accurate predictions of the calcification of stones can be made by computed tomography [10]. Stones of less than 100 HU are with high probability not calcified. Some 10%–20% of gallstones are pigment stones, which – as calcified stones – cannot be dissolved by bile acid treatment. Smaller stones dissolve faster than larger stones [6, 17]. The dissolution of stones with a diameter of over 2 cm may require 3–5 years (Fig. 1), however the dissolution of such stones may nowadays be accelerated by the use of extracorporeal shock waves (ESWL) [22]. Stones with a diameter of over 10 mm should preferably be treated by shock waves before bile acid therapy, in contrast to stones with a diameter of less than 10 mm diameter which may be dissolved with bile acids without prior shock wave therapy.

Differences Between Chenodeoxycholic Acid and Ursodeoxycholic Acid

The efficacy of chenodeoxycholic acid (CDCA) increases with the dose, up to that of 20 mg/kg [8, 29]. Side effects of CDCA administration include diarrhea, elevation of serum transaminases, and alterations in liver histology [7, 8, 19, 24, 26]. Such side effects, occurring in one-third of all patients, are observed mainly at higher bile acid doses [24]. Therefore a dose of 15 mg/kg CDCA is in general recommended when this bile acid is used for gallstone dissolution.

Ursodeoxycholic acid (UDCA) treatment of gallstone patients is not accompanied by side effects [2, 6, 17, 26], and therapy with this bile acid has therefore largely replaced that with CDCA. The efficacy of UDCA increases only up to a dose of 8–10 mg/kg [6, 28]; higher doses do not produce greater effects (Fig. 2). UDCA has the disadvantage of leading to gallstone calcification in 10%–20% of patients, which makes the stones undissolvable [2, 6, 17]. During CDCA treatment gallstone calcification is also observed, but at a lower frequency [24].

The mechanism of action differs considerably between CDCA and UDCA [2, 16, 31]. UDCA acts mainly by decreasing intestinal absorption of cholesterol whereas CDCA decreases hepatic synthesis of cholesterol (Table 2) [1, 12, 14, 18, 31]. Simultaneously decreasing intestinal absorption and reducing hepatic synthesis of cholesterol may repre-

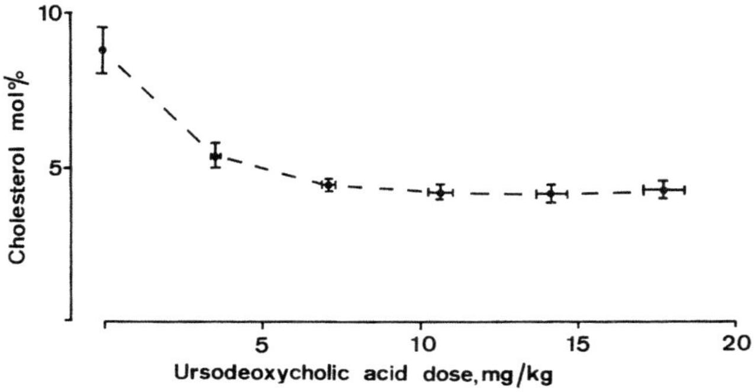

Fig. 2. Biliary cholesterol content during treatment of patients with gallstones with increasing doses of ursodeoxycholic acid. (From Stiel et al. [28])

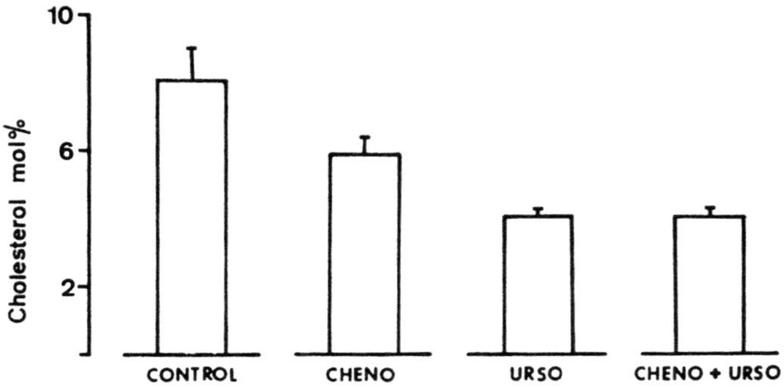

Fig. 3. Effect on the cholesterol content of bile in gallstone patients of treatment with 11.9–15.6 mg/kg ursodeoxycholic acid (*URSO*) chenodeoxycholic acid (*CHENO*), or a combination of both at half dose. (From Stiel et al. [27])

Table. 2. Effect of ursodeoxycholic acid (UDCA) and chenodeoxycholic acid (CDCA) on cholesterol absorption and synthesis

	UDCA	CDCA
Intestinal absorption of cholesterol	Decrease	No effect
Hepatic synthesis of cholesterol	No effect	Decrease

sent a means to accelerate gallstone dissolution (Fig. 3) [27]. Combined treatment with CDCA and UDCA was tested in a prospective controlled cross-over study which showed that the combination of 8–10 mg CDCA and 8–10 mg UDCA decreases biliary cholesterol very markedly and is not followed by side effects [27]. In two prospective controlled clinical studies this combination induced gallstone calcification less often than UDCA alone and also had the advantage of faster gallstone dissolution [4, 5, 17]. At present the combination of UDCA and CDCA seems to be the treatment of choice when bile acid therapy is indicated [4, 5, 17, 20].

How Long Should Bile Acid Treatment Be Continued?

Dissolution efficacy depends very much on adequate selection of patients. Probably 10% of all gallstone patients may be treated by bile acids without additional measures. Following complete dissolution of stones therapy should be continued for 3–6 months in order to achieve dissolution of very small stone residues which cannot be identified by ultrasound or X ray. Such stone residues may lead to rapid stone recurrence.

Bile acid therapy should be discontinued if no reduction in stone diameter can be demonstrated after 6–12 months. With very small stones a reduction in stone size should be seen within 6 months whereas in larger stones a reduction in stone size often cannot be detected before 1–2 years of treatment.

Recurrence

The metabolic defect leading to stone formation continues to exist in most patients after dissolution of gallstones. Therefore it is not surprising that 5 years after complete dissolution approximately 50% of patients have stone recurrence [15, 21]. This figure can be expected to be the same after ESWL and also after direct lysis by methyl *tert*-butyl ether (MTBE). The redissolution rate of gallstones which recur is 80% per year. The measures which probably may help to reduce gallstone recurrence include avoidance of cholesterol-rich diets and of overweight. The benefit of nonsteroidal antiphlogistic drugs (e.g., aspirin), which inhibit cyclo-oxygenase and prostaglandin synthesis, in reducing stone recurrence is not completely clear at present [3, 11]. A benefit with respect to recurrence was observed in one study [11], whereas in patients on low-calory diet gallstone formation was not prevented by these substances [3].

Indication for Bile Acid Therapy

Patients with complications of their gallbladder disease should undergo surgical treatment. Litholysis by bile acids is the method of choice in patients with relatively small stones and relatively minor symptoms. Larger stones should first be fragmented and subsequently dissolved by bile acids. Direct litholysis by a solvent (e.g., MTBE) via a transhepatic catheter placed into the gallbladder is an alternative mode of treatment [13, 30]. After direct lysis of gallstones by MTBE bile acid treatment may be necessary to clear the gallbladder completely of the stone debris. Probably more important than all the methods to dissolve and fragment stones are measures which help to prevent gallstone formation and recurrence.

References

1. Angelin B, Ewerth S, Einarsson K (1983) Ursodeoxycholic acid treatment in cholesterol gallstone disease: effects on hepatic 3-hydroxy-3-methylglutaryl coenzyme A reductase activity, biliary lipid composition, and plasma lipid levels. J Lipid Res 24:461–468
2. Bachrach WH, Hofmann AF (1982) Ursodeoxycholic acid in the treatment of cholesterol cholelithiasis. A review. Dig Dis Sci 27:737–856
3. Broomfield PH, Chopra R, Sheinbaum R, Bonorris GG, Silverman A, Schoenfield LJ (1988) Effects of ursodeoxycholic acid and aspirin on the formation of lithogenic bile and gallstones during loss of weight. N Engl J Med 319:1567–1572

4. Czygan P, Stiehl A, Männer C, Seitz H, Raedsch R, Kommerell B (1982) Significant improvement in cholesterol gallstone dissolution by a chenodeoxycholic acid and ursodeoxycholic acid combination therapy. Abstract No 136, EASL, Göteborg
5. Czygan P, Stiehl A, Männer C, Raedsch R, Seitz H, Kommerell B (1982) Gallensteinauflösung mit Ursodesoxycholsäure versus einer Kombination von Urso-Cheno in reduzierter Dosis. Z Gastroenterol 20:542 (abstr)
6. Erlinger S, Go AL, Husson JM, Fevery J (1984) Franco-Belgian cooperative study of ursodeoxycholic acid in the medical dissolution of gallstones: double blind, randomized, dose-response study, and comparison with chenodeoxycholic acid. Hepatology 4:308–314
7. Fisher RL, Anderson DW, Boyer JL, Ishak K, Klatskin G, Lachin JM, Phillips MJ (1982) A prospective morphologic evaluation of hepatic toxicity of chenodeoxycholic acid in patients with cholelithiasis: the National Cooperative Gallstone Study. Hepatology 2:187–201
8. Gerolami A, Sarles H, Brette RM, Paraf A, Rautureau J, Debray C, Bermann C, Etienne JP, Chaput JC, Petite JP (1977) Controlled trial of chenodeoxycholic acid therapy for radiolucent gallstones. Digestion 16:299–307
9. Gracie WA, Ransohoff DF (1982) The natural history of silent gallstones. The innocent stone is not a myth. N Engl J Med 307:798–800
10. Hickman MS, Schwesinger WH, Bova JD, Kurtin WE (1986) Computed tomographic analysis of gallstones. Arch Surg 121:289–291
11. Hood K, Gleeson D, Ruppin DC, Dowling RH (1988) Prevention of gallstone recurrence by non-steroidal anti-inflammatory drugs. Lancet II:1223–1225
12. Leiss O, von Bergmann K, Streicher U, Strotkoeter H (1984) Effect of three different dihydroxy bile acids on intestinal cholesterol absorption in normal volunteers. Gastroenterology 87:144–149
13. Leuschner U, Hellstern A (1988) Perkutan-transhepatische Litholyse (PTL) mit Methyl-tert-Butyl-Äther (MTBE). Internist 29:788–791
14. Nilsell K, Angelin B, Leijd B, Einarsson K (1983) Comparative effects of ursodeoxycholic acid and chenodeoxycholic acid on bile acid kinetics and biliary lipid secretion in humans. Gastroenterology 85:1248–1256
15. O'Donnell LDJ, Heaton KW (1988) Recurrence and re-recurrence of gallstones after medical dissolution: a longterm follow up. Gut 29:655–658
16. Park Y-H, Igimi H, Carey M (1984) Dissolution of human cholesterol gallstones in simulated chenodeoxycholate-rich and ursodeoxycholate-rich biles. Gastroenterology 87:150–158
17. Podda M, Zuin M, Battezzati PM, Ghezzi C, de Fazio C, Dioguardi ML (1989) Efficacy and safety of a combination of chenodeoxycholic acid and ursodeoxycholic acid for gallstone dissolution: a comparison with ursodeoxycholic acid alone. Gastroenterology 96:222–229
18. Ponz de Leon M, Carulli N, Loria P, Jori R, Zivoni F (1980) Cholesterol absorption during bile acid feeding. Effect of ursodeoxycholic acid administration. Gastroenterology 78:214–219
19. Roda E, Bazzoli F, Morselli L et al. (1982) Ursodeoxycholic acid versus chenodeoxycholic acid as cholesterol gallstone dissolving agents: a comparative randomized study. Hepatology 2:804–810
20. Roehrkasse R, Fromm H, Malavolti M, Tunuguntla K, Ceryak S (1986) Gallstone dissolution treatment with a combination of chenodeoxycholic and ursodeoxycholic acids. Dig Dis Sci 31:1032–1040
21. Ruppin DC, Dowling RH (1982) Is recurrence inevitable after gallstone dissolutin by bile acid treatment? Lancet I:181–185
22. Sackmann M, Delius M, Sauerbruch T, Holl J, Weber W, Ippisch E, Hagelauer U, Wess O, Hepp W, Brendel W, Paumgartner G (1988) Shock-wave lithotrypsy of gallbladder stones. N Engl J Med 318:393–397
23. Sauerbruch T, Stellaard F, Sohendra N, Paumgartner G (1983) Cholesteringehalt von Gallengangssteinen. Dtsch Med Wochenschr 108:1099–1102
24. Schoenfield LJ, Lachin JM et al. (1981) Chenodiol (chenodeoxycholic acid) for dissolution of gallstones: the National Cooperative Gallstone Study. A controlled trial of efficacy and safety. Ann Intern Med 95:257–282
25. Sieg A, Metz W, Stiehl A, Raedsch R, Wysocki S, Kohlmeier M, Kommerell B (1986) Zusammensetzung von Gallenblasen- und Gallengangssteinen. Dtsch Med Wochenschr 111:1760–1762

26. Stiehl A, Czygan P, Kommerell B, Weiss HJ, Holtermüller KH (1978) Ursodeoxycholic acid versus chenodeoxycholic acid. Comparison of their effects on bile acid and bile lipid composition in patients with cholesterol gallstones. Gastroenterology 75:1016–1020
27. Stiehl A, Raedsch R, Czygan P, Götz R, Männer Ch, Walker S (1980) Effects of biliary bile acid composition on biliary cholesterol saturation in gallstone patients treated with chenodeoxycholic acid and/or ursodeoxycholic acid. Gastroenterology 79:1192–1198
28. Stiehl A, Raedsch R, Rudolph G, Walker S (1984) Effect of ursodeoxycholic acid on biliary bile acid and bile lipid composition in gallstone patients. Hepatology 4:107–111
29. Thistle JL, Hofmann AF, Paulina YS, Ott B (1977) Effect of varying doses of chenodeoxycholic acid on bile lipid and biliary bile acid composition in gallstone patients: a dose-response study. Dig Dis 22:1–6
30. Thistle JL, May GR, Bender CE, Williams HJ, LeRoy AJ, Nelson PE, Peine CJ, Petersen BT, McCullough JE (1989) Dissolution of cholesterol gallbladder stones by methyl *tert*-butyl ether administered by percutaneous transhepatic catheter. N Engl J Med 320:633–639
31. Tint GS, Salen G, Shefer S (1986) Effect of ursodeoxycholic acid and chenodeoxycholic acid on cholesterol and bile acid metabolism. Gastroenterology 91:1007–1018

Systemic Litholysis with Bile Acids: Ursodeoxycholic Acid

W. Kurtz

Medizinische Klinik I, Zentralkrankenhaus Reinkenheide, Postbrookstr., D-2850 Bremerhaven, FRG

In 1972 cholesterol gallbladder stones were dissolved for the first time with chenodeoxycholic acid (CDCA) [1, 2]. CDCA induced a rise in transaminases and diarrhea in 20%–30% of patients treated; complete stone dissolution was observed in 60%–70% of cases, depending on stone number and size. In 1973 Nakano and Nakano [3] reported for the first time the successful dissolution of cholesterol gallbladder stones with ursodeoxycholic acid (UDCA). This result was confirmed in a prospective study by Makino et al. [4]. UDCA has the advantage that it can be administered entirely without side effects.

Therapeutic mechanisms of CDCA and UDCA are different. CDCA inhibits HMG-Coenzyme A reductase and 7α-hydroxylase in the liver, inducing a suppression of cholesterol synthesis and a change in bile acid pool composition favoring CDCA. Furthermore, CDCA is a good micelle former. Cholesterol from biliary concrements is carried off in mixed micelles consisting of bile acids and phospholipids. UDCA has little or no effect on HMG-Coenzyme A reductase [5, 6], and because of its high polarity it is a poor micelle former. However, UDCA forms liquid crystals with cholesterol and inhibits the absorption of cholesterol in the gut. It also impairs cholesterol secretion at the biliary side of the sinusoidal cell. Thus, too, a bile undersaturated in cholesterol is secreted which is capable of extricating cholesterol from concretions. As a poor micelle former, UDCA has a somewhat higher choleretic effect than CDCA. Free UDCA has been shown to have a hypercholeretic effect, possibly by inducing bicarbonate secretion into bile [7]. In this respect, however, it probably does not differ much from free CDCA, and it is not established whether the choleretic effect of bile acids has any impact on their cholelitholytic activity.

While CDCA produces some side effects, UDCA has no side effects at all. Its high polarity not only makes it the least toxic of human bile acids but also gives it astonishing healing capacities. UDCA had been used in the therapy of dyspeptic symptoms [8], chronic active hepatitis [9], primary biliary cirrhosis [10], and primary sclerosing cholangitis [11]. UDCA improves hepatic bile acid extraction [12], detoxifies more toxic, less polar bile acids by integrating them into mixed micelles [13], and has a singular specific membrane-protecting effect [14]. In addition, it replaces other, more lipophilic and toxic bile acids in the bile acid pool. The first double-blind study on UDCA therapy of primary biliary cirrhosis has just been completed and gave favorable results [15].

While CDCA is administered in a daily dosage of 15 mg/kg body weight, UDCA is given in a dosage of 10 mg/kg. According to Dowling et al. [16], this is the optimal dosage for gallstone dissolution. Erlinger and colleagues showed in 1983 and 1984 [17, 18] that 2.5 mg/kg per day dissolves gallstones only rarely, but that a dose of only 8.4 mg/kg distinctly improves the dissolution rate. Further dose-response studies were carried out by a group from Japan [19], one from the United States [20], and one from Italy [21]. There is some speculation that doses exceeding 10 mg/kg might induce secondary stone calcification during treatment. However, at present there is no proven correlation between UDCA dosage and calcification [22]. In a study of our own which comprised 145 patients with 10 mg/kg UDCA daily ten patients dropped out for nonmedical reasons; in the remaining 135 patients there was stone dissolution in 62.2% [23]. In 10 of the 51 nonresponders (7.4%) we observed stone calcification. There was no correlation to the UDCA dose. Usually it occurred in young overweight patients with small stones which seemed to dissolve rapidly at first. The effect of UDCA is established by more than 15 open studies with UDCA alone and an equal number of comparative studies (UDCA versus placebo or versus CDCA). Depending on treatment time and stone size, the therapeutic success rate was between 13% [24] and 88% [25], as with CDCA. In stones measuring less than 1.5 cm, the dissolution rate averages 60%–70% [26, 27]. The success rate with UDCA corresponds to that with CDCA.

The mean treatment time with UDCA until dissolution is 16–19 months [23]. To shorten this relatively long treatment time, to improve the mean dissolution rate of only 60%, and to reduce the stone calcification rate of about 10%, there have been attempts to change the administration time of UDCA by giving UDCA with and without a special diet, by combining UDCA with CDCA, by the simultaneous administration of UDCA with the amino acid taurine, and by combining UDCA with terpenes.

A group in the United Kingdom showed for CDCA that bedtime administration [28] of this bile acid induced stone dissolution more rapidly than administration three times a day. Although UDCA also diminished the lithogenic index with bedtime administration [29], there was no accelerated stone dissolution by this regimen. Nevertheless, to date UDCA is also given in a single dose at bedtime since this mode of administration has proven more convenient for the patient.

Since CDCA and UDCA induce gallstone dissolution by different mechanisms, three groups of investigators studied whether the combination of these substances could enhance their effect. In the combination preparation the individual bile acids could be reduced, and it was hoped that side effects such as increase in aminotransferases and diarrhea with CDCA and stone calcification with UDCA would be reduced. A preliminary study by Stiehl et al. [30] in 1980 showed that a combination of CDCA and UDCA reduced the saturation index to a statistically significant extent compared to controls on monotherapy. The amount of the less water-soluble glycoursodeoxycholic acid (GUDCA) decreased from 85.8% (monotherapy) to 34.2% of total bile acids. GUDCA is thought to be responsible for stone calcification. There was no elevation of aminotransferases as seen with CDCA, and there was no diarrhea. In 1985 Czygan et al. [31] and in 1986 Roehrkasse et al. [32] presented clinical data. Czygan et al. treated 24 patients with UDCA and 25 patients with a combination of UDCA and CDCA. The stone dissolution rate in the UDCA group was 40.5% and that in the combination group 58.3%; the difference was statistically not significant. Three out of 25 patients on UDCA showed stone calcification. Roehrkasse et al. [32] treated 16 patients with a combination preparation without convincing results. An assessment of stone calcification is not possible from these two studies. Podda et al. [33] treated 120 patients with gallbladder stones by monotherapy or by combination treatment. After 6 months there was a statistically significant difference between the combination group and the monotherapy group (the former fared batter). After 2 years the difference was statistically not significant.

Another measure to prevent stone calcification was the administration of UDCA plus taurine (TUDCA), which is more water-soluble than GUDCA [34, 35]. Thistle and LaRusso [36] administered 10 mg UDCA plus 2 g taurine and compared their data to that of a combination therapy of 5 mg UDCA plus 10 mg CDCA. The administration of taurine reduced the ratio GUDCA:TUDCA, but no treatment regimen increased the absolute TUDCA concentration. The combination treatment showed the best stone dissolution results and most marked desaturation of bile. The study provided no evidence that stone calcification can be prevented by coadministration of taurine. In 1985 Fraboni et al. [37] reported on investigations covering a total of 262 patients and showing calcifications in 13.2% of patients with UDCA (14/106), in 8.8% with CDCA (11/125), and in 12.9% with TUDCA (4/31); the differences were not statistically significant.

On the basis of investigations by Bell and colleagues [38, 39], who successfully administered a mixture of six terpenes in combination with CDCA to gallstone patients, we performed an investigation with a menthol/UDCA preparation [40]. This preparation proved as effective as monotherapy with UDCA but was considerably cheaper.

On the whole, the theoretical advantages of various combination therapies have not yet produced better clinical results than UDCA therapy alone. The main problem in chemical gallstone dissolution is the recurrence rate of 20%–70% [41–43]. These data are derived from the CDCA treatment; according to recent Italian investigations, they are also valid for UDCA treatment. Stones usually recur without symptoms, and we must therefore perform routine ultrasound investigations in order to detect them. Almost all recurrent stones are cholesterol concretions and are thus amenable to renewed UDCA treatment. There is no general consensus on the means for preventing stone recurrence. Continuous therapy with UDCA in a reduced dosage and the interval treatment have been discussed, as have been therapy with the gel-reducing aspirin and that with low-cost terpene preparations [40].

In comparison to CDCA or various other medicamentous cholesterol gallstone dissolution therapies, UDCA has not been surpassed in final dissolution rate and lack of side effects.

References

1. Danzinger RG, Hofman AF, Schoenfield LJ, Thistle JL (1972) Dissolution of cholesterol gallstones by chenodeoxycholic acid. N Engl J Med 286:1–8
2. Bell GD, Whitney B, Dowling RH (1972) Gallstone dissolution in man using chenodeoxycholic acid. Lancet 2:1213–1216
3. Nakano Y, Nakano K (1973) Some cases of gallstones dissolved by bile acid preparations. J Natl Council Commun Hosp 70:25–32
4. Makino I, Shinozaki K, Yashino K, Nakagawa S (1975) Dissolution of cholesterol gallstones by ursodeoxycholic acid. Jpn J Gastroenterol 72:690–702
5. Nielsell K, Angelin B, Leijd B, Einarsson K (1983) Comparative effects of ursodeoxycholic acid and chenodeoxycholic acid on bile acid kinetics and biliary lipid secretion in humans. Evidence for different modes of action on bile acid synthesis. Gastroenterology 85:1248–1256
6. William G, Hardison M, Grundy SM (1984) Effect of ursodeoxycholic acid and its taurine conjugate on bile acid synthesis and cholesterol absorption. Gastroenterology 87:130–135
7. Dumont M, Erlinger S, Uchmann S (1980) Hypercholeresis induced by ursodeoxycholic acid and 7-ketolithocholic acid in the rat: possible role of bicarbonate transport. Gastroenterology 79:82–89
8. Masuda M, Hosoda S, Baba T, Kashima T, Aki H, Nakagawa M (1980) Double blind trial of ursodeoxycholic acid in maldigestive malabsorption syndrome (chronic biliary tract and pancreatic disease). Clin Rep 10:85–109
9. Leuschner U, Leuschner M, Sieratzki J, Kurtz W, Hübner K (1985) Gallstone dissolution with ursodeoxycholic acid in patients with chronic active hepatitis and two years' follow-up. A pilot study. Dig Dis Sci 30:642–649
10. Leuschner U, Leuschner M, Hübner K (1981) Gallstone dissolution patients with chronic active hepatitis. Gastroenterology 80:1834 (abstr)
11. David R, Kurtz W, Strohm WD, Leuschner U (1985) Die Wirkung von Ursodesoxycholsäure bei chronischen Leberkrankheiten. Eine Pilotstudie. Z Gastroenterol 23:420 (abstr)
12. Kurtz W, Leuschner U, Langhans G (1985) Ursodeoxycholic acid improves hepatic bile acid extraction in the rat. Hepatology 1 [Suppl 2] 270

13. Güldütuna S, Kurtz W, Pelekanos C, Zimmer G, Leuschner U (1988) Mechanismen von Membranschädigung und Membranschutz durch Gallensäuren. In: Kurtz W (ed) Gallensäuren und Magen-Darm-Trakt. Hygieneplan, Oberursel, pp 19–29
14. Güldütuna S (1988) Membranwirkungen von Gallensäuren. Gastroenterologischer Workshop Leber und Gallensäuren, Bad Homburg, 2 Dec 1988
15. Leuschner U, Fischer H, Kurtz W, Güldütuna S, Hübner K, Hellstern A, Gatzen M, Leuschner M (1989) Ursodeoxycholic acid treatment of primary biliary cirrhosis: results of a randomized, controlled double-blind trial. Gastroenterology 97:1268–1274
16. Dowling RH, Ruppin DC, Meredith T, Myszor M, Fogacs I, Murphy GM (1983) Efficacy of bile acid treatment in dissolving gallstones: collateral benefits of CDCA and UDCA therapy; gallstone recurrence and postdissolution management. In: Paumgartner G, Stiehl A, Gerok W (eds) Bile acids and cholesterol in health and disease. MTP Press, Lancaster, pp 345–362
17. Erlinger S (1983) Ursodeoxycholic acid and chenodeoxycholic acid treatment of radiolucent gallstones: follow-up report of a multicentric trial. In: Paumgartner G, Stiehl A, Gerok W (eds) Bile acids and cholesterol in health and disease. MTP Press, Lancaster, pp 365–366
18. Erlinger S, Go AL, Hussen JM, Fevery J (1984) Franco-Belgian cooperative study of ursodeoxycholic acid in medical dissolution of gallstones: a double-blind, randomised, dose-response study, and comparison with chenodeoxycholic acid. Hepatology 4:308–314
19. Tokyo Cooperative Gallstone Study Group (1980) Efficacy and indications of ursodeoxycholic acid treatment for dissolving gallstones. Gastroenterology 78:542–548
20. Salen G, Colalillo A, Verga D, Bagan E, Tint GS, Shefer S (1980) Effect of high and low dose of ursodeoxycholic acid on gallstone dissolution in humans. Gastroenterology 78:1412–1418
21. Podda M, Zuin M, Carulli N, Ponz de Leon M, Dioguardi ML (1982) Gallstone dissolution after 6 months of ursodeoxycholic acid (UDCA): effectiveness of different doses. J Int Med Res 10:59–63
22. Bouchier IAD, Neligan P (1983) Calcification of radiolucent gallstones during ursodeoxycholic acid therapy. In: Paumgartner G, Stiehl A, Gerok W (eds) Bile acids and cholesterol in health and disease. MTP Press, Lancaster, pp 397–398
23. Leuschner U, Baumgärtel H, Kurtz W, Leuschner M, Strohm WD (1987) Medical treatment of cholesterol gallstones: present and future. In: Onkolicsányi L, Csomós G, Crepaldi G (eds) Assessment and management of hepatobiliary disease. Springer, Berlin Heidelberg New York, pp 107–114
24. Schoenfield LJ, Lachin JM, The NCGS Steering Committee, The NCGS Group (1981) National cooperative gallstone study. A controlled trial of the efficacy and safety of chenodeoxycholic acid for dissolution of gallstones. Ann Int Med 95:257–282
25. Barbara L, Bazzoli F, Festi D, Morselli AML, Roda E (1983) A comparative study of chenodeoxycholic acid and ursodeoxycholic acid as cholesterol gallstone dissolving agents. In: Paumgartner G, Stiehl A, Gerok W (eds) Bile acids and cholesterol in health and disease. MTP Press, Lancaster, pp 367–370
26. Maton PN, Murphy GM, Dowling RH (1977) Ursodeoxycholic acid treatment of gallstones. Dose-response study and possible mechanism of action. Lancet II:1297–1301
27. Dowling RH (1983) Cholelithiasis: medical treatment. Clin Gastroenterol 12:125–178
28. Kupfer RM, Maudgal DP, Northfield T (1982) Gallstone dissolution rate during chenid acid therapy: effect of bedtime administration plus low cholesterol diet. Dig Dis Sci 27:1025–1029
29. Northfield TC, Lanzini A, Jazrawi R, Maudgal DP, Kupfer R (1985) Methods of improving the efficacy of litholytic therapy. In: Paumgartner G, Stiehl A, Gerok W (eds) Enterohepatic circulation of bile acids and sterol metabolism. MTP Press, Manchester, pp 335–350
30. Stiehl A, Raedsch R, Czygan P, Götz R, Männer C, Walker S, Kommerell B (1980) Effects of biliary bile acid composition on biliary cholesterol saturation in gallstone patients treated with chenodeoxycholic and/or ursodeoxycholic acid. Gastroenterology 79:1192–1198
31. Czygan P, Stiehl A, Raedsch R, Seitz H, Kommerell B (1985) Dissolution of cholesterol gallstones by combination therapy of urso/cheno versus urso. In: Paumgartner G, Stiehl A, Gerok W (eds) Enterohepatic circulation of bile acids and sterol metabolism. MTP Press, Manchester, pp 351–353
32. Roehrkasse R, Fromm H, Malavolti M, Tunuguntla AK, Ceryak S (1986) Gallstone dissolution treatment with a combination of chenodeoxycholic and ursodeoxycholic acids. Studies of safety, efficacy and effects on bile lithogenicity, bile acid pool, and serum lipids. Dig Dis Sci 10:1032–1040

33. Podda M, Zuin M, De Fazio C, Dioguardi ML, Battezzati PM, Ghezzi C (1987) Comparison of the efficacy and safety of ursodeoxycholic acid alone and in combination with chenodeoxycholic acid in patients with radiolucent gallstones: a randomized controlled trial. In: Paumgartner G, Stiehl A, Gerok W (eds) Bile acids and the liver. MTP Press, Lancaster, pp 347–352
34. Bateson MC, Bouchier IAD, Trash DB (1981) Calcification of radiolucent gallstones during treatment with ursodeoxycholic acid. Br med J 283:645–646
35. Batta AK, Salen G, Shefer SD (1981) The effect of feeding tauroursodeoxycholic acid on biliary bile acid composition. Gastroenterology 80:1106 (abstr)
36. Thistle JL, LaRusso NF (1985) Combination of taurine or chenodeoxycholic acid with ursodeoxycholic acid therapy: effects on biliary lipids, bile acids and gallstones. In: Paumgartner G, Stiehl A, Gerok W (eds) Enterohepatic circulation of bile acids and sterol metabolism. MTP Press, Lancaster, pp 335–339
37. Frabboni R, Bazzoli F, Mazzella G, Festi D, Villanova N, Roda E, Barbara L (1985) Acquired gallstone calcification during cholelitholytic treatment with chenodeoxycholic, ursodeoxycholic and tauroursodeoxycholic acids. Hepatology 5:1004 (abstr)
38. Bell GD, Doran J (1979) Gallstone dissolution in man using an essential oil preparation – Rowachol. Br Med J 1:24
39. Ellis WR, Sommerville KW, Whitten BH, Bell GD (1984) Pilot study of combination treatment for gallstones with medium dose chenodeoxycholic acid and a terpene preparation. Br Med J 289:153–156
40. Leuschner M, Leuschner U, Lazarovici D, Kurtz W, Hellstern A (1988) Dissolution of gallstones with an ursodeoxycholic acid/menthol preparation: a controlled prospective double-blind study. Gut 29:428–432
41. Ruppin DC, Dowling RH (1982) Is recurrence inevitable after gallstone dissolution by bile acid treatment? Lancet I:181–185
42. Iser JH, Dowling RH, Mok HYI, Bell GD (1975) Chenodeoxycholic acid treatment of gallstones – a follow-up report and analysis of factors influencing response to therapy. N Engl J Med 293:378–383
43. Ponz de Leon M, Carulli N, Iori T, Loria P, Smerieri A, Zironi F (1980) Medical treatment of radiolucent gallstones with chenodeoxycholic acid (CDCA): follow-up report at four years. Ital J Gastroenterol 12:17–22

Combination Therapy of Chenodeoxycholic Acid and Ursodeoxycholic Acid

M. Podda, M. Zuin, M. L. Petroni, E. Bertolini, A. Crosignani, and G. Grandinetti

Chair of Internal Medicine, University of Milan, Via A. di Rudini 8, 20142 Milan, Italy

Introduction

Bile acid therapy has become well established as nonsurgical treatment in selected patients with cholesterol gallstones since chenodeoxycholic acid (cheno) and, later on, ursodeoxycholic acid (urso) were introduced in the early 1970s and 1980s, respectively.

Urso is more efficacious than cheno for gallstone dissolution and relatively free from side effects like diarrhoea and hypertransaminasaemia. On the other hand, urso is about twice as expensive as cheno and also causes a higher proportion of acquired gallstone calcifications.

A better understanding of physicochemical and pharmacological properties of bile acids has led to the combined administration of both cheno and urso, with the aim of enhancing their cholesterol solubility capacity and reducing their side effects. In this chapter, the rationale of the combined use of cheno and urso and a review of the effects of the combination on biliary lipids and gallstone dissolution are reported.

Mechanisms of Action of Cheno Plus Urso

The physicochemical and pharmacological properties of cheno and urso are summarised in Table 1.

The combined administration of cheno and urso might create more favourable conditions for cholesterol gallstones dissolution since both mechanisms of cholesterol solubilisation (micellation by cheno and liquid crystals formation by urso) are probably active at the same time. Urso reduces cholesterol secretion into bile even more than cheno [1, 2] and also reduces intestinal cholesterol absorption, but it does not reduce de novo bile acid synthesis [1, 2].

The side effects and disadvantages of cheno and urso monotherapy are summarised in Table 2. Diarrhoea and hypertransaminasaemia are dose-related side effects of

Table 1. Differences in physicochemical and pharmacological properties of cheno and urso

	Cheno	Urso
Detergent capacity	↑↑	↑
Cholesterol solubilisation in micelles	↑↑	↑
Cholesterol solubilisation in liquid crystals	0	↑↑
Cholesterol secretion	↓	↓↓
Bile acid synthesis	↓↓	(↓)
Intestinal cholesterol absorption	0	↓

Table 2. Advantages and disadvantages of treatment with cheno or urso and in combination

	Cheno	Urso	Cheno plus urso
Diarrhoea	+	0	±
Hypertransaminaemia	+	0	0
Plasma triglycerides	↓	0	0
Plasma LDL cholesterol	↑	0	0
Gallstone calcification	±	+	±
Cost of treatment	+	+++	++

chenotherapy [3, 4] and can therefore be reduced when a lower dose of cheno is used in combination with urso. Moreover, urso has been shown to have a specific protective effect against cheno-induced hepatocyte damage [5–8].

On the other hand, the acquired calcification of radiolucent gallstones reported during therapy with urso [9–11], probably due to a decreased calcium solubility in an aqueous bile salt-lecithin mixture at increasing concentrations of urso in the bile [9], might also be reduced with the combination therapy.

Changes in Biliary Lipids with Cheno Plus Urso in Normal Weight and Obese Gallstone Patients

Normal Weight Patients

The effect of combination treatment on biliary lipids in gallstone patients who are not obese has been studied by others [12–14] and by us [15], using different doses of bile acids.

Stiehl et al. [12] carried out a controlled study on 10 patients after a 9-week sequential administration of three regimens, with total daily doses ranging from 11.9 to 15.6 mg/kg. Urso alone and combination treatment resulted in a significantly greater decrease of biliary cholesterol than cheno, whilst the corrected saturation index (CSI) was significantly lower after cheno plus urso and cheno alone than after urso.

In our study biliary lipid composition following 45–60 days of administration of equimolar doses of cheno plus urso (5 mg/kg of each) and of each bile acid alone in the same total dose (10 mg/kg) was investigated in 18 gallstone patients in a controlled, double-blind study with a balanced latin square design. The results showed that the molar percentage of cholesterol in bile (initial value 9.7% ± 2.2%) is significantly lower after combination treatment (5.2% ± 1.2%) and urso alone (5.4% ± 1.3%) than after cheno alone (7.2% ± 1.7%), thus in agreement with Stiehl et al. [13]. However, in our experience, CSI showed a greater decrease after cheno plus urso (0.81 ± 0.12) than on either urso alone (0.94 ± 0.12) and cheno alone (1.00 ± 0.19).

Thistle [16] evaluated the effect on biliary lipids of the two bile acids combined in a different proportion (urso 5 mg/kg plus cheno 10 mg/kg). This regimen was compared with urso alone (10 mg/kg) and with urso plus taurine (urso 10 mg/kg, taurine 2 g/day). The CSI was below 1.0 in six of seven patients after cheno plus urso, in three of seven patients after urso plus taurine and in three of seven after urso alone.

Roehrkasse et al. [13] found a decrease, although not significant, in the mean uncorrected saturation index (SI) from the initial value of 1.49 to 0.99 during treatment with urso, 6.5 mg/kg, plus cheno, 7.5 mg/kg. Within their study population, three subjects

Table 3. Bile acid composition and SI before and during treatment with cheno (15 mg/kg), urso (15 mg/kg) and cheno plus urso (7.5 mg/kg of each) in obese gallstone patients

	Before (mean ± SD)	After (mean ± SD)		
		Cheno	Urso	Cheno + urso
SI	1.7 ± 0.25	1.1 ± 0.19	0.8 ± 0.16[a]	0.74 ± 0.15[a, b]
Urso (%)	0.6 ± 0.4	1.4 ± 1.1	55.4 ± 6.1[a]	32.1 ± 4.7[d]
Cheno (%)	30.7 ± 8.2	84.0 ± 5.4	19.9 ± 4.9	49.0 ± 5.6
Cheno plus urso (%)	31.4 ± 8.2	85.4 ± 4.8	75.3 ± 5.5	81.0 ± 3.4[c]
Deoxycholic acid (%)	28.0 ± 8.8	3.1 ± 2.6	8.3 ± 2.6	5.4 ± 1.3
Lithocholic acid (%)	3.9 ± 1.4	6.8 ± 1.9	4.2 ± 1.4	5.9 ± 1.3
Cholic acid (%)	36.6 ± 7.3	4.6 ± 2.9	12.1 ± 3.5	8.2 ± 3.0

SI; uncorrected saturation index [23]
[a] $P<0.05$ vs cheno. [b] $P<0.05$ vs urso. [c] $P<0.01$ vs urso. [d] $P<0.01$ vs cheno and urso

were obese, and in all of them the SI fell below 1.0 during treatment with the combination.

Lanzini et al. [14] have recently documented the existence of an inverse dose-response relation of combination therapy on the SI: doses as low as 5 mg/kg reduced SI to values less than 1.0 in all patients, while the calculated minimum effective dose for achieving a consistent desaturation of gallbladder bile, i.e. an SI of 0.8 or less, was 7 mg/kg.

Obese Patients

We investigated the effect of treatment with cheno plus urso in a double-blind study with a balanced latin square design, in which 12 obese gallstone patients (mean ideal body weight = 153%) were treated for three consecutive 2-month periods with cheno (15 mg/kg), urso (15 mg/kg) and cheno plus urso (7.5 + 7.5 mg/kg). SI of gallbladder bile was determined before and after each period (Table 3), with and without the correction factor for urso-rich bile.

According to SI values, bile was unsaturated in all patients after cheno plus urso, in 83% (10/12) of patients after urso alone, in 33% (4/12) of patients treated with cheno alone. Bile enrichment in litholitic bile acids (cheno and urso) was significantly higher after cheno alone and cheno plus urso than after urso alone. Combination treatment was well tolerated since only one patient reported mild diarrhoea, while a slight and transient increase in serum transaminases was noted in another patient.

Clinical Use of Cheno Plus Urso

The available data on the clinical efficacy of combination therapy as investigated in preliminary or uncontrolled studies are reported in Table 4.

Safety

All studies, so far [13, 15–18], showed that the urso plus cheno combination is well tolerated since only occasional diarrhoea and a transient rise in transaminases above twice the upper limit in a tiny proportion of patients were reported as side effects. No deleterious changes in serum lipids have been reported.

Table 4. Studies on clinical efficacy of combination therapy

Author	Study design	Total no. of patients	Doses	Results
Thistle et al. [16]	Controlled study. Compared urso plus cheno vs urso plus taurine vs urso alone	25	– 5 mg/kg urso plus 10 mg/kg cheno – 10 mg/kg urso – 10 mg/kg urso plus 2 gr/day tauringe	Higher response rates (partial plus complete dissolution) at 3, 6, 12–24 months after cheno plus urso than the other two regimens (statistical analysis not available)
Kawamoto et al. [17]	Controlled study. Compared different proportions of urso and cheno in combination	53	Urso plus cheno (mg/day) – 200 + 400 (group A) – 300 + 300 (group B) – 400 + 200 (group C)	Response rates at 12 months: group A: 29%; group B: 48%; group C: 72%, Significant difference between the highest and the lowest dose of urso
Czygan et al. [18]	Three distinct controlled studies. Compared urso plus cheno vs urso alone	159	– 5–8 mg/kg urso plus 5–10 mg/kg cheno – 10–12.4 mg/kg urso	Complete dissolution rates in each study (combination vs urso alone): – 53% vs 33% – 80% vs 40% – 59% vs 40%
Roehrkasse et al. [14]	Uncontrolled study	16	– 6.5 mg/kg urso plus 7.5 mg/kg cheno	Response rate: 60% at 1 year. Longer periods of treatment resulted in further improvements
Podda et al. [19]	Controlled study. Compared urso plus cheno vs urso alone	120	– 5 mg/kg urso plus 5 mg/kg cheno – 10 mg/kg urso	Combination significantly more effective at 6 months (68% vs 48% response rate). After longer periods also higher, but no longer significant response rates

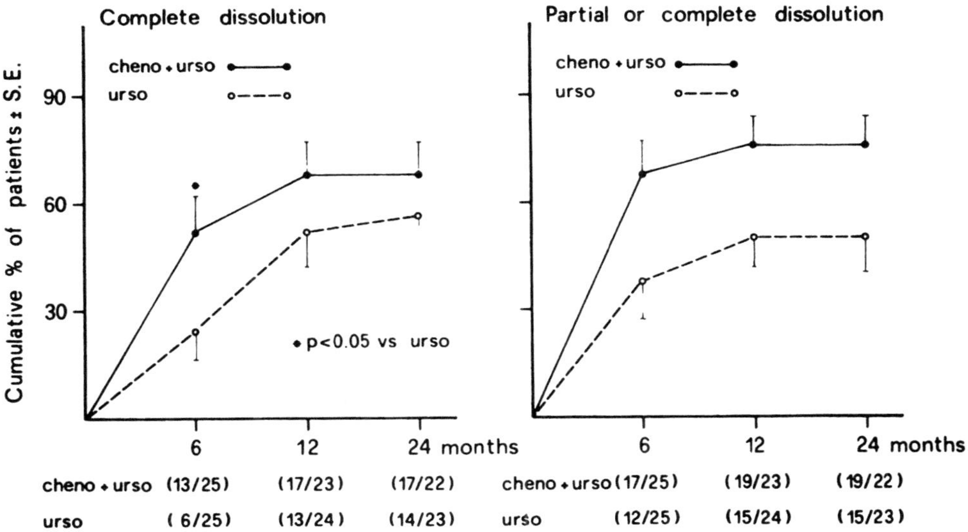

Fig. 1. Cumulative percentages of dissolution (mean ± SE) in patients with small stones. Left panel complete, right panel partial or complete; within brackets are numbers of patients with effect/patients presenting for check-up (reprinted with permission from [19])

Gallstone Dissolution

High dissolution rates are achieved with combination therapy (Table 4). This was particularly true when strict admission criteria were applied (i.e. patients who were not obese with gallstones less than 15 mm in diameter) [19]. In this study combination therapy resulted in a significantly higher dissolution rate than urso alone (Fig. 1).

Acquired stone calcification, an important cause of nonresponse to therapy, was less frequent during treatment with the combination than with urso alone, even if the numbers involved were too small to show a statistically significant difference [13, 15–18].

Moreover, as suggested by Czygan [18], efficacy of combination treatment could be further enhanced by administration of the whole dose at bedtime, rather than in divided doses at mealtimes, as has been demonstrated for treatment with cheno and urso [20–22].

Summary

The validity of the rationale for the combined administration of cheno plus urso has been confirmed by the studies on biliary lipids and stone dissolution. All trials have shown a trend towards a greater efficacy of combination treatment in achieving complete dissolution. Combination therapy is well tolerated by patients, probably because of the low dose of cheno administered. The cost of combination treatment is lower than cost of urso treatment.

References

1. Nilsell K, Angelin B, Leijd B, Einarsson K (1983) Comparative effect of ursodeoxycholic acid and chenodeoxycholic acid on bile acid kinetics and biliary lipid secretion in man. Evidence for different modes of action on bile acid synthesis. Gastroenterology 85:1248–1256
2. Von Bergmann K, Epple-Gutsfeld M, Leiss O (1984) Differences in the effects of chenodeoxycholic and ursodeoxycholic acid in biliary lipid secretion and bile acid synthesis in patients with gallstones. Gastroenterology 87:136–143
3. Mok HYI, Bell GD, Dowling RH (1974) Effect of different doses of chenodeoxycholic acid on bile lipid composition and on frequency of side effects in patients with gallstones. Lancet 2:253–257
4. Thistle JL, Hofmann AF, Ott BJ, Stephens DH (1978) Chenotherapy for gallstone dissolution. I. Efficacy and safety. JAMA 239:1041–1046
5. Miyai K, Toyota N, Jones HM, Gochman N (1982) Protective effect of ursodeoxycholic acid against cholestatic and hepatotoxic effects of lithocholic acid (Abstract). Hepatology 2:705
6. Krol T, Kitamura T, Miyai K, Hardison W (1983) Tauroursodeoxycholate reduces ductular proliferation in bile duct-ligated hamsters (Abstract). Hepatology 3:881
7. Tanikawa K, Kawahara T, Kumashiro R et al. (1986) Effects of bile acids on the cultured hepatocyte and Kupffer cell (Abstract). Hepatology 6:779
8. Poupon R, Chretien Y, Poupon RE et al. (1987) Is ursodeoxycholic acid an effective treatment for primary biliary cirrhosis? Lancet 1:834–836
9. Raedsch R, Stiehl A, Czygan P (1981) Ursodeoxycholic acid and gallstone calcification. Lancet 2:1296
10. Bateson MC (1981) Calcification of radiolucent gallstones during treatment with ursodeoxycholic acid. Br Med J 283:645–646
11. Meredith TJ, Williams GV, Murphy GM et al. (1982) Retrospective comparison of "cheno" and "urso" in the medical treatment of gallstones. Gut 23:382–389
12. Stiehl A, Raedsch R, Czygan P et al. (1980) Effects of biliary bile acid composition on biliary cholesterol saturation in gallstone patients treated with chenodeoxycholic acid and/or ursodeoxycholic acid. Gastroenterology 79:1192–1198
13. Roehrkasse R, Fromm H, Malavolti M, Tunuguntla AK, Ceriak S (1986) Gallstone dissolution treatment with a combination of chenodeoxycholic and ursodeoxycholic acid. Studies of safety, efficacy and effects on bile lithogenicity, bile acid pool and serum lipids. Dig Dis Sci 31:1032–1040
14. Lanzini A, Facchinetti D, Rossi A, Muiesan G (1989) Cheno plus urso (CDCA+UDCA) combination therapy: dose-response effect on cholesterol saturation index (SI) of gallbladder bile (Abstract). 1st International Lugano Symposium on Biliary Physiology and Diseases. Strategies for the treatment of hepatobiliary diseases. 15–17 June 1989, Lugano
15. Podda M, Zuin M, Dioguardi ML, Festorazzi S, Dioguardi N (1982) A combination of ursodeoxycholic acid and chenodeoxycholic acid is more effective than either alone in reducing biliary cholesterol saturation. Hepatology 2:334–339
16. Thistle JL (1987) Dissolution of gallstones using ursodeoxycholic acid with or without chenodeoxycholic acid or taurine. In: Paumgartner G, Stiehl A, Gerok W (eds), Biological effects of bile acids. MTP Press, Lancaster, pp 353–354
17. Kawamoto T, Horiuchi I, Hino F, Okahashi M, Kajiyama G (1984) Combination treatment with different doses of urso (U) and chenodeoxycholic acid (C) in patients with cholesterol gallstones (Abstract). Proceedings of the VIIIth International Bile Acid Meeting, Berne, p 183
18. Czygan P (1987) Efficacy of combined ursodeoxycholic and chenodeoxycholic acid treatment. In: Paumgartner G, Stiehl A, Gerok W (eds) Biological effects of bile acids. MTP Press, Lancaster, pp 343–344
19. Podda M, Zuin M, Battezzati PM, Ghezzi C, De Fazio C, Dioguardi ML (1989) Efficacy and safety of a combination of chenodeoxycholic acid for gallstone dissolution: a comparison with ursodeoxycholic acid alone. Gastroenterology 96:222–229
20. Maudgal DP, Kupfer RM, Northfield TC (1982) Minimum effective dose of chenic acid for gallstone patients: reduction with bedtime administration and a low cholesterol diet. Gut 23:280–284

21 Mazzella G, Labate AMM, Malavolti M, Petronelli A, Roda A, Barbara L (1983) The effect of ursodeoxycholic acid administration on bile lipid composition in man: comparison of bedtime versus mealtime administration. Curr Ther Res 30:551–557

22. Northfield TC, Lanzini A, Jazrawi R, Maudgal DP, Kupfer R (1985) Methods of improving the efficacy of litholitic therapy. In: Paumgartner G, Stiehl A, Gerok W (eds) Enterohepatic circulation of bile acids and sterol metabolism. MTP Press, Lancaster, pp 335–350

23. Carey MC, Ko G (1979) The importance of total lipid concentration in determining cholesterol solubility in bile and the development of critical tables for calculating "percent cholesterol saturation" with a correction factor for ursodeoxycholic-rich bile. In: Paumgartner G, Stiehl A, Gerok W (eds) Biological effects of bile acids. MTP Press, Lancaster, pp 299–308

Results of an Index-Controlled Combination Therapy with Ursodeoxycholic and Chenodeoxycholic Acid

P. Janowitz, W. Swobodnik, J. G. Wechsler, S. Fischer, J. Tudyka, and H. Ditschuneit

Abteilung Innere Medizin II, Gastroenterologie und Ernährungswissenschaften, Universitätsklinik Ulm, Robert-Koch-Str. 8, D-7900 Ulm, FRG

Introduction

Since 1972 chenodeoxycholic acid (CDCA) and since 1977 ursodeoxycholic acid (UDCA) have been used for the in vivo dissolution of cholesterol gallstones [1, 2]. The success of this therapy is dose dependent, with CDCA administered in daily doses of 15 mg/kg body weight and UDCA in daily doses of 10 mg/kg body weight. An increase in dosage above these levels led to no observable change in the efficacy of therapy [3]. While the mechanism of these two bile acids is different, both serve to change the composition of the total bile acid pool as well as to reduce biliary cholesterol saturation. CDCA inhibits HMG coenzyme A reductase together with 7α-hydroxylase. This results in decreased secretion of both cholesterol and bile acid. CDCA is able to dissolve biliary cholesterol in micelles and in this way compensates for decreased bile acid production, so that the total bile acid balance remains intact [4–6]. Hepatotoxicity, diarrhea, and changes in serum lipids and lipoproteins have been reported as side effects of CDCA therapy. Increases in transaminases have been observed in up to one-third of patients. This, however, was correlated with no observable changes in liver morphology [7, 8]. An increase in the level of lithocholic acid, a bacterial degradation product of CDCA, has been discussed as the cause of this increase in transaminases [9]. Diarrhea is usually of short duration and can be mitigated by dose reduction or by administration of the drug q.h.s.

UDCA reduces cholesterol resorption in the intestine and dissolves biliary cholesterol in the form of liquid crystals [10]. To date, no changes in liver parameters have been observed. The serum lipoprotein profile has remained constant [11]. The calcification of cholesterol stones in some 10% of patients during UDCA therapy has been described as a secondary effect [12]. The incidence of colic in the course of UDCA therapy is less than that during CDCA monotherapy, perhaps based on a reduced contractility of the gallbladder. Recently conducted studies have shown that, in comparison with either CDCA or UDCA monotherapy, the combined administration of both these substances leads to more rapid stone dissolution at a lower overall dose and to a higher passage rate [13–16]. The incidence of side effects is also lower.

In selected patients, oral cholelitholysis leads to stone dissolution in 13.5%–65% of cases in the course of 24 months of therapy [3, 7, 11, 17–19]. Because of the suspected cocarcinogenity and comutagenicity, particularly of the secondary bile acids (e.g., lithocholic acid and deoxycholic acid), therapy has seldom been continued for longer than 24 months [20].

Patients and Methods

A total of 55 patients (11 men and 44 women) were included in our clinically controlled prospective study. The average age for this group was 44.0 ± 5.3 years, and mean body weight was 107.5% of the ideal body weight as determined by the Metropolitan Life Insurance Company. The oral cholelitholysis was begun with an initial dose of 500 mg UDCA and 500 mg CDCA. These drugs were administered in split doses at midday and at bedtime together with a glass of milk (bedtime milk).

Patient selection was carried out on the basis of the following criteria:

- Cooperative patients with minor symptoms
- Radiolucent stones with a diameter of <20 mm
- Lithogenic index (LI, CSI) > 1.0
- Normal gallbladder emptying (positive gallbladder function by ultrasound)
- Total stone volume not exceeding two-thirds of total gallbladder volume
- No contraindications to therapy with UDCA or CDCA (pregnancy, underlying malignant or inflammatory conditions, severe colic, obstruction of the cystic duct, gallbladder anomalies, gastric and/or duodenal ulcers)

Patients with an LI value below 1.0 (cholesterol hyposaturation of the bile) were not admitted to the study. Before starting the oral cholelitholysis therapy, patients were subjected to a sonographic examination, X rays of the upper right quadrant of the abdomen, ultrasound evaluation of gallbladder emptying, and the endoscopic removal of bile. The bile was obtained through prepapillar suction after stimulation of the gallbladder with 5 µg ceruletide. The bile was ultracentrifuged at 100 000 *g* for 2 h at 37 °C, and the isotropic phase (cholesterol crystal-free phase) was then incubated at 37 °C. Nucleation time was determined using the method of Holan et al., defined as the earliest time required for the detection of cholesterol monohydrate crystals [21]. Cholesterol was measured enzymatically and gas-chromatographically with 5α-cholestane as an internal standard. Bile acids were determined by HPLC according to the method of Swobodnik et al. with dexamethasone as an internal standard [22]. The LI or CSI was calculated using the method of critical tables for calculating the cholesterol saturation of native bile as elaborated by Admirand and Small [23] and Carey [24].

At 3-month intervals an ultrasound was performed, and the following laboratory values were obtained: complete blood count, blood sedimentation rates, blood glucose, total protein, electrophoresis, urea creatinin, sodium, potassium, uric acid, cholesterol, high- and low-density lipoprotein cholesterol, triglycerides, lipoprotein electrophoresis, apolipoproteins A-I, A-II, and B, serum glutamic oxaloacetic transaminase (SGOT), serum glutamic pyruvic transaminase (SGPT), alkaline phosphatase, gamma-glutamyl transpeptidase (GGT), bilirubin, amylase, and urine status. A second endoscopic removal of bile was conducted 12 months after initiation of therapy. UDCA and CDCA doses were increased in patients showing an inadequate LI decrease (greater than 1.0). Administration of both drugs in unchanged doses was continued for 3 months after complete stone dissolution.

All patients received dietetic counseling and were advised to consume diets rich in fiber and to limit dietary cholesterol to 300 mg per day [25].

Results

Complete dissolution of gallbladder stones was achieved in an average of 13.6 months (range, 3–24 months) in 27.3% of patients ($n = 15$). Incomplete dissolution (approximately 35% reduction in stone volume) was achieved in a further 28 study subjects (50.9%). Treatment of these patients was discontinued after 24 months. Therapy interruption within 24 months of initiation was necessary in 12 patients (21.8%) due to noncompliance (3.6%), failure to respond to therapy (no stone volume reduction, 10.9%), nonfunctioning gallbladder (3.6%), and acute cholecystitis (3.6%). Two patients

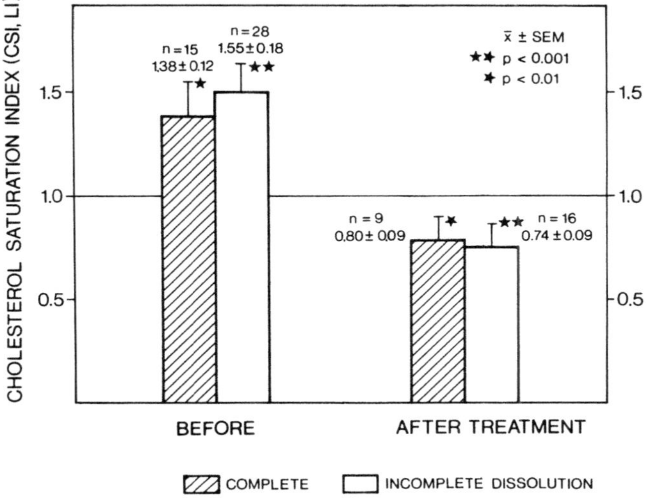

Fig. 1. Lithogenic index (LI, CSI). Mean values for those with complete and those with incomplete dissolution before and after dissolution therapy

(3.6%) experienced transient diarrhea, which resolved spontaneously without dose reduction or discontinuation of treatment. Significant side effects resulting from the oral cholelitholytic therapy were not observed in the course of the study period. Calcification of a solitary stone was observed in two patients (3.6%) showing no tendency toward reduction of stone volume. These calcifications were verifiable only on the computed tomographic scan of the gallbladder.

The LI of the total group was reduced significantly from 1.54 ± 0.12 to 0.82 ± 0.06 ($p < 0.001$). The reduction in the LI of the successfully treated patients from 1.38 ± 0.12 to 0.80 ± 0.09 ($p < 0.01$) was comparable to that of the remaining patients (a reduction from 1.55 ± 0.18 to 0.74 ± 0.09; $p < 0.001$; Fig. 1). This decrease in the LI was correlated with a decrease in the biliary cholesterol from 8.84 ± 0.77 to 4.78 ± 0.43 mol% ($p < 0.001$). The increase in total bile acids from 74.01 ± 1.33 to 77.32 ± 1.26 mol% and that of lecithin from 17.10 ± 0.97 to 17.87 ± 1.02 mol% were not statistically significant. As expected, the total concentration of CDCA and UDCA increased significantly during dissolution therapy in both groups while decreases in the concentration of cholic acid and deoxycholic acid were statistically significant (Table 1).

The elevated levels of transaminases and serum cholesterol described in the literature were not observed in the present study. Serum enzyme levels glutamic oxaloacetic transaminase, glutamic pyruvic transaminase, apolipoproteins, GGT, bilirubin, amylase, cholesterol, high- and low-density lipoprotein cholesterol, triglycerides) showed no tendentially or statistically significant changes during the period of observation (Fig. 2). The nucleation time in the successfully treated group (4.7 ± 0.8 days) was significantly shorter

Fig. 2. Laboratory parameters in patients with complete dissolution (**a**, **c**, **e**, **g**) and those with incomplete dissolution (**b**, **d**, **f**, **h**). **a**, **b** Serum cholesterol, low-density lipoprotein (*LDL*) cholesterol, and high-density lipoprotein (*HDL*) cholesterol. **c**, **d** Serum triglyceride. **e**, **f** Serum glutamic oxaloacetic transaminase (*GOT*) and glutamic pyruvic transaminase (*GPT*). **g**, **h** alkaline phosphatase (*AP*) and gamma-glutamyl transpeptidase (*GGT*)

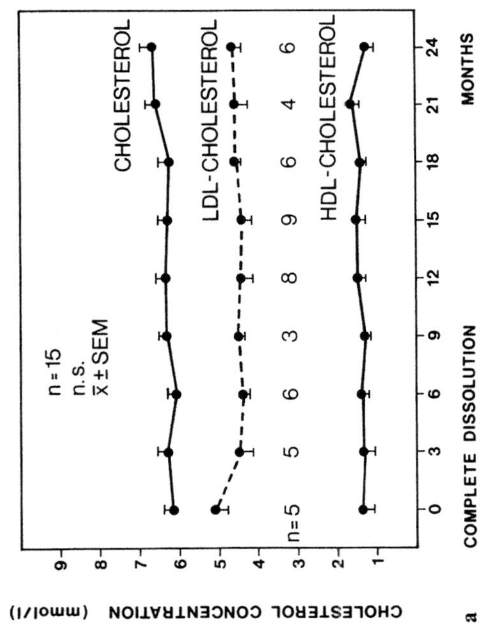
SERUM CHOLESTEROL CONCENTRATION (mmol/l)
n=15
n.s.
x̄ ± SEM
CHOLESTEROL
LDL-CHOLESTEROL
HDL-CHOLESTEROL
n=5 5 6 3 8 9 6 4 6
COMPLETE DISSOLUTION
MONTHS

2 a

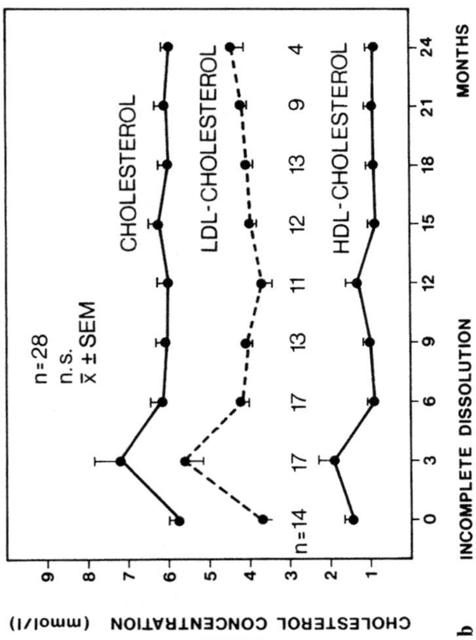
SERUM CHOLESTEROL CONCENTRATION (mmol/l)
n=28
n.s.
x̄ ± SEM
CHOLESTEROL
LDL-CHOLESTEROL
HDL-CHOLESTEROL
n=14 17 17 13 11 12 13 9 4
INCOMPLETE DISSOLUTION
MONTHS

2 b

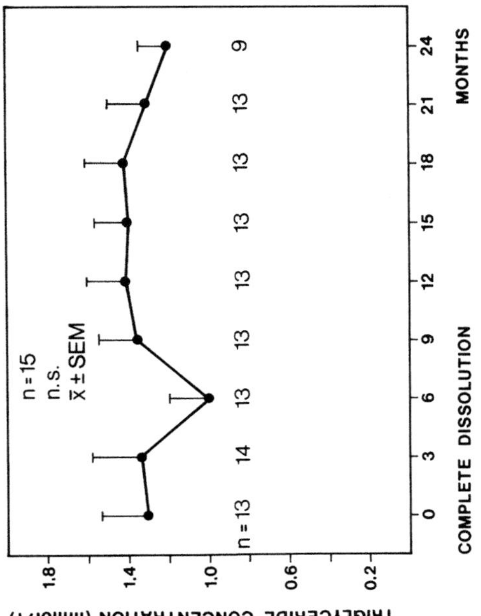
SERUM TRIGLYCERIDE CONCENTRATION (mmol/l)
n=15
n.s.
x̄ ± SEM
n=13 14 13 13 13 13 13 13 9
COMPLETE DISSOLUTION
MONTHS

2 c

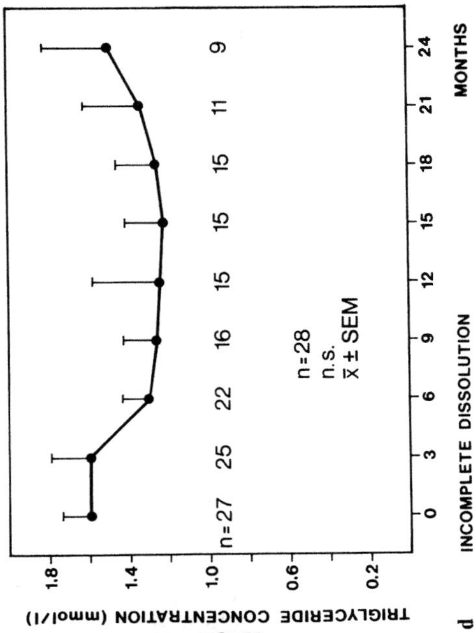
SERUM TRIGLYCERIDE CONCENTRATION (mmol/l)
n=28
n.s.
x̄ ± SEM
n=27 25 22 16 15 15 15 11 9
INCOMPLETE DISSOLUTION
MONTHS

2 d

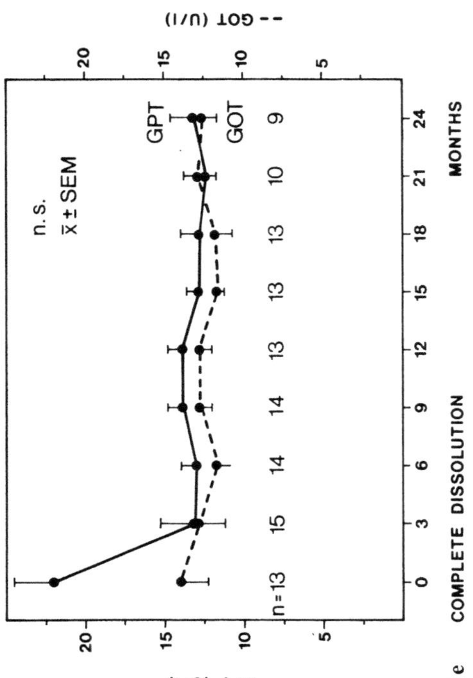
GPT (U/l)
GOT (U/l)
n.s.
x̄ ± SEM
GPT
GOT
n=13 15 14 14 13 13 13 10 9
0 3 6 9 12 15 18 21 24
COMPLETE DISSOLUTION
MONTHS

2e

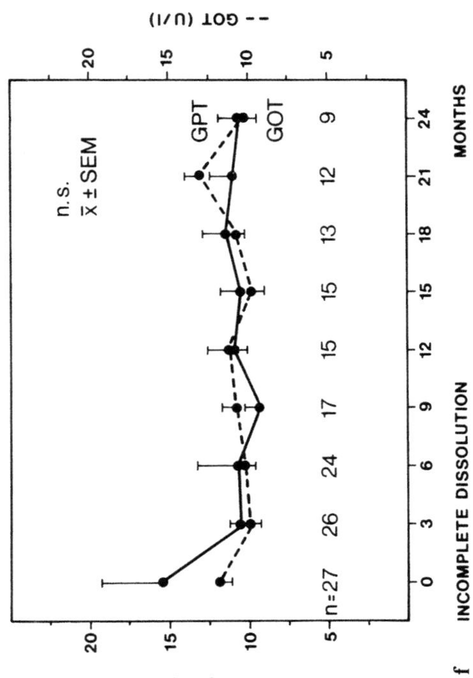
GPT (U/l)
GOT (U/l)
n.s.
x̄ ± SEM
GPT
GOT
n=27 26 24 17 15 15 13 12 9
0 3 6 9 12 15 18 21 24
INCOMPLETE DISSOLUTION
MONTHS

2f

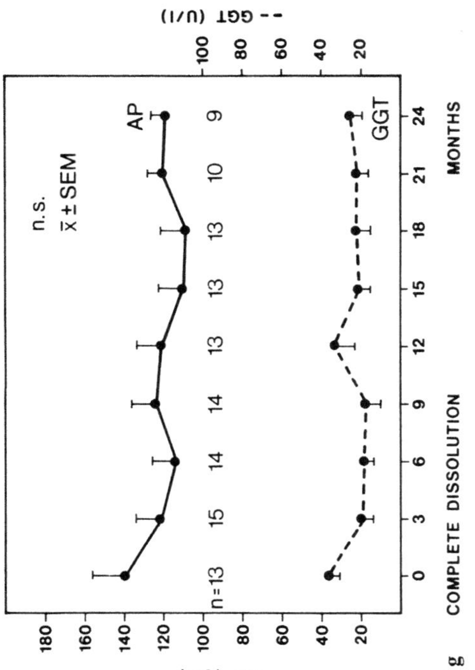
AP (U/l)
GGT (U/l)
n.s.
x̄ ± SEM
AP
GGT
n=13 15 14 14 13 13 13 10 9
0 3 6 9 12 15 18 21 24
COMPLETE DISSOLUTION
MONTHS

2g

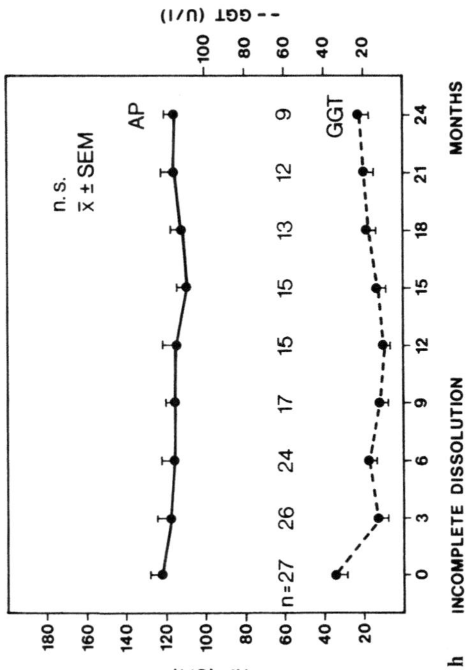
AP (U/l)
GGT (U/l)
n.s.
x̄ ± SEM
AP
GGT
n=27 26 24 17 15 15 13 12 9
0 3 6 9 12 15 18 21 24
INCOMPLETE DISSOLUTION
MONTHS

2h

Table 1. Biliary bile acids (mol%) before and after dissolution therapy ($n=26$)

		Before treatment	After treatment	p
Cholic acid	Total	39.45 ± 9.45	8.86 ± 5.90	0.001
	Glyco-	26.75 ± 7.58	7.02 ± 4.62	0.001
	Tauro-	12.72 ± 6.19	1.83 ± 1.93	0.001
Chenodeoxycholic acid	Total	37.52 ± 9.78	46.89 ± 9.03	0.001
	Glyco-	27.68 ± 9.72	39.96 ± 7.97	0.001
	Tauro-	9.78 ± 3.47	6.88 ± 3.48	0.01
Deoxycholic acid	Total	20.38 ± 10.60	4.99 ± 3.67	0.001
	Glyco-	15.36 ± 8.52	4.01 ± 3.11	0.001
	Tauro-	4.92 ± 2.83	0.94 ± 1.12	0.001
Lithocholic acid	Total	0.81 ± 1.19	1.94 ± 2.14	0.05
	Glyco-	0.68 ± 1.03	1.70 ± 2.09	0.05
	Tauro-	0.13 ± 0.32	0.24 ± 0.33	NS
Ursodeoxycholic acid	Total	1.83 ± 2.32	37.29 ± 9.31	0.001
	Glyco-	1.59 ± 2.19	34.34 ± 9.66	0.001
	Tauro-	0.25 ± 0.57	2.94 ± 1.32	0.001

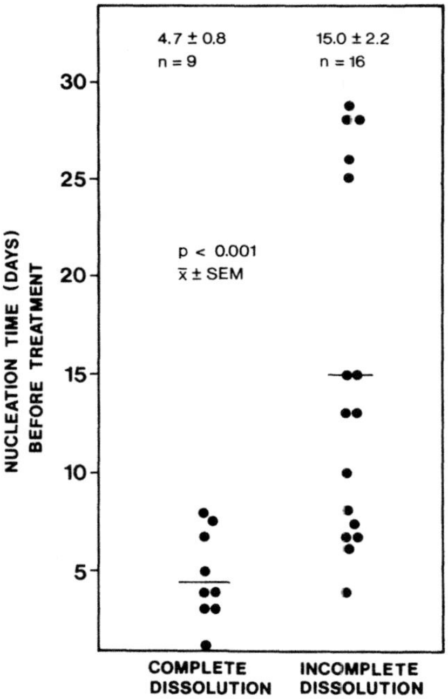

Fig. 3. Nucleation time. Distribution of cases

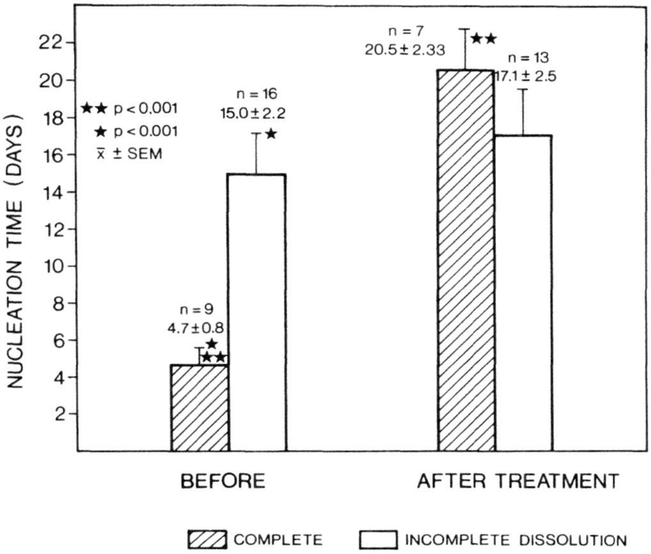

Fig. 4. Nucleation time. Mean values for those with complete and those with incomplete dissolution before and after dissolution therapy

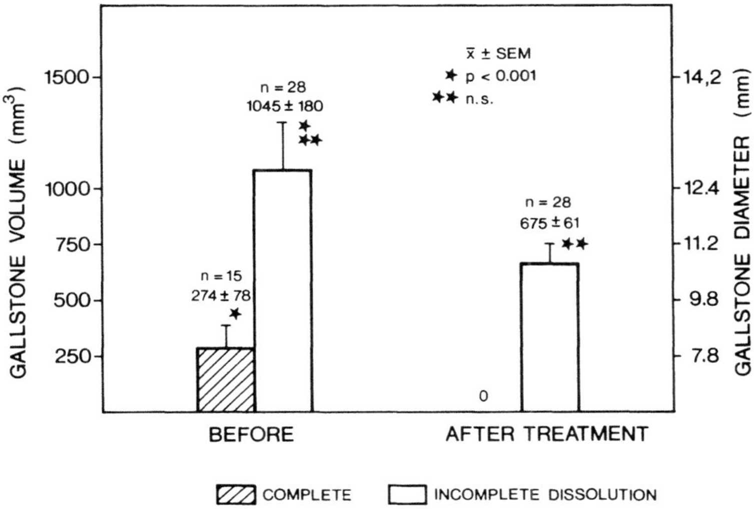

Fig. 5. Initial gallstone volume. Mean values for those with complete and those with incomplete dissolution before and after dissolution therapy

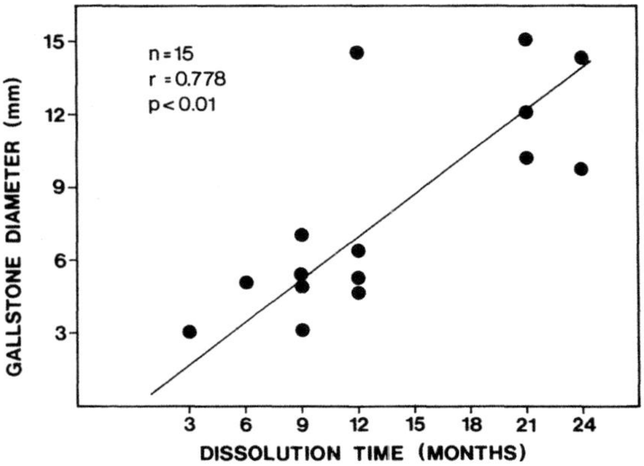

Fig. 6. Relationship between initial gallstone size and dissolution time

than that in the unsuccessfully treated group (15.0 ± 2.2 days; $p < 0.001$; Fig. 3). The biliary total lipid concentration was 5.61 ± 0.76 g/dl and thus well concentrated and reliable for determination of the nucleation time [26, 27]. The nucleation time increased in both groups after treatment (20.5 ± 2.33 days in the successfully treated group, $p < 0.001$; 17.1 ± 2.5 in the other group, n.s.; Fig. 4).

There were no statistically significant differences between patients with complete and incomplete stone dissolution in relation to age, mean body weight, or laboratory parameters. Initial stone volume was significantly smaller in the successfully treated group than in the unsuccessfully treated group (274 ± 78 mm^3 versus 1045 ± 180 mm^3; $p < 0.001$; Fig. 5). At termination of therapy after 24 months, the mean stone volume in the unsuccessfully treated group had been reduced to 675 ± 61 mm^3 (Fig. 5). This represents a decrease in volume of 35.4% and a decrease in median diameter of 13.5%. Figure 6 shows the statistically significant correlation between initial stone size and duration of successful dissolution therapy.

Discussion

Combination therapy with UDCA and CDCA led to complete dissolution of radiolucent gallstones in 27.3% of patients. Duration of therapy ranged from 3 to 24 months. The therapeutic dose of UDCA was 8.5–10.8 mg/kg body weight, and that of CDCA was 7.1–10.7 mg/kg body weight. Nine of the 15 successfully treated patients had an initial stone diameter between 3 and 7 mm. The remaining six had stone diameters between 10 and 15 mm. No instance of complete dissolution was observed in patients with stone diameters above 15 mm in the course of the 24 months of therapy.

These results support the widely accepted belief that oral cholelitholysis should be limited to patients with stone diameters of less than 15 mm. The stone volume of the successfully treated group (274 mm^3 or a diameter of about 8 mm) was significantly smaller than that of patients in whom only incomplete dissolution could be achieved (1045 mm^3 or a diameter of 12 mm; Fig. 5). The median volume reduction of 370 mm^3 (or a diameter of 9 mm) in the unsuccessfully treated group suggests that, at the abovementioned doses of UDCA and CDCA, the dissolution of all stones of a diameter under 9 mm could be achieved within 2 years. That this is, in fact, not the case is probably explained by the probability that many calcifications escape detection through conventional radiologic methods, and that an overly large proportion of mixed bilirubin stones were dissolved. Although the computed tomographic determination of Hounsfield units allows a differentiation of bilirubin and cholesterol stones, its use on a routine basis would greatly increase the total cost of oral cholelitholysis therapy [28, 29]. In another study on 31 patients with radiolucent gallstones, computed tomographic scan of the gallbladder revealed calcification in 17 cases (54.8%) in the form of thin shells or at the center of the stone, while 16.2% of these patients had bilirubin gallstones.

The determination of the lithogenic index as an additional selection criterion (LI > 1.0) did not yield appreciable benefits in the selection process. Although the average LI was lowered significantly from 1.54 ± 0.12 to 0.82 ± 0.06, there was no difference between responders and nonresponders either before or during the therapy period.

The nucleation time of patients with complete stone dissolution (4.7 ± 0.8 days) was significantly shorter than that of patients responding with only incomplete dissolution (15.0 ± 2.2 days; $p < 0.001$; Fig. 3). Determination of nucleation time as an additional selection criterion may lead to more effective patient selection. Patients with shorter nucleation time have cholesterol-containing, easily dissolvable stones, whereas those with a longer nucleation time probably have bilirubin stones or mixed stones with a high bilirubin content, which do not respond to oral cholelitholysis therapy [21, 27, 28, 30]. A final determination of the nucleation time above which patient selection should be conducted must be made through studies with a larger number of patients. In our patient group, the exclusion of patients with a nucleation time of over 8 days would have increased the efficiency of the oral cholelitholysis therapy by approximately 70%.

At the initiation of therapy, all 55 study subjects complained of upper abdominal pain and colic. This number was reduced to 12 of 55 after 6 months, 8 of 53 after 12 months, and 5 of 43 after 18 months. In other words, 88.3% of all patients became symptom free during the course of the combination therapy. The transient diarrhea observed in two patients resolved spontaneously without dose reduction within 3 months. We did not observe an increase in transaminases or serum cholesterol. Other laboratory values did not show any statistically significant or tendential changes. It is therefore possible to regard the combination therapy with UDCA and CDCA as essentially free of side effects.

The success of cholelitholysis therapy is heavily dependent on adequate patient selection methods. A difference between responders and nonresponders in our study could be observed only in the variables of initial stone size and nucleation time. This study lends support to the recommendation to attempt cholelitholysis therapy in cases of radiolucent stones with a diameter of under 15 mm. The question of whether or not computed tomographic evaluation or the determination of nucleation time could be useful as additional selection criteria must be investigated in appropriate studies.

Acknowledgements. We thank Mr. R. Mason and Mrs. H. Wenk for their assistance in preparing the manuscript.

References

1. Danzinger G, Hofmann AF, Schoenfiled LJ, Thistle JL (1972) Dissolution of cholesterol gallstones by chenodeoxycholic acid. N Engl J Med 286:1
2. Nakagawa S, Makino I, Ishizaki T, Dohi I (1977) Dissolution of cholesterol gallstones by ursodeoxycholic acid. Lancet II:367
3. Erlinger S, Go AL, Hüssen JM, Fevery J (1984) Franco-Belgian cooperative study of ursodeoxycholic acid in the medical dissolution of gallstones: a double-blind randomised, dose-response study and comparison with cheno-deoxycholic acid. Hepatology 4:308
4. Ighimi H, Carey MC (1981) Cholesterol gallstone dissolution in bile: dissolution kinetics of crystalline cholesterol with chenodeoxycholate, ursodeoxycholate and their glycine and taurine conjugates. J Lipid Res 22:254

5. Ponz de Leon M, Carulli N, Murphy GM, Dowling RH (1980) Intestinal solubilization, absorption, pharmacokinetics and bioavailability of chenodeoxycholic acid. Eur J Clin Invest 10:261
6. Thistle JL, Hofmann AL, Yu PYS, Ott B (1977) Effect of varying doses of chenodeoxycholic acid on bile lipid and biliary bile acid composition in gallstone patients: a dose-response study. Dig Dis 22:1
7. Schoenfield LJ, Lachin JM et al. (1981) Chenodiol (chenodeoxycholic acid) for dissolution of gallstones: the national cooperative gallstone study. A controlled trial of efficiacy and safety. Ann Intern Med 95:217
8. Koch MM, Giamperi MP, Lorenzini I, Jazequel AM, Orlandi F (1980) Effect of chenodeoxycholic acid on liver structure and function in man: a stereological and biochemical study. Digeston 20:8
9. Stiehl A, Ast E, Czygan P, Fröhling W, Kommerell B (1976) Zur Ursache erhöhter Serumtransaminasen nach Behandlung von Patienten mit Cholesteringallensteinen mit Chenodeoxycholsäure. Innere Medizin 3:75
10. Leiss O, v. Bergmann K, Streicher U, Strotkoetter H (1984) Effect of three different dihydroxy bile acids on intestinal cholesterol absorption in normal volunteers. Gastroenterology 87:144
11. Fromm H, Roat JW, Gonzalez V, Sarva RP, Farivar S (1983) Comparative efficacy and side effects of ursodeoxycholic and chenodeoxycholic acids in dissolving gallstones: a double-blind controlled study. Gastroenterology 85:1257
12. Raedsch R, Stiehl A, Walker S, Kommerell B (1982) Verkalkung von Cholesteringallensteinen unter Ursodeoxycholsäure-Behandlung. Z Gastroenterol 9:542 (Abstr 105)
13. Czygan P, Stiehl A, Raedsch R et al. (1985) Dissolution of cholesterol gallstones by a combination therapy of urso/cheno versus urso. In: Paumgartner G, Stiehl A, Gerok W (eds) Enterohepatic circulation of bile acids and sterol metabolism. MTP, Lancaster, pp 351–354
14. Podda M (1986) Die Kombinationsbehandlung von Gallenblasensteinen mit Ursodesoxycholsäure und Chenodesoxycholsäure. IXth international bile acid meeting, Basel, 1986
15. Roehrkasse R, Fromm H, Malavolti M, Tunuguntla AK, Ceryak S (1986) Gallstone dissolution treatment with a combination of chenodeoxycholic acid and ursodeoxycholic acid. Studies of safety, efficacy and effects on bile lithogenicity. Dig Dis Sci 31:1032
16. Podda M, Zuin M, Dioguardi ML, Festorazzi S, Dioguardi N (1982) A combination of chenodeoxycholic acid and ursodeoxycholic acid is more effective than either alone in reducing biliary cholesterol saturation. Hepatology 2:334
17. Bell CD, Whitney B, Dowling RH (1972) Gallstone dissolution in man using chenodeoxycholic acid. Lancet II:1213
18. Wechsler JG, Swobodnik W, Janowitz P, Tudyka J, Ditschuneit H (1988) Ergebnisse der Kombinationsbehandlung mit Cheno- und Ursodesoxycholsäure bei Cholecystolithiasis. Klin Wochenschr 66 [Suppl 13]:34
19. Stiehl A, Czygan P, Kommerell B et al. (1978) Ursodeoxycholic acid versus chenodeoxycholic acid. Comparison of their effects on bile acid and bile lipid composition in patients with cholesterol gallstones. Gastroenterology 75:1016
20. Reddy BS, Watanabe K, Weisburger JH, Tynder EL (1977) Promoting effect of bile acids in colon carcinogenesis in germ-free and conventional F 344 rats. Cancer Res 37:3238
21. Holan KR, Holzbach RT, Herrmann RE, Cooperman AM, Claffey WL (1979) Nucleation time: A key factor in the pathogenesis of cholesterol gallstone disease. Gastroenterology 77:611
22. Swobodnik W, Klüppelberg U, Wechsler JG, Volz M, Normandin G, Ditschuneit H (1985) Rapid and accurate reversed-phase high-performance liquid chromatographic determination of conjugated bile acids in human bile for routine clinical applications. J Chromatogr 339:263
23. Admirand WH, Small DM (1968) The physiochemical basis of cholesterol gallstone formation in man. J Clin Invest 47:1043
24. Carey MC (1978) Critical table for calculating the cholesterol saturation of native bile. J Res 19:945
25. Wechsler JG, Swobodnik W, Wenzel H, Heuchemer T, Nebelung W, Hutt V, Ditschuneit H (1984) Ballaststoffe vom Typ Weizenkleie senken die Lithogenität der Galle. Dtsch Med Wochenschr 109:1248
26. Kibe A, Dudley MA, Halpern Z, Lynn MP, Breuer AC, Holzbach RT (1985) Factors affecting cholesterol monohydrate crystals nucleation time in model systems of supersaturated bile. J Lipid Res 26:1102

27. Erpecum VKJ, van Berge-Henegouwen GP, Stoelwinder B, Stolk MFJ, Eggink WF, Govaert WHA (1988) Cholesterol and pigment gallstone disease: comparison of the reliability of three bile tests for differentiation between the two stone types. Scand J Gastroenterol 23(8):948
28. Hickmann MS, Schweisinger WH, Bova JD, Kurtin WE (1986) Computer tomographic analysis of gallstones. Arch Surg 121:289
29. Rambow A, Staritz M, Wosiewitz U, Mildenberger P, Meyer zum Büschenfelde KH (1988) Computertomographische Analyse von Gallensteinen: ein unverzichtbarer Selektionsparameter vor oraler Litholyse. Klin Wochenschr 66:34 (abstr)
30. Janowitz P, Wechsler JG, Swobodnik W, Fischer S, Klüppelberg U, Ditschuneit H (1987) Untersuchungen zur Beurteilung der Lithogenität der Galle. Klin Wochenschr 65:124 (abstr)

Extracorporeal Shock-Wave-Lithotripsy

Physical Basis of Lithotriptors

U. Faust

Institut für Biomedizinische Technik, Universität Stuttgart, Seidenstr. 36, D-7000 Stuttgart 1, FRG

Introduction

I will proceed from the assumption that the readers are familiar with the principles of the application of ultrasound as a diagnostic tool. A mechanical impulse produced by a piezoceramic transducer, which is excited by an electrical impulse, enters the body and is reflected by inhomogeneities within the acoustic field. These reflections are received by the same transmitter and are transformed back into an electrical signal, which is rectified and coded to the intensity of the screen. Moving the weakly focused ultrasound beam, we generate a cross-sectional image of the inhomogeneities of the body. The inhomogeneous structure is therefore very important for the reciprocation of ultrasound. We calculate on the basis of a unique traveling velocity of the impulse and transform the traveling time into a distance [7].

The velocity (c_0) of the acoustic wave depends on the properties of the material, its density (ϱ_0), and elasticity (E) for solid materials or compressibility (K) for fluids:

$$c_0 = (E/\varrho_0)^{\frac{1}{2}} \quad \text{or} \quad c_0 = (K/\varrho_0)^{\frac{1}{2}}$$

where E is defined as pressure divided by relative change of length and K is defined as pressure divided by relative change of volume.

In fact, a wave of compression and decompression is propagated. It is accompanied by a density and a temperature wave. If the generator has a sinusoidal excitation, these waves also follow a sinusoidal function (Fig. 1). This equation holds for a one-dimensional propagation in a loss-free medium. Table 1 demonstrates the relationships among the various mechanical parameters, with A representing the displacement of a mass

Table 1. Relationships among various oscillation parameters in a plane sinusoidal acoustic wave: $A = A_{max} \sin(\omega t - kx + \phi)$; $k = \omega/c_0$

Physical quantity	Symbol	Unit	Amplitude	Phase
Particle displacement	ξ	m	v_{max}/ω	$-\Pi/2$
Particle velocity	v	m/s	v_{max}	0
Particle acceleration	a	m/s^2	ωv_{max}	$+\Pi/2$
Pressure	p	$Pa = N/m^2$	$\varrho_0 c_0 v_{max}$	0
Density	ϱ_0	g/cm^3	$\varrho_0 v_{max}/c_0$	0
Relative deformation	s	–	v_{max}/c_0	0
Energy/volume*	W	J/cm^3	$\varrho_0 v_{max}^2$	0
Intensity/area*	I	W/cm^2	$\varrho_0 c_0 v_{max}^2$	0

* Energy and intensity are a function of $\sin^2$; their mean or effective values are calculated by multiplying the maximum amplitude by 0.5.

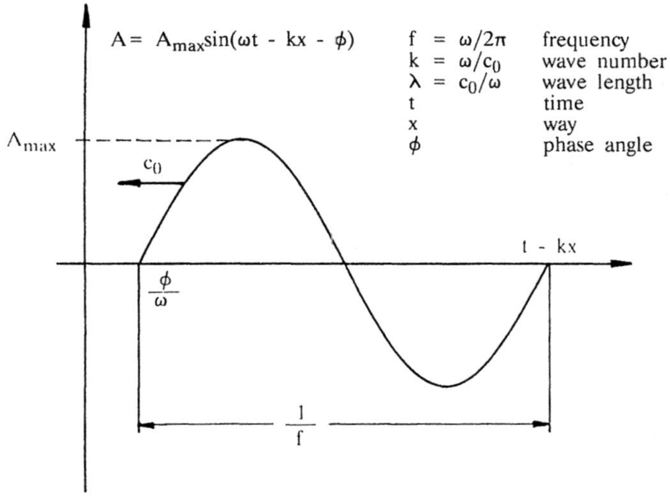

Fig. 1. Loss-free sinusoidal wave traveling with the velocity c_0 in direction x

Table 2. Values calculated from Table 1 for a sinusoidal excitation in distilled and degassed water under standard atmosphic conditions

p_{max} Pa	ξ_{max} (m)	v_{max} (m/s)	a_{max}/g	$\frac{\varrho_{max}-\varrho_0}{\varrho_0}$	W (J/cm^3)	I (W/cm^2)
10^4	1.1×10^{-9}	6.7×10^{-3}	$4.3\times10^{+3}$	4.5×10^{-6}	4.5×10^{-8}	6.7×10^{-3}
10^6	1.1×10^{-7}	6.7×10^{-1}	$4.3\times10^{+5}$	4.5×10^{-4}	4.5×10^{-4}	$6.7\times10^{+1}$
10^8	1.1×10^{-5}	$6.7\times10^{+1}$	$4.3\times10^{+7}$	4.5×10^{-2}	4.5×10^{0}	$6.7\times10^{+5}$

$f=1$ MHz; $\varrho_0=0.998$ g/cm^3; $c_0=1490$ m/s; $g=9.81$ m/s^2

point, its velocity, acceleration, the density, deformation, pressure, and energy. Given, for example, the pressure (p) or intensity (I) and the frequency (f), all other parameters can be calculated if the density and elasticity or compressibility of the material are known. Considering a sinusoidal excitation of 1 MHz in degassed and distilled water, we can calculate values for the mechanical parameters. The presumption is that there exists a plane wave front, and that the behavior of the medium is linear. This means that force and displacement are proportional. The pressure or intensity range (Table 2) contains diagnostic applications at the lower energy level and therapeutic applications at the higher level. As can be seen from these values, pressure and intensity are in a quadratic relationship. The acceleration of particles is related to gravity and rises to very high values.

Shock Wave Generation

We know that the linear approximation does not hold for pressure values above 1 MPa. In using a second-order approximation between the pressure or force applied and the relative compressibility of the material, we have a theory to describe the generation of shock waves [10].

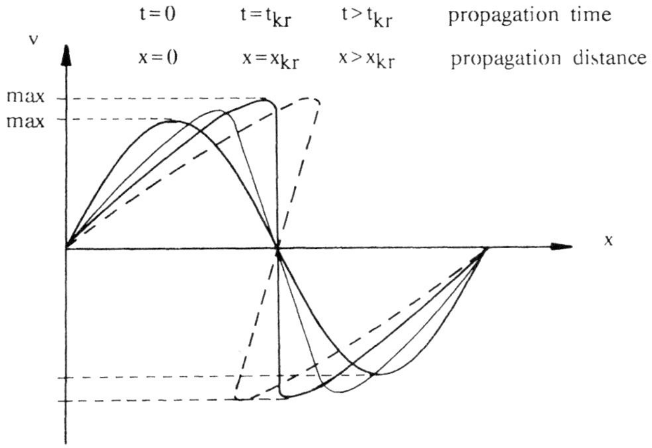

Fig. 2. Loss-free propagation of a plane acoustic wave with sinusoidal excitation at $x=t=0$. Nonlinear effects occurring at high pressure amplitudes. The wave is distorted. After a propagation time (t_{kr}) or distance (x_{kr}) a critical value is reached. (See [10], p. 96)

Although the propagation of the acoustic wave is at a level much higher than the velocity of the point oscillation, we can take their sum or difference into account and find an evident explanation. The velocity of propagation is higher than c_0 during the positive pressure phase and lower during the negative phase. As a consequence the front of the wave becomes steeper and the back flatter during the propagation. After a certain wave length – depending on the pressure amplitude and the frequency – a critical value is reached. The wave looks like a tooth saw (Fig. 2). All shock waves are followed by a negative pressure wave. If no loss of energy occurs, the pressure amplitude of the shock wave increases during its formation. Beyond this point this simple theory no longer holds. The loss of energy due to nonadiabatic conditions, the generation of shear waves, and other factors must be taken into consideration. If not, instability is the result, as can be seen in Fig. 2. At an identical point three different pressures must exist at the same time, which is physically impossible. With the distortion of the sinusoidal wave which takes place the energy is transferred to higher harmonics.

When using an exciting impulse with a frequency of 10 MHz and an intensity of 5 W/cm^2, the critical distance in water rises to 5 cm, which is about 30 times the wave length.

Generating the ultrasound impulse by an underwater explosion, for example, a shock wave is generated immediately. Very high pressure amplitudes exist, accompanied by nonlinear conditions from the beginning. Using other generators, where the pressure amplitude is not as high, the pressure increases by superimposition when employing a focusing device. The shock wave is formed during the propagation in the surroundings of the focus and is full developed in the focus. In the further course the shock wave is destroyed by dissipation processes and energy absorption.

Boundary Surfaces

Special conditions exist on boundary surfaces of two different media. These are characterized by their acoustic impedance and their propagation velocity. Both depend on the density and on the elasticity of the material or an the compressibility in case of fluids.

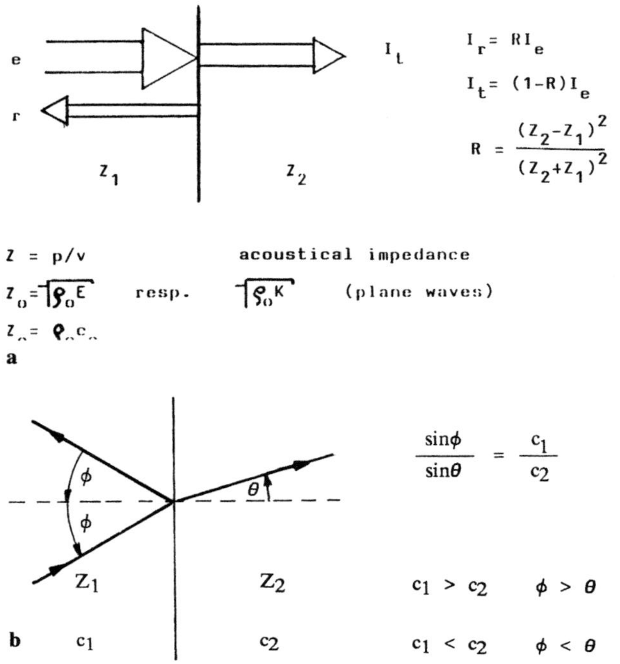

Fig. 3. **a** Reflected and transmitted energy are dependent on the acoustic impedance of both materials. In a field of plane waves it has a real value, in other cases it is a complex value. **b** Diffraction occurs if the incident acoustic beam forms an angle with the perpendicular

The incident acoustic wave is partly reflected. The portion of reflected energy can be calculated by multiplying the incident energy by the coefficient of reflection (R) and the transmitted part by multiplying it by the factor of $1-R$ (Fig. 3a). The reflected or transmitted nonenergetic parameters, such as pressure, must be calculated by multiplying the input values by $R^{1/2}$ or by $(1-R)^{1/2}$. If the acoustic impedance (Z_1) is less than Z_2, the pressure of these reflected waves have the same sign as the incident, and they superimpose upon each other positively; if Z_1 is greater than Z_2, the reflected wave has a negative sign.

In soft tissues the reflected energy on such border surfaces is about 1%. From air to water there is a loss of over 99% and from water to gallstones one of about 10%. In the case of nonrectangular angles between the direction of the acoustic wave and the reflector plane the coefficient of reflection is also dependent on the incident angle. The direction of the reflected and transmitted waves is dependent on both acoustic velocities. This is described quantitively by Snellius's law (Fig. 3b) and the coefficient of reflection by:

$$R = \frac{(Z_2 \cos \Phi - Z_1 \cos \theta)^2}{(Z_2 \cos \Phi + Z_1 \cos \theta)^2} .$$

As with electromagnetic waves, the ultrasound waves produce a radiation pressure on boundary surfaces, characterized by the coefficient of reflection, acoustic velocity, and energy. This value, however, is very small compared with the alternating pressure amplitude generated by the oscillation. It is always directed from that medium with the lower acoustic impedance into that with the higher one, independently of the direction of the sound velocity.

Assuming a plane wave front and a border surface in this plane, we can calculate this radiation pressure on the surface if the coefficient of reflection and the acoustic velocity are known, by:

$$\Pi = \bar{I}[(1+R)\,c_{02} - (1-R)\,c_{01}]/c_{02}$$

where $\bar{I}$ is the effective energy. Using the transformation from Table 2, we obtain:

$$\frac{\Pi}{p} = \frac{v_{\max}}{2\,c_{02}}\,[(1+R)\,c_{02} - (1-R)\,c_{01}].$$

Looking at the values in Table 4 for $v_{\max}$ and assuming the maximum value for the expression in brackets, which is 1 for $R=1$, it is obvious that the quotient of the pressures is always very small. This is also true if one calculates using nonlinear properties of the medium, as is necessary with shock waves.

Cavitation

Cavitation is defined as the generation of cavities in a fluid. These are produced during the underpressure phase of the wave. The longer this condition exists, and the lower the pressure is, the more cavitation bubbles are produced. The existence of cavitation nuclei enhance this effect. The bubble is filled with saturated steam. During the compression phase it condenses. Pressure and temperature increase to very high levels immediately before the collapse of the bubble, which is accompanied by the generation of a secondary shock wave.

Theoretical considerations [10, p. 126–143] show that cavitation occurs in water if a negative pressure of 0.1–1 MPa and cavitation nuclei with a radius of 1.0–0.1 μm exist. This is in accordance with experimental results. Negative pressure of 100 MPa is necessary for nuclei which have a radius of only about 0.01 μm. This is in accordance with the theoretical limit for cavitation in calculations using the strength factor for water. The theory also yields values for the time interval in which the collapse of the bubbles takes place. For a negative pressure of 0.1 MPa and a nuclei radius of 1 μm it takes about 0.01 μs. Cavitation is accompanied by another effect, the acoustic streaming. From many experiments it is known that cavitation is generated in all existing lithotripters. Effects on aluminium foils have been demonstrated by Coleman et al. [3].

Measuring Devices

Microphones are used to measure pressure. These are called hydrophones in the case of measurements in fluids. It is not easy to produce such sensors with a high mechanical stability and the necessary short response time. The sensor material successfully used is a plastic foil, called PVDF, which shows the piezoelectric effect [4]. The calibration procedure is complicated. Therefore the results of many measurements are given in relative numbers. A new device proposed by Staudenraus and Eisenmenger [9] consists of a thin optical fiber. Its effect depends on the change in diffraction of the fluid as a function of the pressure (Fig. 4). These sensors determine the pressure without any delay. The device is small and can be sterilized. There is some hope that it can be used within the body.

Acoustic Wave Generation

For diagnostic application ultrasound is generated by the piezoelectric effect. By applying a high voltage to a cristalline material – in general, piezoceramics – a mechanical

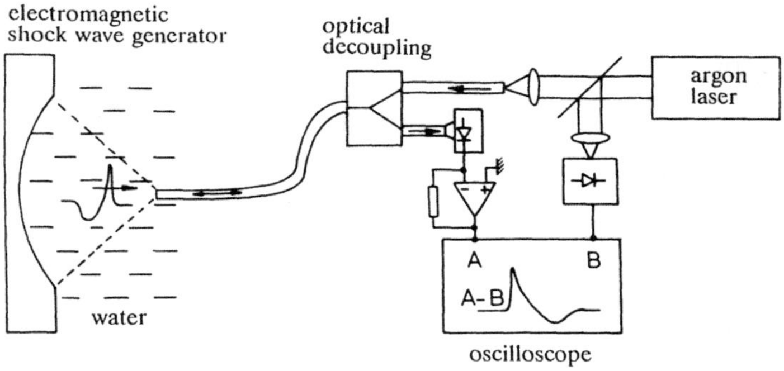

Fig. 4. Optical device for the delay-free measurement of pressure in fluids. It is based on the change of the fraction index as a function of the pressure. (From [9])

contraction or distraction occurs. To generate shock waves a multitransducer arrangement is used which has a focusing characteristic (Fig. 5a). Up to 3000 piezoelectric elements are located on a spherical shell. Another device uses the electromagnetic force which is generated by an electric current flowing through a flat coil. This current produces eddy currents in an isolated copper membrane opposite it (Fig. 5b). As a consequence the membrane is pushed off. Either by using shaped membranes or by an acoustical lens the wave is focused [5]. A third possibility is the use of explosives which directly generate a shock wave; this has been tried in Japan. The same principle is applied when generating an underwater spark discharge. When this is done in one focus of a spherical ellipsoid, the energy is concentrated in the other (Fig. 5c).

Through its course the generated acoustic impulse is distorted, as described above. With the electromagnetic or piezoelectric principle shock waves are not generated primarily at the transducer. In Fig. 6a the formation of shock waves becomes clear. With the increase in steepness the amplitude rises. Spark discharge generates primarily shock waves, as can be seen in Fig. 6b. Although the resolution of this measurement is insufficient, it can be supposed that the front becomes steeper because the amplitude increases, and the energy content must be constant in a loss-free medium, which does not really exist. For this device the local maximal pressure distribution within the focus is shown in Fig. 7. It is clear here that the focus is not a real point but is extended over an area of several square centimeters. In all principles described here – except that involving the use of explosives – the electrical energy to be applied is stored in a battery of condensers.

A comparison of characteristic properties of existing lithotriptors has been made [1, 4, 8] and the essential results are presented in Table 3. It can be seen here that there are essential differences in the amplitudes of positive and negative pressures as well as in the focus dimension.

Of great importance is the coupling of the acoustic energy to the body with a minimal loss of energy. No air bubbles between the shock wave applicator and surfaces in the patients are allowed. Usually a gel with the acoustic properties of water is applied between the applicator and the body, guaranteeing good coupling.

Adjustment of the Focus in the Stone

The adjustment of the stone in the focus of the device is a three-dimensional problem. It can be solved by using biplane imaging techniques. Either X-ray projections from two different directions or ultrasound cross-section imaging may be employed. The advan-

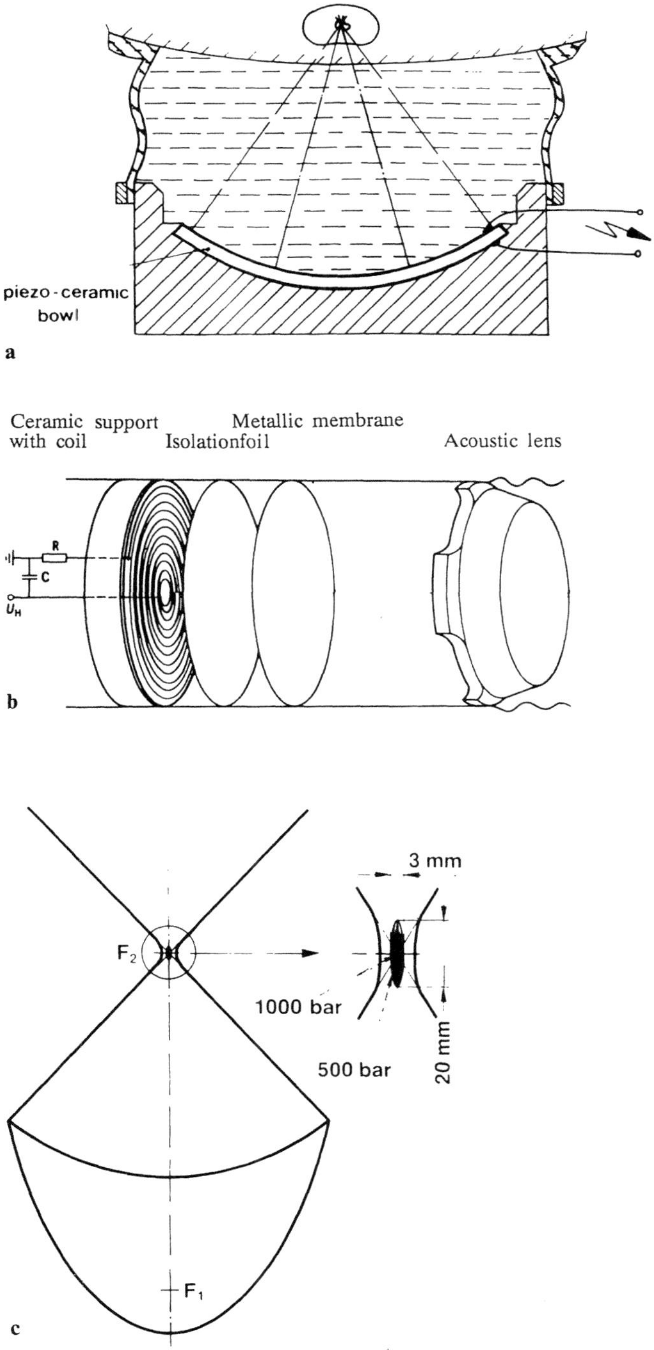

Fig. 5a–c. Principles of shock wave generators. **a** Piezoceramic multielement transducer on a spherical surface. **b** Electromagnetic transducers with a focusing lens. **c** Underwater spark discharge in one focus (F_1) of a spherical ellipsoid (1 bar $= 10^5$ Pa)

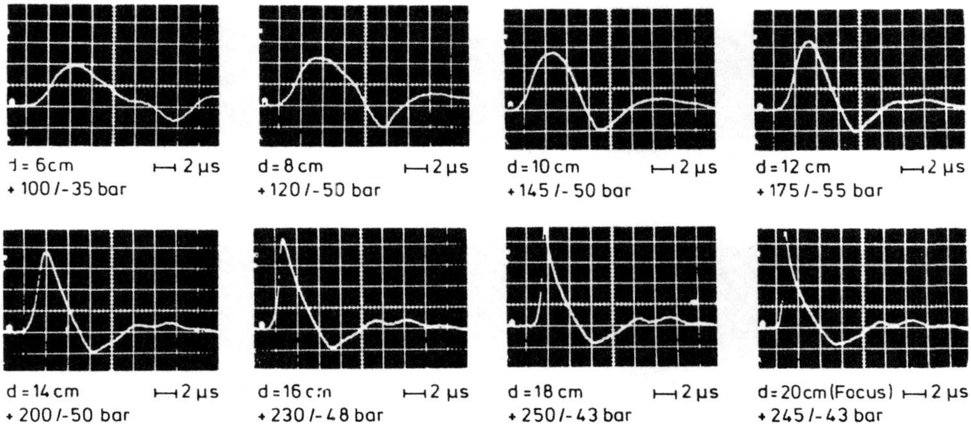

a

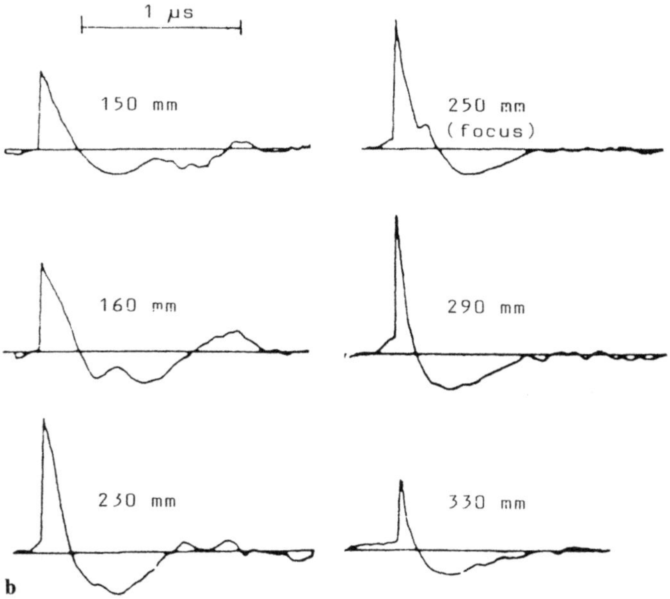

b

Fig. 6 a, b. Distortion of acoustic impulses as a function of distance. **a** Impulse generated by electromagnetic principle with a spherically shaped self-focusing membrane (1 bar = 10^5 Pa). **b** Impulse generated by spark discharge in one focus of spherical ellipsoid. Values represent distances from focus. The focal length is 250 mm [2]

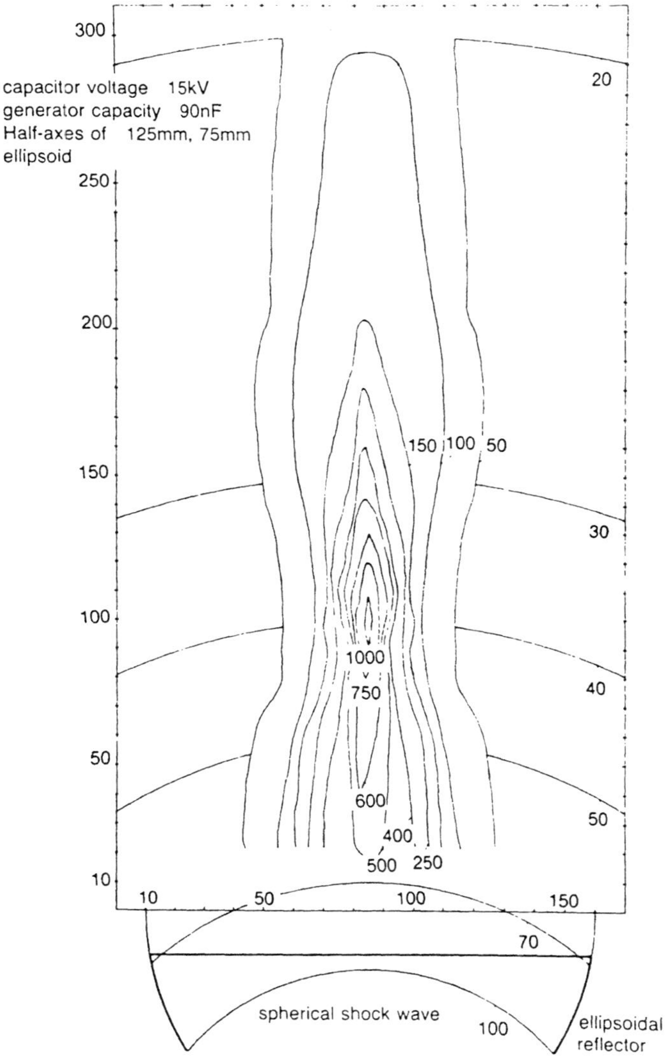

Fig. 7. Peak pressure distribution in the central plane of a spherical ellipsoid generated by spark discharge in water in one focus. Scaling of the axis is in millimeters; values of the isobars are $\times 10^5$ Pa. (From [6])

Table 3. Performance of second-generation lithotriptors. (From Coleman and Saunders [1])

Producer	Type	Working principle	Pressure peak MPa		Rise time (ns)	Focus dimension		Pressure gain [a]
			Positive	Negative		Axial (mm)	Radial (mm)	
Dornier	HM3	Spark discharge	38.6±9	9.5± 1	<30	12	2.1	10
Technomed	Sonolith 2000	Spark discharge	21.4±4	3.6± 0.5	50	16	2.4	1
Wolf	Piezolith 2200	Piezoelectric	62.5±3	9.5± 1	300	1.1	0.17	200
EDAP	LF 01	Piezoelectric	0–100	<10	600	2.0	0.5	100
Siemens	Lithostar	Electromagnetic	22	4	200	7.0	0.8	15

[a] Pressure gain is defined as the quotient of maximum pressure in the focus divided by that at the source

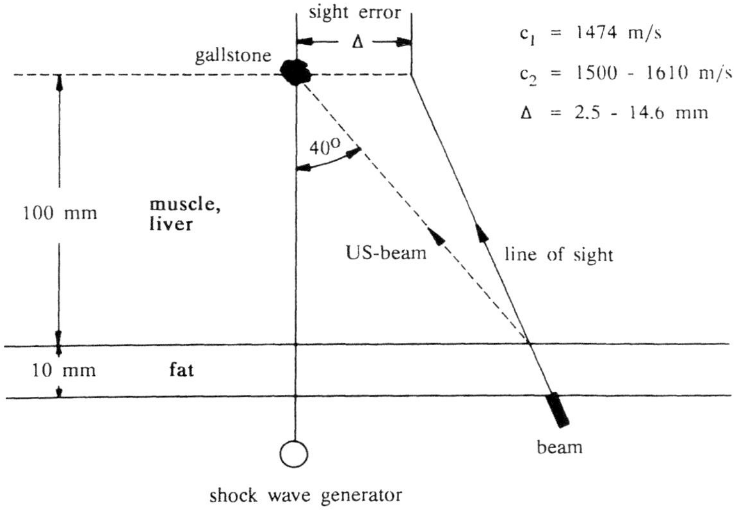

Fig. 8. Example of inaccuracy in ultrasonics. Deflection of the beam by border surfaces leads to a significant sighting error

tage of the ultrasound technique is that it is not destructive however this is compensated by the disadvantage that the beam is deflected at internal boundary surfaces (Fig. 3b). The beam must pass various tissues such as skin, fat, muscle, liver, and kidney under different angles. Each of these has different acoustic impedances and velocities. A typical arrangement of the transducers and the resulting sighting error are shown in Fig. 8. From experiments it is known that the sighting error can be as great as 20 mm.

Mechanical Properties of Gallstones

Gallstones can be characterized by their acoustic impedance and velocity. Studies on these properties have been carried out by us and others. It can be shown that their acoustic velocity and impedance differ remarkably from that of water, and that they differ among various types of stones. Results of our measurements are demonstrated in Table 4. The values for the pure cholesterol stone show only small differences to those for water.

Most of the stones are inhomogeneous. For example, the picture of a cross-section and the local acoustic velocity of a slice from the same plane of the stone are shown in Fig. 9. This type has been classified as a pigmented-calcified-cholesterol stone. The lines of constant velocity reflect the structure very well. The shell structure is evident.

The mechanisms of destruction are not yet well understood. A question now under discussion is which of the following effects is the most effective:

- The shock wave front when reaching the stone
- The shock wave front when leaving the stone
- The oscillations of the stone, excited by the shock impulse and the internal inhomogeneities
- The negative pressure phase following the shock wave
- The numerous secondary shock waves related to the cavitation

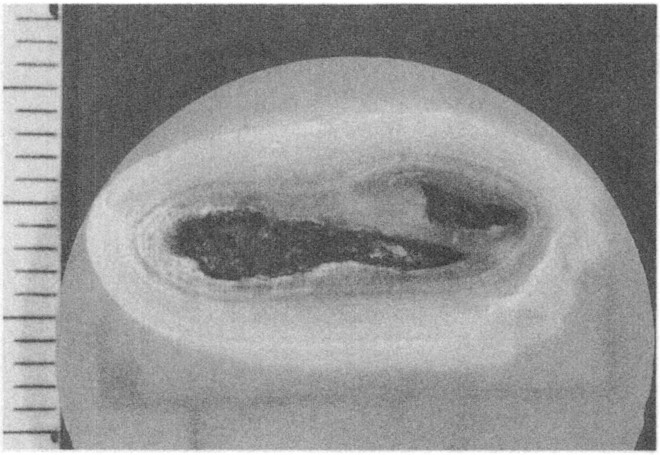

a

b

2,44	2,44	2,44	2,44	2,44	2,43	2,44	2,43	2,42	2,44	2,44
2,44	2,44	2,45	2,44	2,41	2,40	2,39	2,37	2,37	2,37	2,36
2,45	2,45	2,45	2,43	2,41	2,38	2,35	2,34	2,34	2,34	2,33
2,46	2,42	2,37	2,34	2,28	2,27	2,27	2,29	2,28	2,28	2,28
2,45	2,42	2,39	2,20	2,18	2,16	xxxx	xxxx	xxxx	xxxx	xxxx
2,36	2,19	2,14	xxxx	1,92	1,88	1,86	1,83	2,14	xxxx	xxxx
2,42	2,35	2,20	2,15	2,11	xxxx	xxxx	xxxx	xxxx	xxxx	xxxx
2,38	2,37	2,29	2,22	xxxx	1,87	1,71	1,96	1,95	xxxx	xxxx
1,50	1,51	2,45	2,43	2,37	2,31	2,27	2,25	2,23	2,21	xxxx
1,50	1,51	1,50	1,50	1,50	1,51	2,44	2,45	2,45	2,37	2,31
xxxx	xxxx	xxxx	xxxx	xxxx	xxxx	xxxx	2,42	2,40	2,36	2,35
1,50	1,51	1,51	1,47	1,51	1,52	2,43	2,42	2,42	2,42	2,41

2,43	2,42	2,43	2,42	2,43	2,41	2,43	2,44	2,44	2,44	2,44
2,38	2,36	2,37	2,36	2,36	2,37	2,37	2,38	2,41	2,42	2,42
2,33	2,33	2,33	3,34	2,35	2,36	2,35	2,36	2,41	2,42	2,45
2,27	2,27	2,28	2,27	2,27	2,27	2,26	2,26	2,29	2,26	2,31
xxxx	xxxx	1,70	2,18	xxxx	2,19	xxxx	xxxx	xxxx	2,18	2,20
xxxx	xxxx	1,80	2,01	1,93	2,31	1,62	2,51	xxxx	xxxx	xxxx
xxxx	xxxx	1,85	1,79	1,63	2,28	2,43	xxxx	xxxx	2,38	2,34
xxxx	xxxx	1,86	2,13	1,98	xxxx	xxxx	2,21	2,22	2,25	2,29
xxxx	xxxx	xxxx	xxxx	xxxx	2,22	2,22	2,24	2,26	2,27	2,27
2,28	2,27	2,26	2,27	2,27	2,27	2,28	2,27	2,27	2,29	2,33
2,34	2,35	2,35	2,35	2,35	2,39	2,37	2,39	2,40	2,41	2,42
2,42	2,42	2,41	2,41	2,40	2,39	2.39	2,36	2,37	2,38	2,38

Fig. 9 a, b. Calcified pigmented cholesterol (pearl) stone. **a** Photograph of a cross section. **b** Acoustic velocity in a slice; values represent the velocity (km/s); *lines* connect points of identical velocity

Table 4. Measured values for density, acoustic velocity, acoustic impedance, and reflectivity of various types of gallstones

Type of stone	Density (g/cm^3)	Acoustic velocity (m/s)	Acoustic impedance [10^6 kg/(m^2 s)]	Reflectivity in water
Cholesterol	1.11	1679	1.9	0.01
CPC, pearl	1.06	2267	2.4	0.05
CPC	1.35	2273	3.1	0.12
CPC, faceted	1.06	2277	2.4	0.05
Pigment	1.47	2112	3.1	0.12
Water	0.998	1490	1.5	0.00

CPC, calcified-pigmented-cholesterol

Further questions have also been raised for which answers are not yet available. Therefore research is necessary to understand this mechanism better. Such research may help to identify the "ideal" shock wave form which would produce small fractions of the stones with a minimum of pain and other side effects.

References

1. Coleman AJ, Saunders JE (1987) Comparison of extracorporeal shock-wave lithotripters. In: Coptcoat M, Miller RA, Wichham FJ (ed) Lithotripsy II. BDI Publishing, London
2. Coleman AJ, Saunders JE, Preston RC, Bacon DR (1987) Pressure waveforms generated by a Dornier extracoporeal shock-wave lithotripter. Ultrasound Med Biol 13 (10):651–657
3. Coleman AJ, Saunders JE, Crum LA, Dyson M (1987) Acoustic cavitation generated by an extracorporeal shockwave lithotripter. Ultrasound Med Biol 13 (2):69–76
4. Eisenmenger W (1988) Methoden der Stoßwellenerzeugung und -messung. Biomed Tech 33 [Suppl 2]:1–6
5. Heine G (1987) Alternative Stoßwellenerzeugungsverfahren. In: Ziegler M (ed) Die extrakorporale und laserinduzierte Stoßwellenlithotripsie bei Harn- und Gallensteinen. Springer, Berlin Heidelberg New York
6. Heine G (1986) Physical aspects of shock wave treatment. In: Gravenstein JS, Peter K (eds) Extracorporeal shock-wave lithotripsy for renal stone disease. Butterworth, Boston
7. Hill CR (1986) Physical principles of medical ultrasonics. Ellis Horwood, London
8. Rassweiler J, Westhauser A, Bub P, Eisenberger F (1988) Second-generation lithotripters: a comparative study. J Endourol 2 (2):193–202
9. Staudenraus J, Eisenmenger W (1988) Optisches Sondenhydrophon. Biomed Tech 33 [Suppl 2]:105–106
10. Sutilov VA (1984) Physik des Ultraschalls. Springer, Vienna New York

Extracorporeal Shock-Wave Lithotripsy of Gallstones

G. Paumgartner, M. Sackmann, J. Holl, and T. Sauerbruch

Department of Medicine II, Klinikum Grosshadern, University of Munich, D-8000 Munich 70, FRG

The success rate of gallstone dissolution by oral bile acid treatment has been limited by stone size [1, 2]. Even in patients in whom dissolution therapy is effective it takes a relatively long time until the stones are completely dissolved. Therefore, a method for fragmentation of gallstones by extracorporeally generated shock waves has been developed by an interdisciplinary group at the Grosshadern Clinic in Munich in cooperation with Dornier Medizintechnik [3–5]. In 1985 we treated the first patients with gallstones by extracorporeal shock-wave lithotripsy. Since then, more than 500 patients with gallbladder stones and more than 80 patients with bile duct stones have been treated by this novel therapeutic modality in our hospital.

The lithotriptor used by our group is the model MPL 9000 of Dornier. In this lithotriptor the shock waves are generated by underwater spark discharge. The electrode is located in one focus of an ellipsoidal metal reflector and the stone in the other focus (Fig. 1). The shock waves are transmitted into the body by a compressible water bag which is interfaced with the skin by an ultrasonic coupling gel. When they hit the stone, energy is liberated due to a change in acoustic impedance and to cavitation phenomena on the surface of the stone. These mechanisms lead to stone destruction.

Gallbladder Stones

In general, the patient is treated in the prone position. The shock waves enter the abdomen from the ventral side. Ultrasound is used for location of the stones, positioning

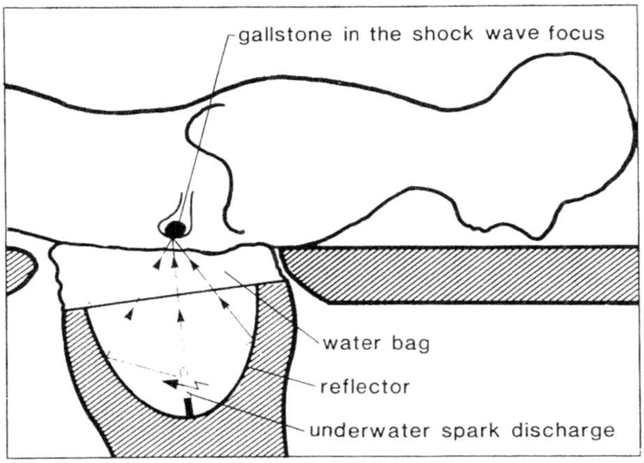

Fig. 1. Shock-wave lithotripsy device

of the patient, targeting, and monitoring of the process of fragmentation. Since our first report on extracorporeal shock-wave lithotripsy of gallbladder stones [3], general and peridural anesthesia have been abandoned. In 1988 about half of treatments were performed under intravenous analgesia with alfentanil [6] and the rest without medication.

Even fragments smaller than 3 mm in diameter cannot be expected to be entirely discharged from the gallbladder. Many patients with gallstone disease have a motility defect of the gallbladder [7, 8], which may be responsible for the long residence time of fragments in the gallbladder in some patients. Therefore, we have combined extracorporeal shock-wave lithotripsy of gallbladder stones with oral bile acid treatment and have selected only patients with radiolucent stones. All patients received adjuvant litholytic therapy consisting of a combination of ursodeoxycholic acid (7–8 mg/kg per day) and chenodeoxycholic acid (7–8 mg/kg per day) given as a single bedtime dose [4, 9].

Patients with gallbladder stones were selected for treatment according to the criteria listed in Table 1. About 20% of the patients seen in our Department were eligible according to these selection criteria. More than 500 patients have been treated in our hospital. In 97% of these patients the stones could be fragmented. Fragmentation efficacy was related to the size and the number of stones. In patients with solitary stones less than 20 mm in diameter, 88% of the patients had fragments with a diameter of 3 mm or smaller. By contrast, only 63% of patients with solitary stones 21–30 mm in diameter and only 31% of the patients with two or three stones had fragments with a diameter of 3 mm or smaller.

The success rate, defined as complete clearance of fragments (stone clearance efficacy), also depended on the size and the number of stones. About 70% of patients with solitary stones smaller than 20 mm in diameter and 40% of patients with solitary stones 21–30 mm in diameter but only 20% of patients with two or three stones were free of fragments 4–8 months after lithotripsy. Twelve to 18 months after lithotripsy about 85% of patients with smaller solitary stones, 75% of patients with larger solitary stones, and 60% of patients with two or three stones were free of fragments.

Adverse effects directly related to shock-wave lithotripsy were minimal. In less than 10% of patients petechiae were seen on the skin at the site of shock-wave entry. Three percent of patients had transient gross hematuria.

Thirty-seven percent of patients reported one or more episodes of biliary colic. Once the gallbladder was free of fragments, no more attacks of biliary pain were observed. Passage of stone fragments caused mild pancreatitis in about 1% and cholestasis in about 0.5% of our patients. These complications occurred weeks to months after lithotripsy in patients who still harbored fragments in their gallbladder. Only rarely, endoscopic

Table 1. Selection of patients with gallbladder stones for extracorporeal shock-wave lithotripsy

Inclusion criteria
History of biliary pain
Solitary radiolucent stone with a diameter up to 30 mm or two to three radiolucent stones with similar total stone volume
Gallbladder visualization by oral cholecystography
Exclusion criteria
Acute cholecystitis or cholangitis
Biliary obstruction or bile duct stone
Acute pancreatitis
Coagulopathy or current medication with anticoagulant effects
Vascular aneurysms in the shock-wave path
Pregnancy

sphincterotomy was necessary to remove prepapillary stone fragments from the common duct. In only a small percentage of patients was elective cholecystectomy necessary because of insufficient stone fragmentation and/or incomplete clearance of fragments within a follow-up period of about 2 years [10]. No emergency operations were necessary. No short-term or long-term effects of extracorporeal shock-wave lithotripsy on gallbladder motility could be detected [8].

Actuarial analysis showed that the risk for stone recurrence was 11% per year in the 1st year after stopping bile acid treatment [11]. It appeared to level out in the 2nd and 3rd years.

Bile Duct Stones

Patients with bile duct stones were treated in a Dornier kidney lithotriptor in the supine position. The shock waves entered the body from the back. Fluoroscopy and retrograde filling of the bile ducts with X-ray contrast medium via a nasobiliary catheter were used to visualize the bile ducts and to position the calculi into the shock-wave focus [3, 12, 13]. Antibiotics were administered prophylactically prior to all recent treatments because of the risk of septic complications after shock-wave lithotripsy.

More than 80 patients with bile duct stones fulfilling the selection criteria listed in Table 2 have been treated by extracorporeal shock-wave lithotripsy in our hospital. Endoscopic procedures for extraction of the stones had failed in these patients because the stones were impacted or too large, or because a bile duct stenosis was present. About 75% of patients had extrahepatic and 25% intrahepatic stones. Stone clearance was achieved in 82% of patients. This result was achieved with a retreatment rate of about 20%. There were relatively few adverse effects or complications in these patients: 4% of the patients had transient hemobilia and 17% transient hematuria. In one patient a septic cholecystitis that required cholecystectomy developed after shock-wave lithotripsy. Two other complications were related to the endoscopic procedure rather than to the shock-wave treatment. In a multicenter study conducted by Sauerbruch and Stern [13] including 113 patients with bile duct stones similar results were obtained. Fragmentation efficacy was 91% and stone clearance efficacy 86% after one or more lithotripsy sessions. Thirty-day mortality was 0.9%. Thus, complications and mortality after extracorporeal shock-wave lithotripsy in these elderly patients are probably lower than after open abdominal surgery.

Fig. 2. Selection of patients with bile ducts stones for extracorporeal shock-wave lithotripsy

Inclusion criteria

Failure of routine endoscopic measures including mechanical lithotripsy
Access to the bile ducts via nasobiliary tube or transhepatic catheter
Orifice of the common bile duct in the intestine large enough for spontaneous passage or extraction of fragments

Exclusion criteria

Coagulopathy or current medication with anticoagulant effects
Lung tissue, vascular aneurysms or bowel loops in the shock-wave path

References

1. Erlinger S, Le Go A, Husson JM et al. (1984) Franco-Belgian cooperative study of ursodeoxycholic acid in the medical dissolution of gallstones: a double-blind, randomized, dose-response study, and comparison with chenodeoxycholic acid. Hepatology 4:308–314
2. Podda M, Zuin M, Battezzati PM, Ghezzi C et al. (1989) Efficacy and safety of a combination of chenodeoxycholic acid and ursodeoxycholic acid for gallstone dissolution: a comparison with ursodeoxycholic acid alone. Gastroenterology 96:222–229
3. Sauerbruch T, Delius M, Paumgartner G et al. (1986) Fragmentation of gallstones by extracorporeal shock waves. N Engl J Med 314:818–822
4. Sackmann M, Delius M, Sauerbruch T et al. (1988) Shock-wave lithotripsy of gallbladder stones: the first 175 patients. N Engl J Med 318:393–397
5. Paumgartner G (1987) Fragmentation of gallstones by extracorporeal shock waves. Semin Liver Dis 7:317–321
6. Sackmann M, Weber W, Delius M et al. (1987) Extracorporeal shock-wave lithotripsy of gallstones without general anesthesia: first clinical experience. Ann Intern Med 107:347–348
7. Pomeranz IS, Shaffer EA (1985) Abnormal gallbladder emptying in a subgroup of patients with gallstones. Gastroenterology 88:787–791
8. Spengler U, Sackmann M, Sauerbruch T et al. (1989) Gallbladder motility before and after extracorporeal shock wave lithotripsy. Gastroenterology 96:860–863
9. Paumgartner G, Sauerbruch T (1989) Lithotripsy of gallstones. In: Zakim D, Boyer TD (eds) Hepatology. A textbook of liver disease, 2nd edn. Saunders, Philadelphia
10. Teichmann RK, Sauerbruch T, Sackmann M et al. (1989) Surgical intervention following fragmentation of gallstones by extracorporeal shock waves. World J Surgery 13:317–320
11. Sackmann M, Ippisch E, Sauerbruch T et al. (1988) Early gallstone recurrence after successful shock-wave therapy. Hepatology 8:1221 (abstr)
12. Sauerbruch T, Holl J, Sackmann M et al. (1987) Treatment of bile duct stones by extracorporeal shock waves. Semin Ultrasound CT MR 8:155–161
13. Sauerbruch T, Stern M, The Study Group for Shock-Wave Lithotripsy (1989). Fragmentation of bile duct stones by extracorporeal shock waves. A new approach to biliary calculi after failure of routine endoscopic measures. Gastroenterology 96:146–152

Administration of Second-Generation Extracorporeal Shock Waves without Waterbath for Fragmentation of Extra- and Intrahepatic Bile Duct Stones

M. Staritz [1], A. Rambow [1], A. Floth [2], P. Mildenberger [3], M. Goebel [3], T. Junginger [4], R. Hohenfellner [3], M. Thelen [3], and K.-H. Meyer zum Büschenfelde [1]

[1] Medical Department I, [2] Urological Department, [3] Radiological Department, [4] Surgical Department, University of Mainz, Langenbeckstr. 1, D-6500 Mainz, FRG

Introduction

First-generation extracorporeal shock-wave sources disintegrate 97% of kidney stones [1, 2]. Recently, in selected patients gallbladder and common bile duct stones were also treated. The technique available so far, however, requires immersion of the patient's body in a tank of degassed water. The procedure is therefore inconvenient, time consuming, and relatively expensive. The high pressure of shocks (up to 1000 bar) generated by underwater spark discharge causes pain, and general anesthesia is necessary in most patients [3, 4].

Second-generation shock-wave devices do not require the use of a waterbath. New techniques for the generation of shock waves have been incorporated into these machines, for example, shock-wave generation by piezocrystals [5] or an electromagnetic coil [6] (Fig. 1). In our Department, a first-generation device (HM 3, Dornier, Munich, FRG) and a second-generation device (Lithostar, Siemens, Erlangen, FRG) were used simultaneously. Clinical experience in the treatment of kidney stones had proven the second-generation lithotriptor to be safe and effective in 97% of patients [6].

After successful in vitro disintegration of gallstones [7] we started treatment of patients with extra- and intrahepatic bile duct stones. The present paper reports on our clinical experience gathered during 51 treatments.

Methods

Patients and Patient Selection

Between October 1986 and December 1987 a total of 174 patients with common bile duct stones were admitted to our Department. Approximately half of these were preselected

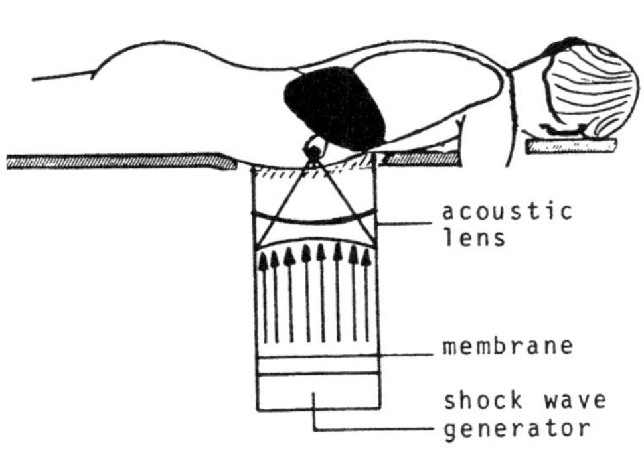

Fig. 1. Second-generation lithotriptor (Siemens Lithostar) generating shock wave energy by discharging an electromagnetic coil

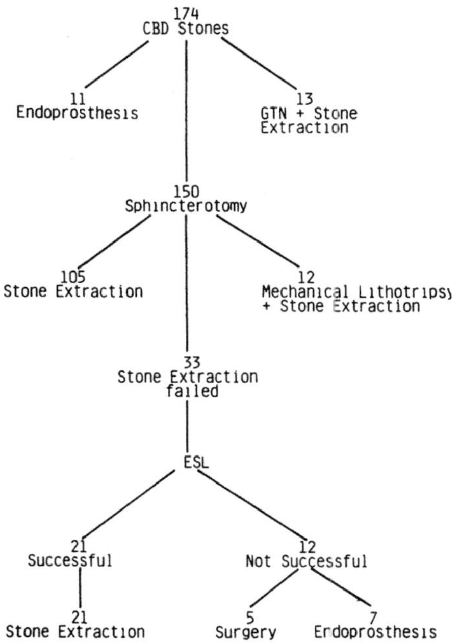

Fig. 2. Therapeutic experience with common bile duct (*CBD*) stones (Department of Medicin I, University of Mainz; October 1986 to December 1987). *ESL*, Extracorporeal shock-wave lithotripsy; *GTN*, glyceryl trinitate

by other gastroenterologists who considered endoscopic treatment of these patients to be too difficult or too risky to be performed in a municipal hospital.

Typical problems were intrahepatic calculi ($n = 4$), large or impacted bile duct stones, bile duct stenosis with concrements proximal to the stenosis, patients with juxtapapillary diverticulum and previous Billroth II resection of the stomach. Of 174 patients (Fig. 2) a total of 150 received conventional endoscopic sphincterotomy, 11 patients were treated by transpapillary endoprothesis because they were unfit for further procedures, and in 13 cases small calculi could be removed following nitroglycerin relaxation of the bile duct sphincter [8]. The remaining 33 patients, aged between 32 and 91 years, were treated by extracorporeal shock waves. They presented with bile duct stones which were too large (18–30 mm) to be snared by a Dormia probe or too hard for mechanical lithotripsy [9, 10]. In seven patients sphincterotomy was considered to be very risky due to juxtapapillary duodenal diverticulum ($n = 4$) or because of Billroth II resection (two-thirds resection) of the stomach ($n = 3$). Four patients had stones in the intrahepatic bile ducts which could not be removed endoscopically, and in whom our surgeon expected an operative approach to be risky, difficult, and presumably not successful.

Endoscopy, Computed Tomography, and Administration of Extracorporeal Shock Waves

In all patients endoscopic retrograde cholangio-pancreaticography (ERCP) was performed using standard techniques. Patients selected for lithotripsy underwent computed tomography to measure radiological stone density. During a second ERCP investigation a nasobiliary probe was advanced into the common bile duct for injection of contrast material (Rayvist, Schering, West Berlin). Prior to shock-wave lithotripsy patients received premedication with 10–15 mg diazepam and 100 mg tramadol (Tramal,

Grünenthal, Aachen, FRG). The concrements were visualized by two-dimensional fluoroscopy after injection of contrast material via the nasobiliary probe. Then, shock waves were applied continuously until stone disintegration was visible or up to a maximal number of 2500 discharges. If necessary, a second or third session of lithotripsy followed 1 day thereafter.

Endoscopic removal of the fragments was attempted in all patients 1 day after administration of shock waves. Endoscopy (ERCP) was also performed in patients without visible stone disintegration.

Follow-Up Investigations

All patients underwent follow-up investigations for at least 3 days after shock-wave administration. Follow-up consisted of an immediate physical examination, laboratory tests including serum glutamic oxaloacetic transaminase, serum glutamic pyruvic transaminase, alkaline phosphatase (AP), γ-glutamyl transpeptidase (gamma-GT), pancreas enzymes, lipase, amylase, and creatinin tests, complete blood count on the day of therapy and on the 1st and 2nd days, thereafter, ultrasonography of the abdomen, particularly of liver and pancreas, and chest X ray.

Results

Shock-Wave Lithotripsy

All patients tolerated shock-wave lithotripsy very well. No complications caused by endoscopies or administration of extracorporeal shock waves were observed. Intrahepat-

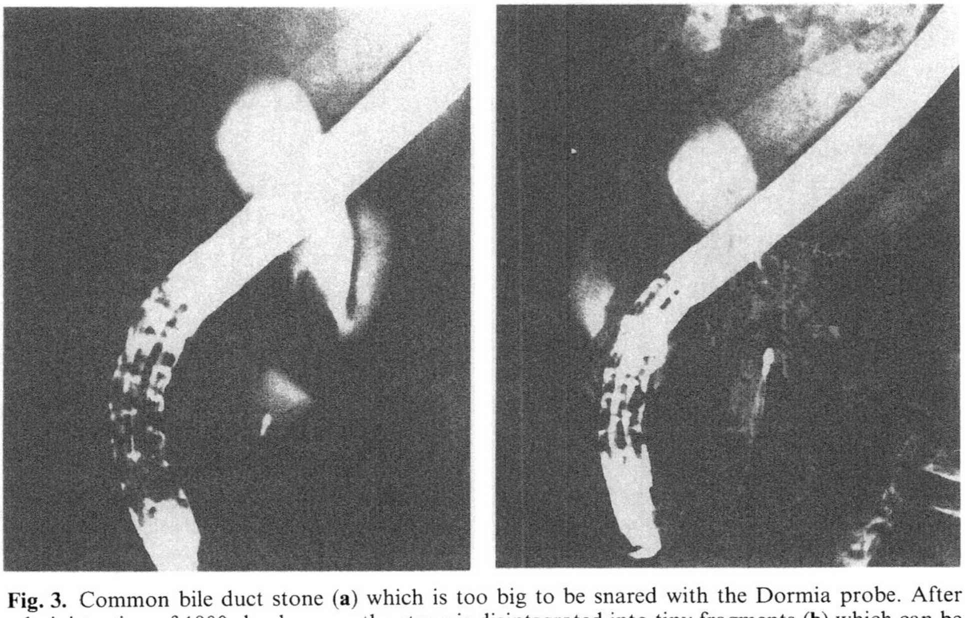

a b

Fig. 3. Common bile duct stone (**a**) which is too big to be snared with the Dormia probe. After administration of 1800 shock waves the stone is disintegrated into tiny fragments (**b**) which can be removed easily by a Dormia probe

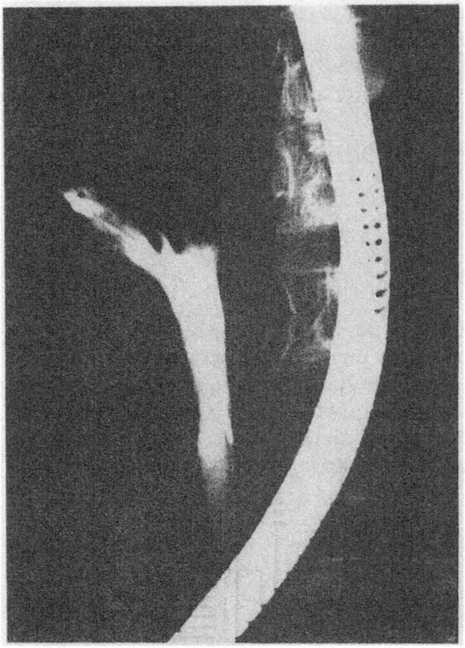
a

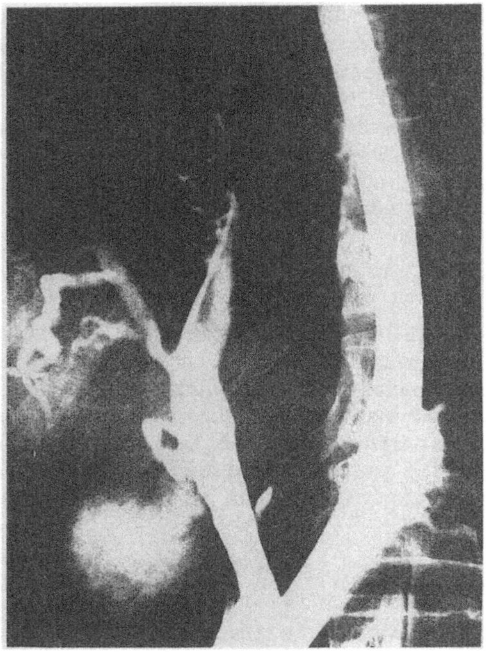
b

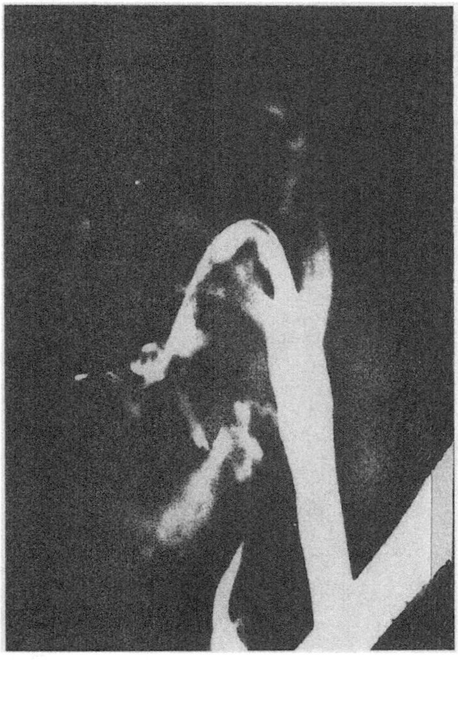
c

Fig. 4a–c. Intrahepatic bile duct stones. Before therapy (**a**) all intrahepatic bile ducts are filled with stones, and contrast material cannot advance into the intrahepatic bile ducts. After two sessions (**b**) and a third session (**c**) the bile ducts are nearly clear, and removal of fragments remaining in the bile duct is possible by means of endoscopy ic concrements could be disintegrated in all patients after two or three sessions. Common bile duct stones were treated successfully in 21 out of 29 patients (70%). Fragments remaining after lithotripsy measured between 1 and 8 mm in diameter and could be removed endoscopically. The X rays of one patient presenting with choledocholithiasis (Fig. 3) and of another with intrahepatic concrements (Fig. 4) are presented here as samples. Minor stone particles from stones which could not be disintegrated after three sessions also passed through the nasobiliary probe. Surprisingly, four impacted stones which at first were considered not to have been affected by the shocks disintegrated upon being touched with the Dormia probe.

Success of Lithotripsy and Radiological Stone Density

Stones which could not be disintegrated had a radiological density between 0 and 40 HU as assessed by computed tomography. Successful lithotripsy was achieved in stones with 60–190 HU, except in two patients who had Billroth II resection, and in whom the duodenal stump was filled with air which probably interposed between shock-wave source and stone.

Side Effects of Therapy

None of the patients presented clinical complications. In only one female patient was elevation of the transaminases observed from twice the normal value before to 400 U/l after lithotripsy; despite these laboratory findings the patient experienced no clinical symptoms. Characteristically, however, shock-wave administration always caused mild fleabite-like petechiae of the skin at the side of shock-wave penetration.

Discussion

Second-generation extracorporeal shock-wave generators have proven effective for the treatment of renal stones [5, 6]. Our previous in vitro experience [7] and the results reported here demonstrate that gallstones can also be disintegrated.

Gallstone fragmentation is, however, much more difficult than disintegration of kidney stones. This fact is demonstrated by the disintegration rate, energy required for disintegration, and size of fragments remaining after lithotripsy. Whereas kidney stones were fragmented with our electromagnetically generated shock waves in 97% of patients [6], gallstone disintegration was achieved in only 70%. According to our cinical experience [6], kidney stones were easily broken up at 15 kV while gallstones were not, not even in vitro [7]. Energy required for fragmentation was at the upper range of the available capacity of the device (discharge voltage 20 kV). When it is administered with the present technology, the disintegration rate can be improved by better selection of patients since, according to the present results, stones with low radiological density (below 40 HU) – as determined by computed tomography – are likely to resist shock waves. The fragmentation pattern of gallstones is also quite different from that of kidney stones. While the latter can be broken up into nothing but tiny particles, gallstones were disintegrated also into larger fragments of up to 8 mm in diameter.

Our experience proves shock-wave administration to be harmless. Side effects affecting the liver, pancreas, or other intra-abdominal organs could not be detected. Also, the tissue of the stomach and duodenum, which was inspected endoscopically after each shock-wave therapy, was not affected.

Thus, after 1.5 years of clinical experience we consider electromagnetically generated second-generation shock waves to be safe and easy to administer. In selected patients risky surgical procedures could be avoided and replaced by conservative treatment. The clinical value of the new procedure could be substantiated, and further application can be recommended.

Acknowledgement. The authors wish to thank Ms. Barbara Paus for careful secretarial assistance.

References

1. Chausy C, Brendel W, Schmiedt E (1980) Extracorporeally induced destruction of kidney stones by shock waves. Lancet ii:1265–1268
2. Challah S, Mays NB (1986) The randomised controlled trial for the evaluation of new technology: a case study. Br Med J 292:877–879
3. Sauerbruch T, Delius M, Paumgartner G, Holl J, Wess O, Weber W, Hepp W, Brendel W (1986) Fragmentation of gallstones by extracorporeal shock waves. N Engl J Med 314:818–822
4. Sackmann M, Delius M, Sauerbruch T, Holl J, Weber W, Ippisch E, Hagelauer U, Wess O, Hepp W, Brendel W, Paumgartner G (1988) Shock-wave lithotripsy of gallbladder stones. The first 175 patients. N Engl J Med 318:393–397
5. Philip T, Kellett MJ, Whitfield HN, Wickham JEA (1988) Painless lithotripsy: experience with 100 patients. Lancet I:41–43
6. Wilbert DM, Riedmiller H, Alken P, Hohenfellner R (1987) Zweite Generation der extrakorporalen Stoßwellenlithotripsie (Lithostar). Dtsch Med Wochenschr 112:1637–1640
7. Staritz M, Floth A, Buess G, Rambow A, Wilbert D, Goebel M, Schild F (1987) Extracorporeal shock waves (ESW) for gallstone fragmentation. First in-vitro-experience with a second generation device working without waterbath. Gastroenterology 92:1652 (A)
8. Staritz M, Poralla T, Dormeyer HH, Meyer zum Büschenfelde KH (1985) Endoscopic removal of common bile duct stones through the intact papilla following medical sphincter dilation. Gastroenterology 88:1807–1811
9. Demling L, Seuberth K, Riemann JF (1982) A mechanical lithotripter. Endoscopy 14:100–101
10. Staritz M, Ewe K, Meyer zum Büschenfelde KH (1983) Mechanical gallstone lithotripsy in the common bile duct – in-vitro and in-vivo experience. Endoscopy 15:316–317

Piezoelectric Lithotripsy of Gallbladder Stones

C. Ell, W. Kerzel, H. T. Schneider, W. Domschke, and E. G. Hahn

Department of Medicine, University of Erlangen-Nuremberg, D-8520 Erlangen, FRG

Introduction

Non-surgical procedures for the treatment of gallbladder stones must be measured against the effectiveness of cholecystectomy, with its low morbidity and mortality rates. For non-invasive alternative procedures to cholecystectomy, however, apart from adequate effectiveness, freedom from anaesthesia and analgesia is a requirement that needs to be met. This latter feature applies in particular when partial successes on initial treatment, or with recurrent stones, make renewed lithotripsy necessary.

Piezoelectric shock-wave lithotripsy has stood the test and has established itself as an anaesthesia- and analgesic-free method in the field of kidney stones [1]. Only preliminary reports exist [2, 3] on the fragmentation of gallbladder stones with subsequent chemical litholysis. After wide-ranging in vitro and in vivo experiments on the feasibility of gallstone fragmentation and the tissue reactions under piezoelectric shock waves [4, 5] we have used piezoelectric lithotripsy for the treatment of symptomatic gall bladder stones since the beginning of 1988.

We report here on our initial experience and preliminary follow-up results with the use of piezoelectric lithotripsy of gallbladder stones combined with oral bile salts.

Material and Methods

Piezoelectric Lithotriptor

The equipment used was a piezoelectric lithotriptor manufactured by R. Wolf, Inc. (Federal Republic of Germany; Piezolith 2300) Here, the shock waves are produced by a self-focussing piezoelectric acoustic generator, which comprises a "bowl" lined on its concave surface with more than 3000 ceramic elements. For transmission of the shock wave, the bowl is filled with degassed water warmed to body temperature. The patient is in the prone position, the skin over the region of the gallbladder being immersed in the water contained within the device. The stones are localized ultrasonographically in two planes with the aid of one of the two real-time ultrasonic B scanners arranged in the longitudinal axis of the transducer (4 MHz). The acoustic path can be selected that is the most favourable for the anatomical situation presenting. For focussing purposes, the acoustic generator can be moved in three planes under continuous ultrasonic control from the electronic operating panel until the gallstone has been positioned exactly within the shock-wave focus (Fig. 1).

The shock-wave pulse sequence can be varied in four steps between 1 and 2.0 Hz, the energy per pulse being adjustable also in four steps. Depending upon the power step selected, the pressures built up in the shock-wave focus vary between 400 and 1200 bar.

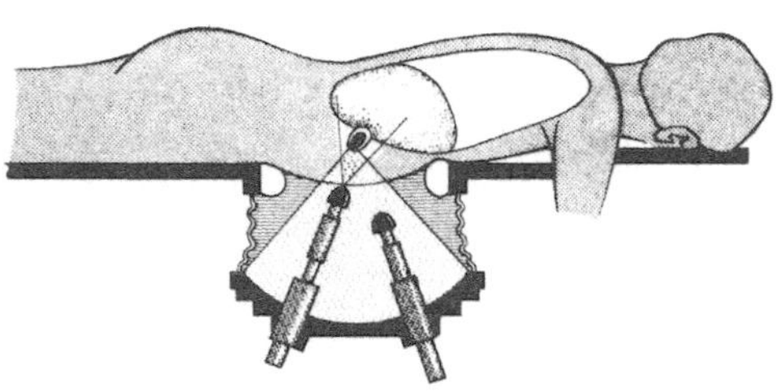

Fig. 1. Patient prior to piezoelectric lithotripsy in prone position over the self-focussing bowl-shaped shock-ware generator with the dual scanner system for targeting the gallstone

Selecting Patients – Prior Examinations

The criteria for selection of patients corresponded to those established by the Munich group [6]. The tests carried out prior to fragmentation included ultrasound imaging before and after fatty meal, plain X ray of the abdomen, and the usual laboratory tests. In the beginning, we also required computed tomography, magnetic resonance imaging, ECG and X ray of the thorax. We report here on 75 patients (59 women and 16 men) with a mean age of 45 years (range, 19–74 years). About 80% of patients had only a solitary calculus (mean diameter 18 ± 5.5 mm; range, 6–30 mm).

Treatment

All the patients in the study were treated in prone position without premedication. After localizing the stone ultrasonographically, the pulse energy was raised slowly to the maximum tolerable level. In general, intensity level 3 was used; in slender patients treatment could also be carried out at level 2 and, in exceptions, at level 1. An ECG triggering is not necessary with the piezoelectric system; we therefore generally worked at a therapy frequency of two shocks per second. A retreatment was scheduled in the study programme if ultrasound re-examinations showed fragments larger than 4 mm. A maximum of two retreatments were allowed.

Lithotripsy was terminated when ultrasonographically no obvious individual fragments with an acoustic shadow were recognizable or after a maximum of 3000 discharges. This upper limit was chosen on the basis of prior in vitro and in vivo investigations [4, 5].

Drug Therapy Prior to and After Lithotripsy

For an average of 7 days prior to lithotripsy and for up to 3 months after reaching complete freedom from stones, each patient received 7.5 mg/kg body weight of ursodeoxycholic acid and chenodeoxycholic acid (Urso Falk, Cheno Falk), respectively. These drugs were administered in a single dose at bedtime.

Diagnostic Evaluation After Lithotripsy

Based on the positive experience concerning adverse side effects of the treatment methods after the first 50 treatments, the test routine was changed. Control tests after lithotripsy then comprised only ultrasound imaging, blood tests (amylase, glutamic oxaloacetic transaminase, (GOT), glutamic pyruvic transaminase (GPT) and gamma-glutamyl transpeptidase (GGT)) 12–24 h after lithotripsy as well as analysis of the first urine after lithotripsy. Patients were examined regularly after their first treatment as to their freedom from stones, and there were clinical tests (ultrasound and, if indicated, laboratory tests) and history taking concerning any side effects.

Results

The results regarding fragmentation efficiency, treatment period and localization time are given in Table 1. On average 2100 shock waves were applied for the first treatment and about 1700 for the second and third treatments. In about 50% of patients (37/75) a second treatment was necessary and in nearly 25% (22/75) a third one. Side effects are presented in Table 2. None of the patients needed any analgesics or sedatives, nor was anaesthesia required. In the majority of cases retreatments were done on an out-patient basis. The number of patients who are completely free of stones is given in Table 3. To date, seven patients have been re-examined for stones or relative freedom from stones 12 months after treatment. In five of the seven cases the gallbladder was completely free of stones after 12 months. A typical sequence in a patient with a solitary stone prior to, immediately after 1500 pulses and 2 months after lithotripsy is shown in Figs. 2–4.

Table 1. Fragmentation efficiency, fragment size (measured 12–16 h after lithotripsy) and times required for localization and treatment (means and ± SD).

Successful fragmentation	74/75 (98%)
Percentage of maximum fragment size < 50% of initial stone diameter	88%
Maximum fragment size	4 mm ± 3
Time required for localization	7 ± 3 min
Treatment time	32 ± 16 min

Table 2. Side effects and serious untoward reactions after piezoelectric lithotripsy in 75 patients

Microhaematuria	8/75 (11.0%)
Mild pancreatitis	1/75 (1.4%)
Increase in liver enzymes	4/75 (5.3%)
Increase in amylase (without symptoms)	2/75 (2.7%)
Gallbladder wall thickening	14/75 (18.6%)
Petechial skin bleeds	4/75 (5.3%)
Biliary colic (in the follow-up period)	24/75 (32%)

Table 3. Stone-free rate in relation to follow-up periods

0–1 month	12%	(9/75)
0–2 months	22%	(15/70)
2–4 months	42%	(25/60)
4–6 months	53%	(27/51)
6–8 months	59%	(17/29)

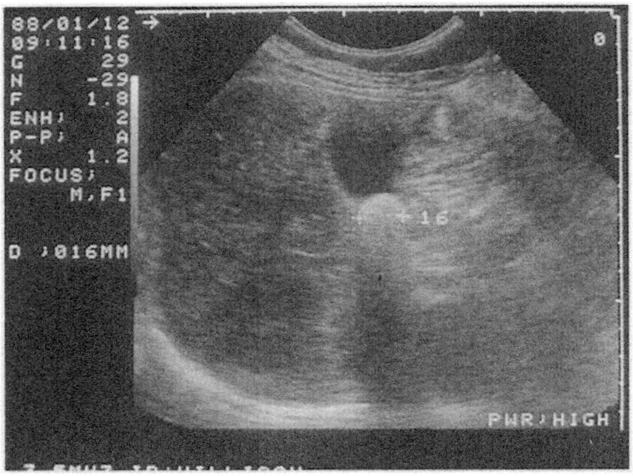

Fig. 2. Solitary radiolucent stone (16 mm in diameter) prior to piezoelectric lithotripsy

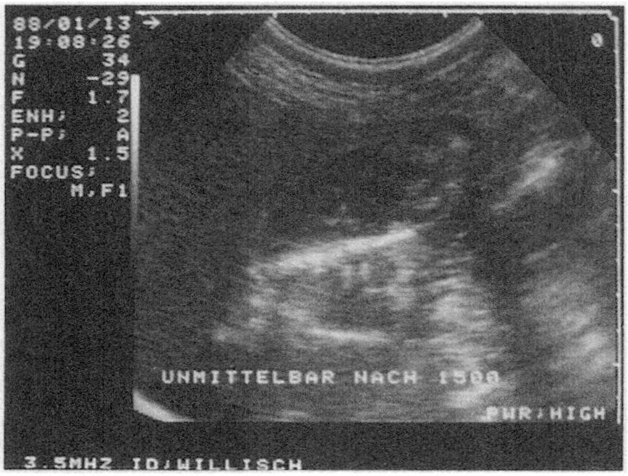

Fig. 3. Immediately after 1500 shockwaves, complete fragmentation with a cloud of tiny fragments

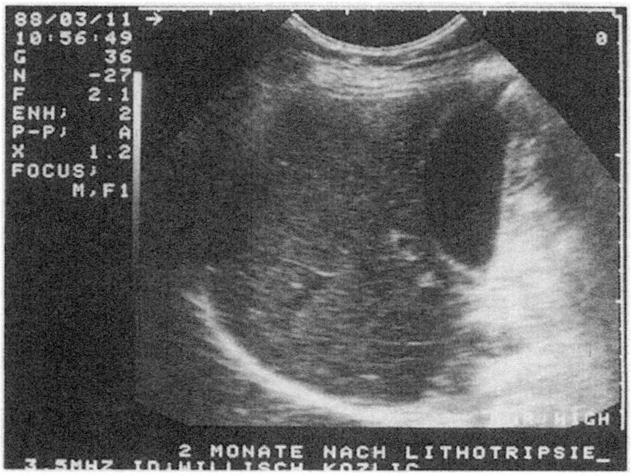

Fig. 4. Two months after lithotripsy, a complete fragment-free gallbladder could be shown ultrasonographically

Discussion

The positive property of the piezoelectric lithotriptor that we used (Piezolith 2300) is that analgesics or anaesthesia are not necessary. In contrast to another report (see the paper by Staritz et al., this volume), none of our patients needed any form of sedative or analgesic during therapy. Owing to this analgesic-free type of lithotripsy this form of shock-wave therapy is also suitable for application under out-patient conditions in the scope of mobile lithotriptor units or in private practice. The procedure has hardly any side effects in the acute post-lithotripsy phase, which makes a clinical follow-up for 24–48 h after lithotripsy unnecessary.

The anaesthesia- and analgesia-free application of piezoelectric shock-waves even in the case of organs with visceral innervation, is, indeed, of decisive clinical advantage vis-a-vis electrohydraulic and electromagnetic principles of shock-wave generation. This advantage can, however, be of importance only when fragmentation efficiency and the stone-free rate achieved with the piezoelectric mechanism are comparable with those associated with the other physical principles.

While the efficiency of extracorporeal shock-wave lithotripsy of gallbladder stones following oral litholysis has been proved only for the electrohydraulic prototype produced by Dornier [6], similar data are not yet available for the piezoelectric system. Only two teams have reported on first preliminary experiences with the piezoelectric shock-wave principle in gallbladder stone fragmentation [2, 3]. As in the in vitro test [4], a good fragmentation efficiency could also be shown clinically. However, fragmentation efficiency is not a very reliable measure when comparing the various systems; the decisive criterion is the number of patients who are free of stones. Concerning this factor no figures have been published yet for a comparison with other second-generation extracorporeal lithotriptors. We can therefore refer only to the figures presented at two meetings on biliary lithotripsy in Boston (1988) [7] and Vancouver (1989) [8, 9]. Considering results presented there, our figures are comparable to those obtained with other electrohydraulic lithotriptors of the second generation (MPL 9000 by Dornier; Sonolith 3000 by Technomed). The best results can be obtained for solitary stones of a size of up to 2 cm – a fact that was similarly described by the Munich and Lyon teams. The results for larger concrements of up to 3 cm and for multiple concrements are not yet satisfactory [6–9].

Use of the Piezolith 2300 in clinical routine was easy. The prone position proved the ideal position in almost all the cases, just as for the electrohydraulic principle. The treatment and localization period was relatively short, 30–40 min on average, which makes the piezoelectric systems very economical; moreover the patient also benefits thereby, especially in repeat treatments. No building or construction measures are necessary to install this mobile lithotriptor, which is another advantage in terms of economics, and the follow-up and maintenance costs are lower than for other systems.

In summary, the piezoelectric system that we use (Piezolith 2300) represents an important step forward in the search for a reliable, economical compromise between patient comfort and therapeutic efficiency.

References

1. Philip T, Kellet MJ, Whitefield HN, Wickham JEA (1988) Painless lithotripsy: experience of 100 patients. Lancet I:41–43
2. Ell C, Kerzel W, Günter E, Heyder N, Rödl W, Flügel H, Domschke W (1988) Piezoelektrische Lithotripsie von Gallensteinen – erste klinische Erfahrungen. Dtsch Med Wochenschr 113:1503–1507
3. Hood K, Keightley A, Dowling RH et al. (1988) Piezoceramic lithotripsy of gallbladder stones: initial experience in 38 patients. Lancet 1:1322–1324

4. Ell C, Kerzel W, Rödl W, Langer H, Heyder N, Foerster E, Domschke W (1989) Fragmentation of biliary calculi by means of extracorporeally generated piezoelectric shockwaves. Dig Dis Sci 34:1006–1010
5. Ell Ch, Kerzel W, Heyder N, Langer H, Mischke U, Giedl J, Domschke W (1989) Tissue reactions under piezoelectric shockwave application for the fragmentation of biliary calculi. Gut 30:680–685
6. Sackmann M, Delius M, Sauerbruch T, Holl J, Weber W, Ippisch E, Hagelauer U, Wess O, Hepp W, Brendel W, Paumgartner G (1988) Shock-wave lithotripsy of gallbladder stones. N Engl J Med 318:393–397
7. Ponchon T, Martin X, Mestas JL, Krawitt E, Lambert R (1989) Dissolution of gallstones following extracorporeal lithotripsy of the gallbladder: preliminary clinical data. In: Ferrucci JT, Delius M, Burhenne JH (eds) Biliary lithotripsy. Year Book, Chicago, pp 79–82
8. Ponchon T (1989) Lithotripsy experience in Lyon. Second international symposium on biliary lithotripsy, Vancouver, Canada, April 25, 1989
9. Sackmann M (1989) Evaluation of fragment clearance. Second international symposium on biliary lithotripsy, Vancouver, Canada, April 25, 1989

Biliary Shock-Wave Lithotripsy: Experience of the First 3 Years in 612 Patients

L. Greiner and C. Jakobeit

Clinic of Gastroenterology, Municipal Hospitals, Wuppertal, FRG

Introduction

The performance of the first cholecystectomy by Langenbuch [1] in 1882 constituted a fundamental step forward in the management of gallstone disease. For decades efforts towards the development of non-surgical forms of treatment for symptomatic cholecystolithiasis took second place to the surgical procedure, but they experienced a certain renaissance with the advent of oral dissolution treatment with chenodeoxycholic acid and later with ursodeoxycholic acid. The limited indications for chemical dissolution and the necessary long duration of treatment particularly in the case of large calculi at first stood in the way of more widespread application of this therapeutic concept. The restriction of this treatment to stones with small or at most medium diameters (up to 15 mm) was particularly limiting. When the disintegration of kidney stones [2] using extracorporeally generated shock waves (extracorporeal shock-wave lithotripsy, ESWL) proved within only a few years to be an extremely successful form of treatment, it was only logical to attempt to apply this non-surgical principle to the treatment of gallstones (biliary ESWL). After extensive pre-clinical studies particularly in experimental animals [3], clinical application of biliary ESWL was begun in 1985 [4], and the results of treatment in the initial studies have since been reported [5, 6].

This chapter describes the physical principles of ESWL, the available shock-wave sources, and the procedures and indications for biliary ESWL. The risks and complications of the treatment are also presented as well as the results obtained by us to date in the clinical management of ductal and gallbladder stones.

Physical Principles

Focussable high-energy shock waves are suitable for the fragmentation of kidney stones [7] and gallstones [3]: they pass through soft tissue and fluid-filled cavities without causing clinically relevant tissue damage (assuming a limited number of pulses) and release their energy only at interfaces with properties of acoustic conductivity differing considerably from those of water or soft tissue. Such interfaces are described as 'highly impedant' and occur between stone and surrounding fluid or surrounding soft tissue. The mechanism by which the repeated impact of numerous shock-wave pulses causes fragmentation of calculi is not fully understood; it is likely that so-called cavitation phenomena and reflected shock waves play a significant role [8]. The shock waves are transmitted into the body with the help of a water bag which moulds itself elastically to fit the surface of the body; ultrasound gel prevents the formation of an impedant interface between the water bag and the skin surface.

Shock-Wave Sources

The extracorporeal generation and focussing of the shock waves can be based on one of three different principles: (a) underwater spark-gap discharge (electrohydraulic principle) [7, 9] (Fig. 1); (b) synchronised impulse emission by numerous piezo-ceramic elements directed towards a single focus [10, 11]; and (c) the electromagnetic principle of shock-wave generation [12]. The spark-gap principle of shock-wave generation is the method hitherto generally used in urology [2, 7] and that which was first applied to the treatment of gallstones; the shock wave is produced by high-temperature vaporisation of a small compartment of water between the two tips of an electrode across which a high-capacitance capacitor is discharged. The shock waves are focussed using a metal ellipsoid [9]. The focussing in the piezo-ceramic system is achieved by the exact positioning of numerous small acoustic generators on the inside surface of a bowl; the high-energy shock-wave effect results from the summation of the acoustic impulses meeting simultaneously at the point of focus [10].

The electromagnetic generation of shock waves works on the 'loudspeaker' principle: switching on a strong magnet deflects a metal membrane at the bottom of a water-filled tube and produces a wave front in the tube. This wave front is focussed by an acoustic lens [12]. The spark discharge systems are considered comparatively powerful shock-wave generators with relatively good focussing. In the piezo-ceramic systems the focal area is small and in the electromagnetic shock-wave generator the focussing by the acoustic lens appears to be relatively poor. The latter disadvantage is circumvented by an ingenious modification of the electromagnetic principle presented recently but not yet clinically tested. In place of a flat membrane, waves are created by the electromagnetical-

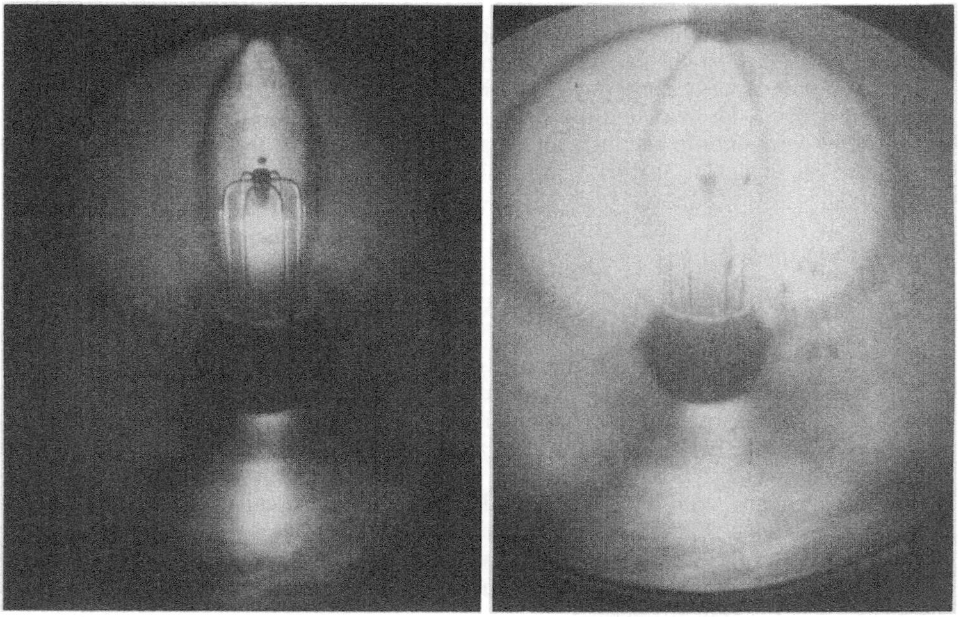

a b

Fig. 1 a, b. Underwater spark-gap method: firing phase of the electrode. (By courtesy of Prof. J. Thüroff, Director of the Urology Unit, Municipal Hospitals, Wuppertal, FRG) ly induced deflection of a cylindrical metal membrane resembling a tin can. This "tin can" is positioned centrally on the bottom of a bowl in a water-bath; the focussing of the waves is determined by the geometry of the bowl. This new shock-wave source is reported to create relatively strong pulses; it remains to be seen whether the modulation of the shock-wave properties permitted by this system will have clinical advantages.

The exact alignment of the shock-wave focus with the calculus to be destroyed – the positioning and targeting procedure – can be performed under either radiological or ultrasonographic guidance. This applies to both indications of biliary ESWL, i.e. fragmentation of bile-duct and of gallbladder stones by extracorporeal shock waves. The different methods of localisation result in essential differences in procedure.

Procedures of Biliary ESWL

The number and intensity of the shock-wave pulses and the duration of an individual session vary depending on the type of machine used; for spark-discharge units limitation of the number of shock-wave pulses to about 2000 is recommended, which means that the treatment lasts about 30 min when the discharges are ECG triggered. The other ESW sources (considered to be weaker) require more pulses, and the treatment takes correspondingly longer. Anaesthesia is not required although in individual cases sedo-analgesia may be appropriate. In this respect the procedures at present adopted by the individual working groups differ considerably. General preconditions for treatment are an intact coagulation system and discontinuation of any anti-platelet medication 10–14 days prior to ESWL [6]. Pregnancy must be excluded.

Bile Duct Stones

It is usually difficult and sometimes impossible to locate bile duct stones by ultrasound. Particularly when there is gas in the biliary tree after endoscopic sphincterotomy (EST), it is almost impossible to distinguish retained bile duct stones from air bubbles by ultrasonography. Ductal stones must therefore as a rule be located radiologically; in the special biliary lithotriptors and in most combination units this is not possible, as they are guided by ultrasound. ESWL of ductal stones must therefore be performed in kidney stone lithotriptors which possess a two-dimensional X-ray system for localisation and positioning of the stones [13, 14]. For visualisation of the bile duct contrast medium is injected via a nasobiliary drain left in situ after EST and failure of extraction by the usual endoscopic operative method. Bile duct ESWL thus follows immediately on the unsuccessful attempt at stone removal by the conventional endoscopic operative technique. Occasional extrahepatic stones and most intrahepatic bile duct stones can be readily localised by ultrasound; in these cases a lithotriptor with ultrasound guidance is used in preference to a unit with radiological guidance. This procedure has proved particularly successful in the case of (intrahepatic) cholangiolithiasis.

When disintegrating bile duct stones, it is usually sufficient to produce fragments of moderate size (10–15 mm) as such fragments can be extracted without difficulty through the papillostoma or even pass spontaneously [13, 15] (Fig. 2).

Gallbladder Stones (Combined with Oral Dissolution Treatment)

Gallbladder stones – known to be ideal targets for ultrasonographic diagnosis – are also optimally suited for ultrasound localisation in shock-wave treatment [5]; radiological

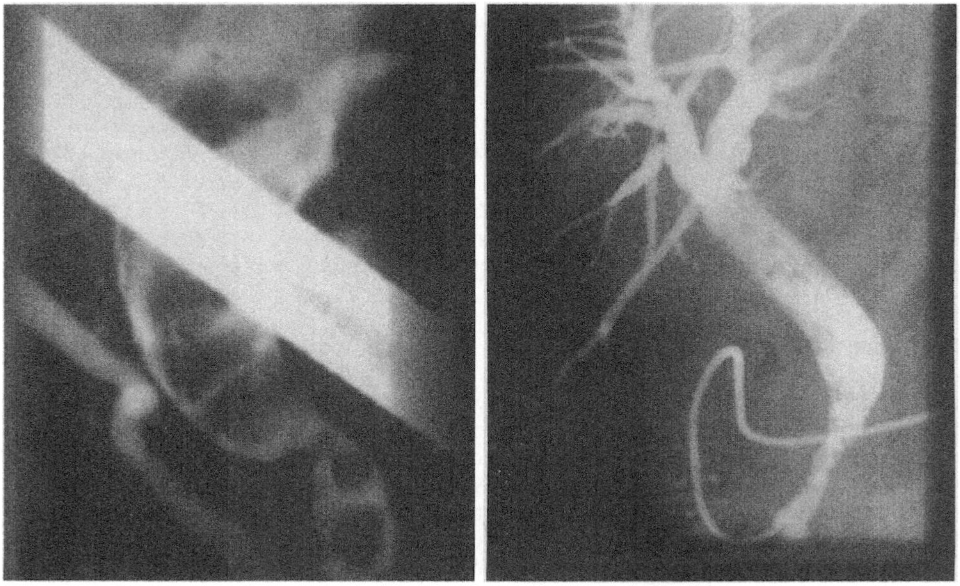

a b

Fig. 2 a, b. Large calculi situated proximal to a common bile duct stricture and not accessible to endoscopic operative measures. **a** Before ESWL. **b** After ESWL

techniques are of no relevance here. Real-time ultrasound observation permits continuous monitoring of the disintegration process. The technique for positioning the patient differs according to the equipment used; in the case of fixed shock-wave sources the calculus can be moved into the focal area of the shock-wave source only by moving the patient (and thus the stone). Some devices have a movable shock-wave source with correspondingly better, individually adaptable possibilities for targeting the stone and the fragments [5]. The extent to which computer-aided partial automation represents a genuine help to the physician well trained in ultrasonography remains to be seen.

The aim of the fragmentation of gallbladder stones is to produce fragments all of which are as small as possible and able, ideally, to pass spontaneously through the papilla via the cystic duct and the common bile duct. At present this is the exception as the fragments produced during the disintegration process increasingly interfere with the focussing of the shock waves (self-limiting effect [16]). This problem of stone fragments retained in the gallbladder can be dealt with in two ways: firstly, by repeated shock-wave exposure in repeat ESWL sessions after the tiny fragments responsible for the interference have been passed [16] and, secondly, by additional oral dissolution treatment of the fragments remaining in the gallbladder [4–6, 16, 17]. The second procedure–which utilises the increased surface area created by the ESWL–is that usually preferred at present. Most working groups perform ESWL-adjuvant oral dissolution treatment with a combination of ursodeoxycholic and chenodeoxycholic acid (500 mg of each substance at bedtime for body weights $\leq$80 kg, in heavier patients 750 mg of each [5, 6]).

Indications

There are important differences between bile duct ESWL and gallbladder ESWL, not least with respect to the urgency of establishing the indication; gallbladder ESWL is an elective method [4–6] while that of bile duct stones is often part of a graded plan for emergency treatment [13, 15], for example, in biliary pancreatitis or lithogenic obstructive jaundice with or without cholangitis.

Bile Duct Stones

Bile duct ESWL can be used – as the last non-operative possibility – to treat all intra- and extrahepatic bile duct stones which cannot be removed by the usual endoscopic operative methods including mechanical lithotripsy [4, 13, 15]. This applies particularly in the case of large stones, calculi proximal to strictures and stones which cannot be reached by endoscopy (for example after Billroth surgery or Roux-en-Y anastomosis of the bile ducts; Table 1). It remains to be seen whether, in the case of common bile duct stones which can be located by ultrasound, ESWL will in future increasingly be carried out before the performance of EST and consequent entry of gas into the biliary tract. An important advantage of such a procedure would be that the length of the sphincterotomy could be reduced and the EST risk would be correspondingly smaller. With optimum disintegration of the ductal stones EST could – at least theoretically – be dispensed with completely.

Gallbladder Stones

While we can say that the indications for bile duct ESWL are on the whole clearly defined, this is by no means the case for gallbladder ESWL. In the initial phase of clinical testing [4–6] it was meaningful to define the indication range as narrowly as possible (Table 2). Further developments will show to what extent it is possible to broaden the range of indications. Initial results in calculi with narrow radio-opaque rims [18] and calculi with discrete central calcification which otherwise fulfil the criteria for inclusion

Table 1. Indications for ESWL of extra- and intrahepatic bile-duct stones

Failure of endoscopic-operative treatment because
Stone too large
Stone too hard
Dormia basket fails to open
EST incision too short
Impossibility of endoscopic operative treatment because
Stone inaccessible
Intrahepatic position
Bile duct strictures
Biliary tree inaccessible
(Partial) gastrectomy
Biliodigestive anastomosis
Large juxtapapillary diverticulum

Table 2. Admission and exclusion criteria for ESWL (plus dissolution) of gallbladder stones

Admission criteria	Exclusion criteria
Symptomatic stones	Asymptomatic stones
Non-calcified stones	(Grossly) calcified stones
Stone size:	Stones too large
Single stone up to 30 mm	Stones too numerous
2 or 3 stones up to 15 mm	Non-functioning gallbladder
≥4 stones up to 10–12 mm	Acute/chronic inflammatory changes of gall-blader
Functioning gallbladder	Pregnancy
Sonomorphologically normal gallbladder wall	Coagulation not intact (including medication with antiplatelet drugs)
Sonomorphologically normal common bile duct	

have been quite promising. With regard to the number [19] and diameter of the stones, too, changes in indication can be expected in the near future, particularly with the help of repeat ESWL sessions.

Risks and Complications

As shock waves in animal experiments caused tissue damage (haemorrhage, necrosis) at the highly impedant boundaries of minute air bubbles, lung tissue must be kept outside the focal area [6]. Larger air bubbles are apparently without clinical relevance, as has been shown by bile duct ESWL performed after EST; entrapment of air in distended intrahepatic bile ducts does not produce relevant side effects, evidently on account of the size of the air bubbles. In the case of gas in non-distended intrahepatic bile ducts a liver haematoma was observed after ESWL in one case. In our own experience bacteriaemia after bile duct ESWL is not infrequent [13, 15] and can be explained by the often pre-existent latent cholangitis or stone infection. Provided there is close clinical surveillance of the patients, this does not lead to an increased clinical risk as a result of ESWL. Experience to date shows that, after gallbladder ESWL, macroscopic haematuria is to be expected in individual cases, and that we can expect biliary complaints and pain or even colics in 20%–30% of the patients treated. As a rule, however, such episodes occur only once or sporadically. In a subjective comparison of pain and complaints before and after ESWL about 75% of the patients do, after all, report (considerable) improvement after fragmentation. Fragment-associated biliary pancreatitis is to be expected as complication in about 2%. The rate of EST necessary after gallblader ESWL to date is less than 1% [5, 6]. In some patients transient fragment-related obstruction of the cystic duct is to be expected but as a rule resolves spontaneously [5, 6]. In two cases acute cholecystitis developed, in one case with obstruction of the common bile duct by a fragment. One liver haematoma – probably resulting from the presence of small gas bubbles in non-distended bile ducts after EST – was managed conservatively. ESWL of bile duct and gallbladder stones, performed to date in over 10000 patients worldwide, has thus proved to be a relatively safe procedure.

Results

Bile Duct Stones

Since 1985 we have used ESWL to treat 73 patients with extrahepatic bile duct stones which could not be managed by endoscopic operative methods [15]. The patient group represented about 8% of all cases in which non-surgical treatment of ductal stones was performed or attempted. There were twice as many women as men, and the average age of the patients was 73.7 years (range, 29–90 years); in half the patients treated the calculous gallbladder was in situ. The ESWL sessions were initially performed under intubation anaesthesia, later under sedo-analgesia and in the past 1.5 years largely without medication. The average duration of treatment was 25 min (range, 10–55 min), the mean number of ESW pulses 1793 (ranges, 430–2100) and the mean generator voltage 18.6 kV (range, 16–24 kV). ESWL disintegration with complete elimination of the stones was achieved in 97.3% (71/73) of those treated (Figs. 2, 3). The two patients in whom the effect of ESWL fragmentation was inadequate had impacted prepapillary calculi. On account of serious concomitant illness we did not refer them for surgery; satisfactory long-term management was possible using a biliodudenal endoprosthesis [20].

We have so far used ESWL to treat nine patients with intrahepatic stones [15] (Fig. 4); freedom from stones was achieved in 55.6% [5, 9]. In the remaining four patients the intrahepatic ducts still contained small fragments which did not pass spontaneously and could not be extracted endoscopically; however, in these patients, too, the clinical symptoms and the biochemical signs of biliary obstruction reverted to normal after ESWL [15].

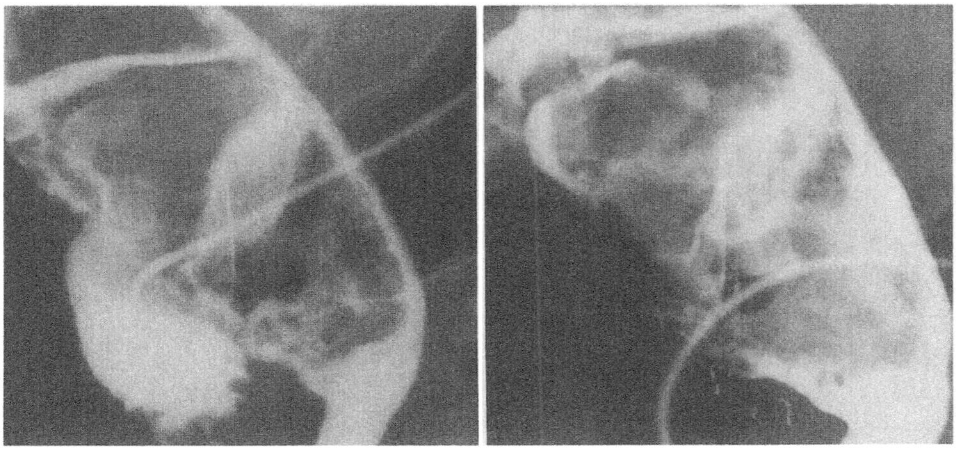

a b

Fig. 3 a, b. Very large common bile duct stones. **a** Before the first ESWL. **b** After the first ESWL. Freedom from stones and/or fragments after a total of three ESWL sessions and endoscopic extraction

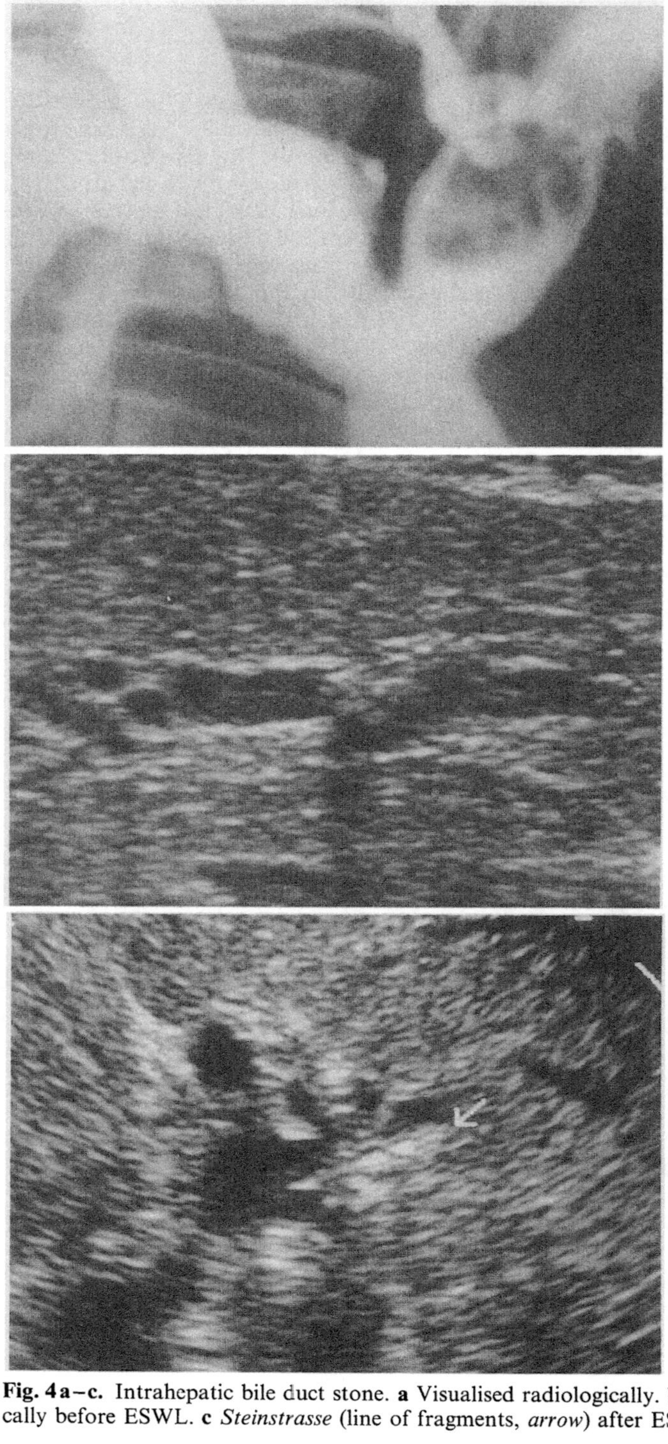

Fig. 4a–c. Intrahepatic bile duct stone. **a** Visualised radiologically. **b** Visualised ultrasonographically before ESWL. **c** *Steinstrasse* (line of fragments, *arrow*) after ESWL

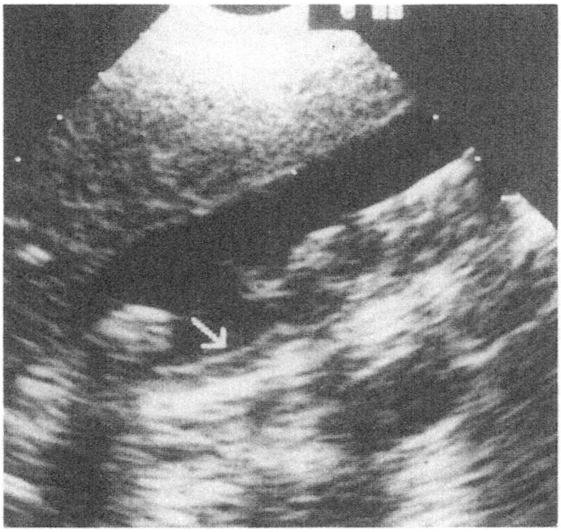

Fig. 5. Circumscribed, inflammatory-scarred thickening of the gallbladder wall (arrow) several months after cholecystitis. No ESWL

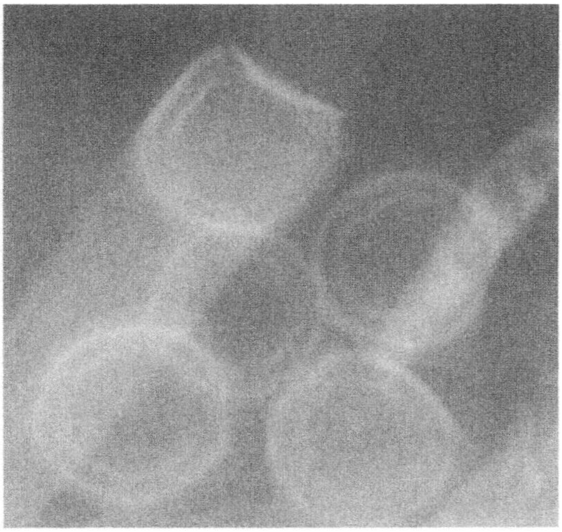

Fig. 6. Several calculi with considerable calcification. No ESWL

Gallbladder Stones

Adequate data on gallbladder ESWL is at present available only for equipment using electrohydraulic shock-wave generation (underwater spark-gap discharge) [4–6, 19]. In our experience in, to date, 530 patients almost all gallbladder calculi could be disintegrated in vivo (Figs. 7, 8). Of our cases, 2.3% (12/530) proved refractory to ESWL. Both the degree of stone fragmentation (Fig. 9a, b) and the rate of complete elimination of stones or fragments from the gallbladder depend on the total stone volume. We monitor the post-ESWL course during continuous dissolution treatment using ultrasound only; adequate evaluation of fragment size or of the volume of retained fragments in the gallbladder is possible only after passage of the small and tiny fragments (Figs. 10, 11). It is noteworthy that after the passage of these fragments, which is almost always asymp-

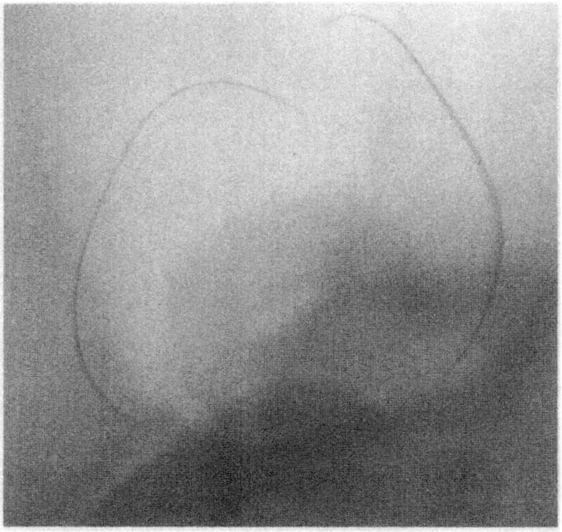

Fig. 7. Small calcified nucleus. Successful ESWL plus dissolution; freedom from fragments 6 months after a single ESWL session

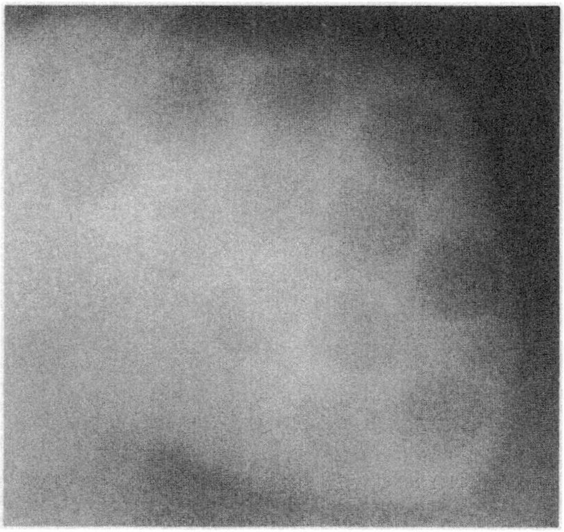

Fig. 8. Twelve calculi measuring 9–11 mm in diameter. Successful ESWL; freedom from fragments 9 months after a single ESWL session

tomatic (Fig. 9), they can be recovered from the stools as fragments measuring 1–5 mm in diameter [16] (in individual cases up to 8 mm in diameter; Fig. 12). Macroscopic examination and infrared spectroscopic analysis [21, 22] showed that the altogether 555 fragments which we recovered from 21 patients were by no means always 'pure' cholesterol fragments (Fig. 12 a). Rather, we found numerous mixed cholesterol-pigment fragments (Fig. 12 b) and also not infrequently mixed cholesterol-calcium fragments (Fig. 12 c). The calcification had evidently escaped radiological detection prior to ESWL.

The success of oral dissolution treatment of the fragments increases with the degree of fragmentation; this can be explained by the improvement in the volume/surface area ratio which benefits dissolution [23]. The longer the time since ESWL the more the chemical dissolution treatment becomes the salient therapeutic principle; in 12% of our patients with single stones measuring up to 20 mm we were able to document freedom

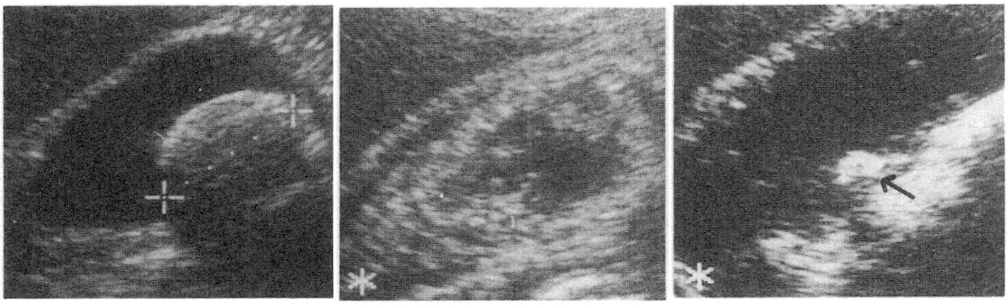

a b c

Fig. 9 a–c. Single 25 mm calculus with homogeneous internal reflex pattern. **a** Before ESWL. **b** Immediately after ESWL. **c** Ultrasonography 1 day after ESWL shows that most of the fragments have been passed (without clinical symptoms). One residual fragment measuring 5 mm remains in the gallbladder (*arrow*)

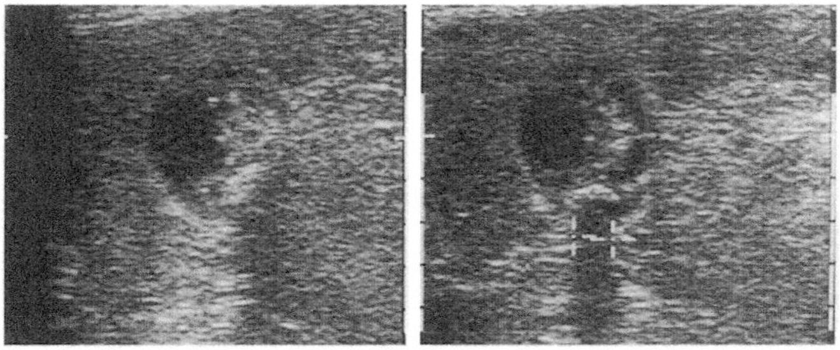

a b

Fig. 10 a, b. One day after ESWL of a single 18-mm stone. **a** Small fragments. **b** One 10-mm fragment detectable only by ultrasound with the patient in a left decubitus position. Repeat ESWL

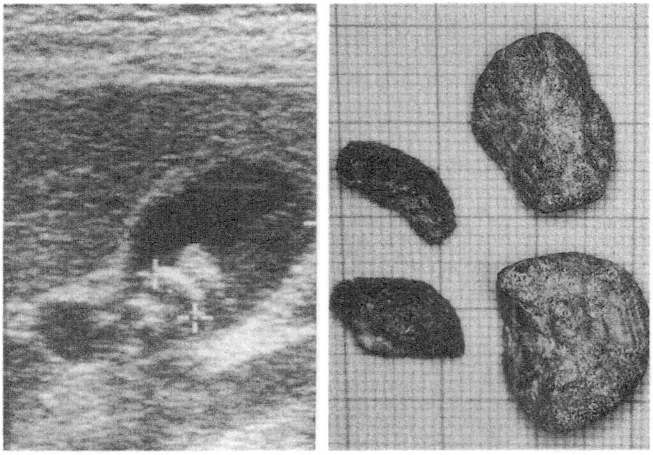

a b

Fig. 11 a, b. Inadequate fragmentation of a single 20 mm stone. **a** Ultrasonogram 4 weeks after ESWL. **b** Surgically removed fragments

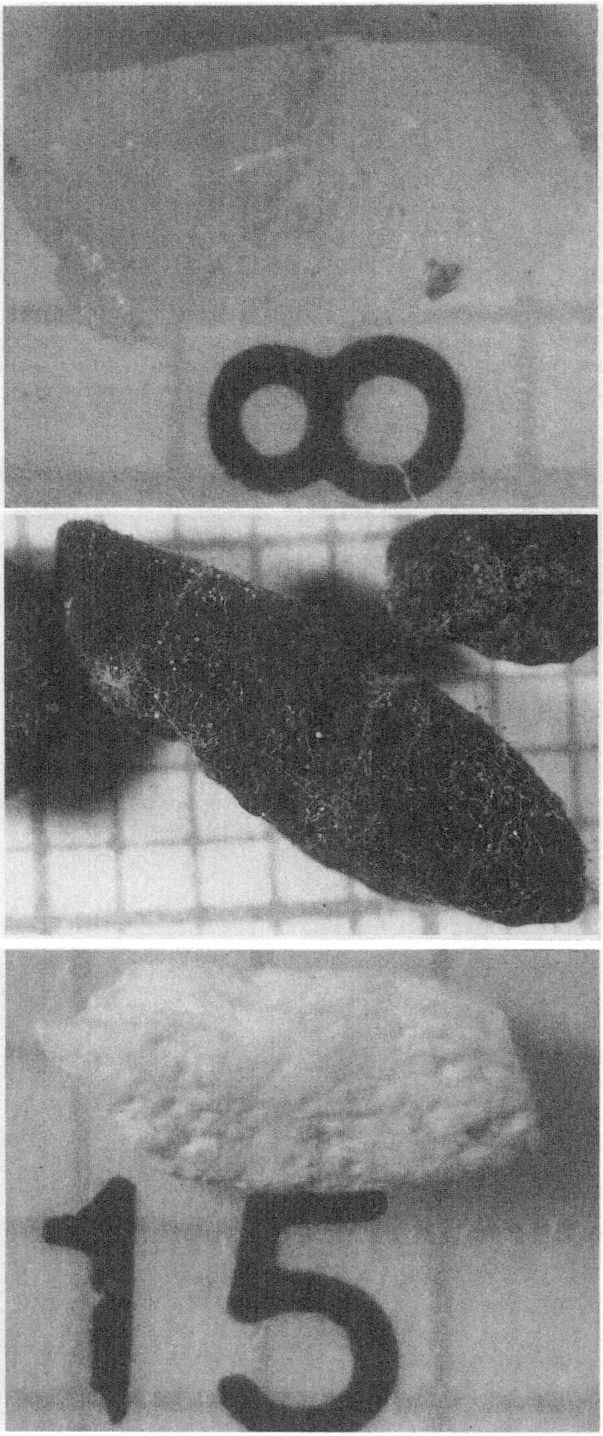

Fig. 12 a–c. Typical gallbladder stone fragments recovered from faeces 1–3 days after ESWL. **a** "Pure" cholesterol fragment. **b** Mixed stone fragments with high pigment contents. **c** Calcium contents. These fragments passed through the biliary tract without symptoms (scale in millimetres)

Table 3. Results in small to medium-sized single stones (8–20 mm; $n=231$)

	Month					
	1	3	6	12	18	24
Stone free	12%	32%	41%	68%	72%	73%
Almost stone free[a]	5%	8%	12%	11%	8%	9%

Lost to follow-up, 8%–15%; failures 3%–12%.
[a] Number of fragments ≤10; fragment size ≤3 mm

Table 4. Results in large single stones (21–32 mm; $n=62$)

	Month					
	1	3	6	12	18	24
Stone free	5%	13%	27%	38%	41%	47%
Almost stone free[a]	–	–	3%	5%	6%	6%

Lost to follow-up, 8%–18%; failures 2%–29%.
[a] Number of fragments ≤10; fragment size ≤3 mm

Table 5. Results in several (2–5) stones ($n=198$)

	Month					
	1	3	6	12	18	24
Stone free	3%	7%	12%	25%	31%	42%
Almost stone free[a]	–	–	–	3%	6%	5%

Lost to follow-up, 12%–27%; failures 8%–45%.
[a] Number of fragments ≤10; fragment size ≤3 mm

Table 6. Results in numerous (>5) stones ($n=39$)

	Month					
	1	3	6	12	18	24
Stone free	–	–	3%	13%	22%	31%
Almost stone free[a]	–	5%	8%	5%	11%	10%

Lost to follow-up, 7%–25%; failures 10%–37%.
[a] Number of fragments ≤10; fragment size ≤3 mm

from stones within the first 4 weeks after ESWL – here the shock-wave disintegration was undoubtedly the more important therapeutic principle. Extensive ultrasound follow-up examinations (5 MHz transducer, multiple positions) showed freedom from stones 6 months after ESWL in 41% of our patients with small to moderate ($\leq$20 mm) single gallbladder stones and 12 months after ESWL in 68% (Table 3). After 1 year we classed about 12% as failures (no reduction under dissolution treatment), the remaining patients had to be classed as lost to follow-up. After only one ESWL session the results for large single stones (21–32 mm) (Table 4) and for several/numerous stones (Tables 5, 6) were distinctly poorer; here freedom from stones was recorded in only 30–40% after 1.5 years, although in about 60% of the patients there was a steady reduction in the volume of the remaining fragments under continued dissolution treatment. Here repeat ESWL sessions will have to be included in future non-operative strategies.

Discussion

Bile Duct Stones

Biliary ESWL is undoubtedly an important addition to our armamentarium of non-operative techniques in the management of bile duct stones [13–15]; it is of particular value in elderly patients as in these patients (re-)laparotomy and common bile duct exploration carry a not inconsiderable morbidity and mortality. Bile duct ESWL, on the other hand, is gentle, safe and efficient; it is probably superior to the often described and seldom performed laser lithotripsy [24] because it does not require direct contact between the calculus and the laser fibre. Hitherto ESWL of extrahepatic bile duct stones has been employed only after failure of endoscopic operative techniques. Perhaps ESWL disintegration of ultrasonographically locatable bile duct stones will in future come to be performed even before EST. The particular value of biliary ESWL for intrahepatic cholangiolithiasis must be especially stressed.

Gallbladder Stones

Initial results of biliary ESWL combined with adjuvant oral dissolution treatment in the management of gallbladder stones are on the whole encouraging [4–6, 10, 11], although it is already evident that the success of this therapeutic principle will never quite match that of non-surgical treatment of kidney stones using ESWL. This is due mainly to the numerous limitations and contraindications for gallbladder ESWL. In our experience, too, only about 15% of symptomatic gallbladder stones can at present be considered for ESWL in combination with dissolution treatment [25, 26]. Additional invasive measures such as instillation of methyl *tert*-butyl ether into the gallbladder via a catheter [27, 28] appear relatively aggressive. Their value alone [28, 29] or in combination with ESWL [27] has yet to be established. Single gallbladder stones up to about 20 mm in diameter which fulfil the admission criteria named can be considered a particularly suitable and increasingly accepted indication for biliary ESWL. An extension of the indication is nevertheless to be expected in the coming years with increasing improvement in the methodological procedures (more specific shock-wave qualities, optimised ultrasound components, less problematic repeat ESWL sessions; more efficient dissolution agents?). An extension of the indication to include non-cholesterol stones is conceivable particularly when ESWL fragmentation of the calculi becomes so efficient that it regularly produces only fragments small enough to be passed spontaneously – if necessary with the help of repeated ESWL exposure. Gallbladder motility and the spontaneous 'clearance' of gallbladder

13 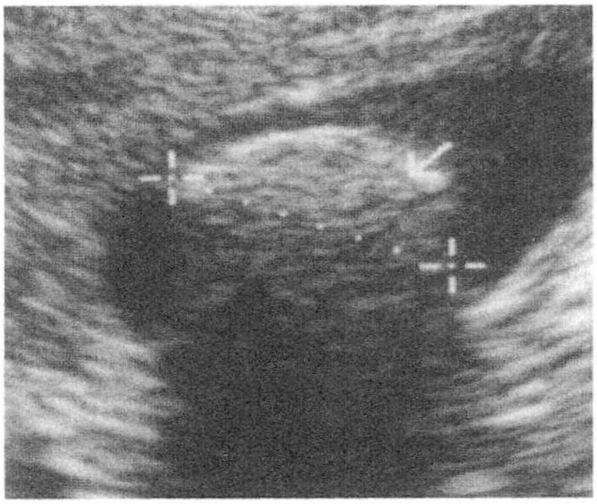

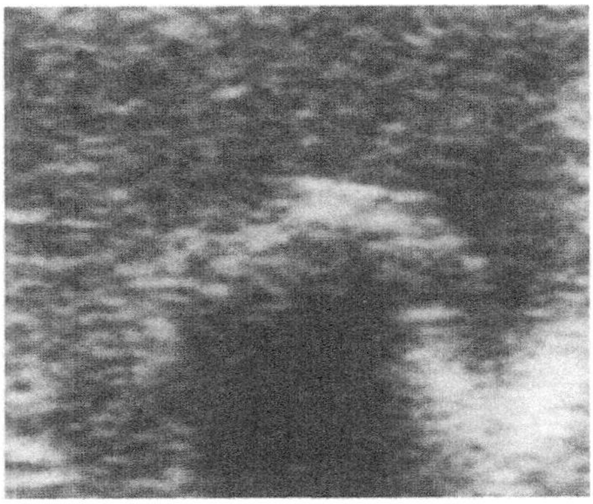 14

Fig. 13. Calculus with uniform internal reflex pattern (*arrow*) probably indicative of homogeneous (cholesterol) crystalline composition. Good fragmentation by ESWL is to be expected

Fig. 14. Calculus with inhomogeneous, stratified internal reflex pattern probably indicative of inhomogeneous (mixed stone) composition. Poorer distintegration by ESWL is the be expected

fragments will then become the limiting factor of the procedure. The fact that even today this concept is already – unintentionally – to some extent reality is shown by our investigation of faecal fragments in which we detected mainly mixed stone fragments [30]. Furthermore, we can expect that in the future the increasingly widespread use of abdominal ultrasound will mean that more gallbladder stones will be discovered and subjected to shock-wave treatment at an earlier stage in their development. In our experience ESWL disintegration is most successful in gallbladder stones with a homogeneous internal echo structure in the ultrasonogram [31] (Figs. 13, 14). A homogeneous structure of this kind is well compatible with a uniform crystalline (cholesterol) composition of the stones. In addition, it is probable that this type of stone corresponds to an earlier stage of stone development at which no recrystallisation or deposit, for example, of pigment has yet taken place [32]. Further systematic investigations will be required to permit assessment of a stone's suitability for ESWL disintegration on the basis of the specific information obtained by ultrasound examination [33]. Ultrasonography also permits unproblematic detection of recurrent stones after successful ESWL. We have so far found such recurrences in only six cases (in which dissolution treatment had not been terminated before exact definition of freedom from stones by careful ultrasound examination). Based on the experience in studies with dissolution treatment alone, recurrent stones are to be expected in 30%–50% (the large majority of the recurrences occurring within the first 2–3 years). These studies are, however, open to the criticism that they are based almost only on radiological follow-up examinations. Ultrasound, a considerably more sensitive method with regard to detection of residual stones, was not employed so that in many cases it was assumed either prematurely or erroneously that dissolution treatment had been effective [34]. It is, therefore, possible that the gallstone recurrences in these studies were not genuine recurrences in the sense of formation of new stones but were the result of renewed growth of residual stones which had been overlooked after only partially effective dissolution ('pseudo-recurrence'). This problem must be dealt with by careful employment of ultrasound for exact ascertainment that the gallbladder is free of stones or fragments.

The expected relativisation of the contraindication silent gallbladder stones for biliary ESWL also points in the direction of more widespread use of the method.

In summary, biliary ESWL is undoubtedly a valuable addition to the non-operative techniques available for the management of extra- and intrahepatic bile duct stones. In the case of gallbladder stones biliary ESWL will become established as an alternative to cholecystectomy in a limited indication range not yet completely defined. Surgical removal of the gallbladder [1] is a good therapeutic procedure but, as the saying goes, the best is the enemy of the good.

References

1. Langenbuch C (1882) Ein Fall von Exstirpation der Gallenblase wegen chronischer Cholelithiasis. Heilung. Berl Klin Wochenschr 19:725
2. Chaussy C, Brendel W, Schmiedt E (1980) Extracorporeally induced destruction of kidney stones by shock waves. Lancet i:1265–1268
3. Brendel W, Enders G (1983) Shock waves for gallstones. Animal studies. Lancet i:1054
4. Sauerbruch T, Delius M, Paumgartner G et al. (1986) Fragmentation of gallstones by extracorporeal shock waves. N Engl J Med 314:818–822
5. Greiner L, Wenzel H, Jakobeit C (1987) Biliary shock-wave lithotripsy. Fragmentation and lysis – a new method. Dtsch Med Wochenschr 112:1893–1896
6. Sackmann M, Delius M, Sauerbruch T, Holl J, Weber W, Ippisch E, Hagelauer U, Wess O, Hepp W, Brendel W, Paumgartner G (1988) Shock-wave lithotripsy of gallbladder stones. The first 175 patients. N Engl J Med 318:393–397
7. Forssmann B, Hepp W, Chaussy C, Eisenberger F, Wanner K (1977) Eine Methode zur berührungsfreien Zertrümmerung von Nierensteinen durch Stoßwellen. Biomed Tech (Berlin) 22:164
8. Delius M, Brendel W, Heine G (1988) A mechanism of gallstone destruction by extracorporeal shock waves. Naturwissenschaften 75:200–201
9. Mueller M (1987) Experimental investigations on focusing of weak spherical shock waves in water by shallow ellipsoidal reflectors. Acustica 64:85–93
10. Hood KA, Dowling RH, Keightley A, Dick JA, Mallinson CN (1988) Piezo-ceramic lithotripsy of gallbladder stones: initial experience in 38 patients. Lancet i:324–325
11. Ell C, Kerzel W, Heyder N, Günter E, Rödl W, Flügel H, Domschke W (1988) Piezoelektrische Lithotripsie von Gallensteinen. Erste klinische Erfahrungen. Dtsch Med Wochenschr 113:1503–1507
12. Staritz M, Floth A, Rambow A, Wilbert D, Meyer zum Büschenfelde KH (1987) Behandlung großer Gallengangssteine durch extrakorporale Stoßwellenlithotripsie mit einem Gerät der zweiten Generation. Z Gastroenterol 25:570
13. Sauerbruch T, Stern M and the study group for shock wave lithotripsy of bile duct stones (1989) Fragmentation of bile duct stones by extracorporeal shock waves. A new approach to biliary calculi after failure of routine endoscopic measures. Gastroenterology 96:146–152
14. Johlin FC, Loening SA, Maher JW, Summers RW (1988) Electrohydraulic shock wave lithotripsy (ESWL) fragmentation of retained common duct stones. Surgery 104:592–599
15. Wenzel H, Greiner L, Jakobeit C (1989) Extracorporeal shock wave lithotripsy in problematic bile duct stones. Dtsch Med Wochenschr 114:738–743
16. Fromm H, Greiner L (1988) Combination of extracorporeal shock-wave fragmentation and bile acid dissolution treatment of gallstones: further data and experience. Gastroenterology 94:1512–1513
17. Podda M, Zuin M, DeFazio C, Dioguardi ML, Battezatti PM, Ghezzi C (1987) Comparison of the efficacy and safety of ursodeoxycholic alone and in combination with chenodeoxycholic acid in patients with radiolucent gallstones: a randomized controlled trial. In: Paumgartner G, Gerok W (eds) Bile acids and the liver with an update on gallstone disease. MTP, Lancaster, pp 347–352
18. Sackmann M, Sauerbruch T, Holl J, Delius M, Ippisch E, Brendel W, Paumgartner G (1987) Results of ESWL in gallbladder stones with radioopaque rim compared to radiolucent calculi. J Hepatol 7:74 (abstr)

19. Greiner L (1989) Whither gallstone? J Abdom Surg 31:22
20. Cotton PB, Forbes A, Leung IWC, Dineen L (1987) Endoscopic stenting for long-term treatment of large bile duct stones, 2–5 years follow-up. Gastrointest Endosc 33:411–412
21. Edwards JD, Adams WD, Halpert B (1959) Infrared spectrums of human gallstones. Am J Clin Pathol 29:236–238
22. Trotmann BW, Morris TA, Sanchez HM, Soloway RD, Ostrow ID (1977) Pigment versus cholesterol cholelithiasis: identification and quantification by infrared spectroscopy. Gastroenterology 72:495–498
23. Neubrand M, Sauerbruch T, Stellaard F, Paumgartner G (1986) In vitro cholesterol gallstone dissolution after fragmentation with shockwaves. Digestion 34:51–53
24. Ell C, Lux G, Hochberger J, Müller D, Demling M (1988) Laser lithotripsy of common bile duct stones. Gut 29:746–751
25. Brink JA, Simeone JF, Mueller PR, Richter JM, Prien EL, Ferruci JT (1988) Physical characteristics of gallstones removed at cholecystectomy: implications for extracorporeal shock wave lithotripsy. AJR 151:927–931
26. Rambow A, Staritz M, Klose P, Meyer zum Büschenfelde KH (1987) Shock-wave lithotripsy of gallbladder stones: how many patients are suitable? J Hepatol 7:71
27. Peine CJ, Petersen BT, Williams HJ, Bender CE, Patterson DE, Segura JW, Nagorney DM, Thistle JL (1987) Fragmentation and dissolution of calcified cholesterol gallstones (CCGS) using extracorporeal shock wave lithotripsy (ESWL) and methyl *tert*-butyl ether (MTBE) in humans. Hepatology 7:1113
28. Allen MJ, Thomas J, Borody TJ, Bugliosi TF, May GR, LaRusso NF, Thistle JL (1985) Rapid dissolution of gallstones by methyl-*tert*-butyl ether. Preliminary observations. N Engl J Med 312:217–220
29. Leuschner U, Hellstern A (1989) Perkutan-transhepatische Litholyse (PTL) mit Methyl-tert-Butyl-Äther. Aktueller Stand und Zukunftsperspektiven. Internist (Berlin) 29:788–791
30. Greiner L, Münks C, Jakobeit C, Wenzel H (1988) Gallenblasenstein-Fragmente im Stuhl nach biliärer ESWL. Z Gastroenterol 26:515
31. Swobodnik W, Ortmann H, Wechsler JG et al. (1986) Sonographie von Gallenblasensteinen. Möglichkeiten und Grenzen der Auswahl konservativ lysierbarer Steinträger. Ultraschall 7:117–122
32. Wolpers C (1986) Gallenblasensteine. Ihre Morphogenese und Auswahl zur Litholyse. Karger, Basel
33. Greiner L, Rebensburg S, Wenzel H, Jakobeit C (1988) Sonographische Gallenstein-Binnenreflexmuster – Artefakt oder reale Information? Z Gastroenterol 26:467
34. Lanzini A, Jazrawi RP, Kupfer RJ, Maugdal DP, Joseph AEA, Northfield TC (1986) Gallstones recurrence after medical dissolution – an overestimated threat? J Hepatol 3:241–244

Laser Lithotripsy

Laser Lithotripsy: Basic Physics

R. Steiner and Th. Meier

Institut für Lasertechnologien in der Medizin, Universität Ulm, 7900 Ulm, FRG

Extracorporeal shock-wave (ESWL) lithotripsy is a useful method for fragmentation of stones in the urinary tract. Its application can be extended to gallstone diseases, where it competes with other conventional techniques. A new technology is now emerging which uses a laser and fiber-optic devices for disaggregation of gallstones (Fig. 1). Some clinical results have already demonstrated that laser systems may provide an important alternative in the therapy of gallstone disease in the future.

In contrast to the ESWL, in which the pressure wave is generated outside the body and must penetrate the body to be refocused on the stone, the laser energy is guided through thin optical fibers directly to the stone. This can be done either transureteroscopically, for fragmentation of ureteral calculi, endoscopically through the gastrointestinal tract, or even percutaneously. The fibers have a diameter of 200–400 μm and are highly flexible. The energy of the laser pulse must be below the damage threshold of the fiber material. The reliability of the laser system involves the coupling of the laser pulse to the transmission system, the production of an optical breakdown, and generation of a shock wave with high reproducibility. The handling of the system should be as simple as possible.

Three types of lasers are in use today: the Nd:YAG laser in Q-switch mode with 15-ns pulse duration, the flashlamp-pumped dye laser, and the Alexandrite laser. The typical

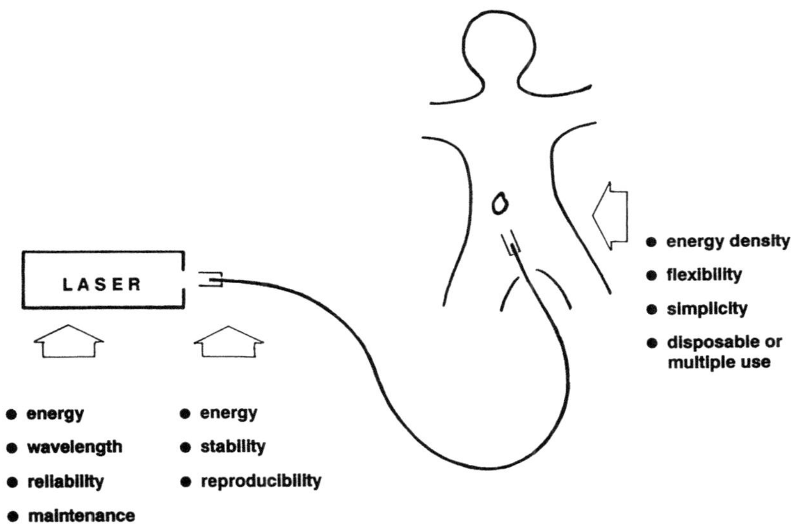

Fig. 1. The laser lithotripsy system

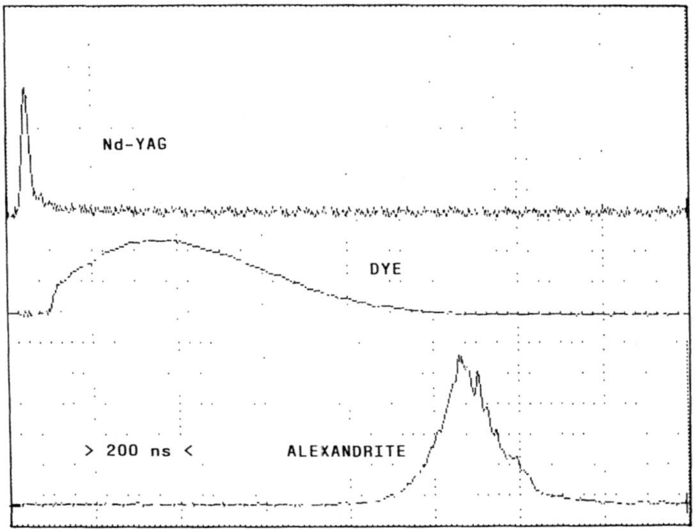

Fig. 2. Laser pulses of the Nd:YAG laser, dye laser, and Alexandrite laser correspond to the form and duration of the shock waves produced

Table 1. Laser parameters of the three types of lasers used in lithotripsy

	Nd:YAG	Dye	Alexandrite
Wave length	1.06 μm	500–700 nm	700–900 nm
Pulse	15 ns	1 μs	250 ns
Energy/pulse	60 mJ	300 mJ	300 mJ
Power	4 MW	0.3 MW	1 MW

parameters of these lasers are listed in Table 1. The wavelengths vary from 500 to 1060 nm. The energy per pulse transmitted through the fiber is typically 60 mJ, which leads to an average peak power of 1 MW, or a power density of GW/cm^2. The shape of the laser pulses are compared in Fig. 2, and the shock waves have a similar time course.

Depending on the pulse duration, two reaction mechanisms for stone fragmentation are observed. The Nd:YAG laser pulse, refocused at the distal fiber tip, leads to an optical breakdown even in water (Fig. 3). By the high-power densities of the electromagnetic field, a plasma formation is accompanied by a growing cavitation bubble which collapses after the laser pulse is over. Local shock waves are produced with an initial pressure amplitude in the range of kilobars. The other type of reaction, with long laser pulses in the range of microseconds, is initiated in the dye laser and Alexandrite laser by light absorption at the stone surface (Fig. 3). Here the power density of the laser pulse is not insufficient to produce an optical breakdown. In the place of a flashlamp-pumped dye laser an Alexandrite laser can be used.

To compare the efficiency of the different lasers in fragmentation experiments the pressure amplitudes of the shock waves were measured with polyvinylidenefluoride (PVDF) sensors (Fig. 4). A fast registration unit measured the rise time (in nanoseconds)

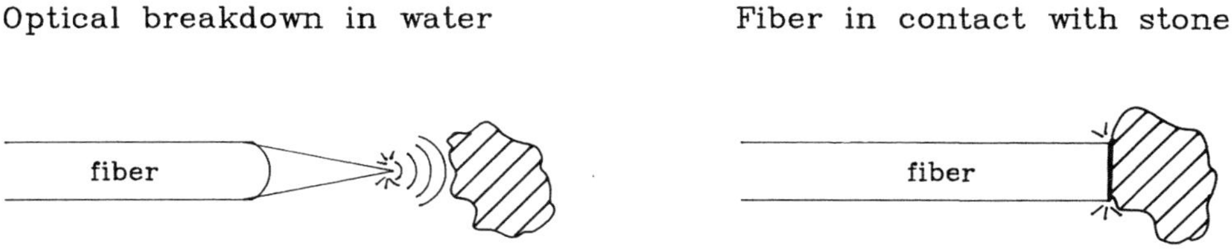

Fig. 3. Two types of reaction mechanism for stone fragmentation. *Left*, optical breakdown in water – in the Nd:YAG laser; *right*, fiber in contact with stone – in dye laser and Alexandrite laser

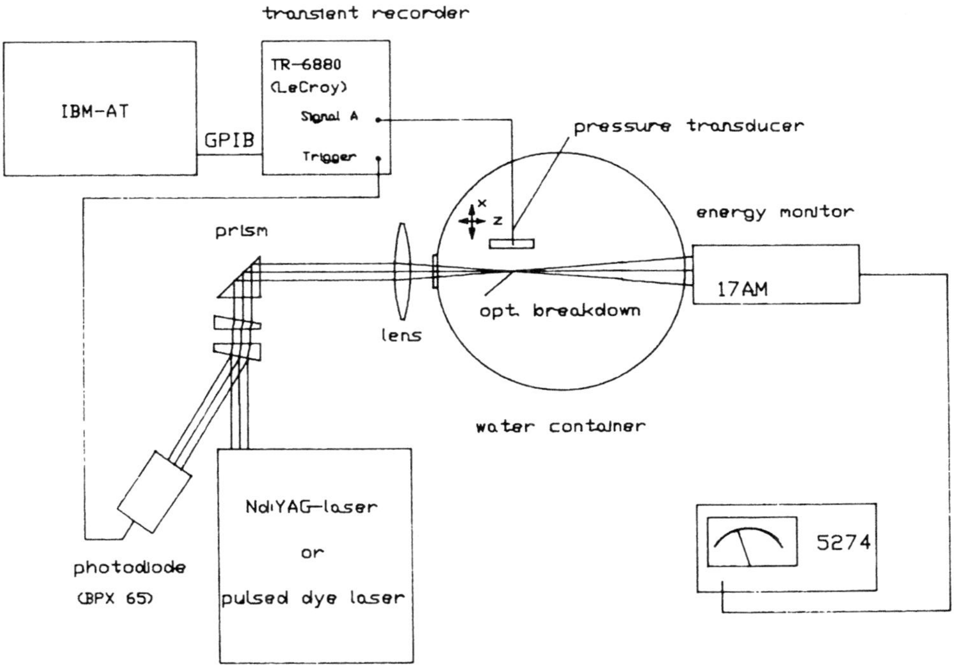

Fig. 4. Experimental scheme for the measurement of shock waves. The pressure transducer is a polyvinylidenefluoride (PVDF) foil. The transient recorder is fast enough to follow the shape of the shock waves

of the supersonically traveling shock wave. The question arises as to whether the energy of the shock wave penetrates the stone or is absorbed at the stone–water interface. To answer this question, different types of stones were cut and then rejoined with the sensor in between. The result is demonstrated in the pressure-time signals of Fig. 5. After a short traveling distance inside the stone, a shock wave was no longer detected for kidney stones, gallstones, or some artificial "soft stones;" on the other hand, in hard and crystalline stones the shock wave travels through the stone and can be measured inside the stone. The consequence is that fragmentation of the former type of stone is rather good because virtually the total energy is absorbed at the stone surface; fragmentation is poor for the latter type.

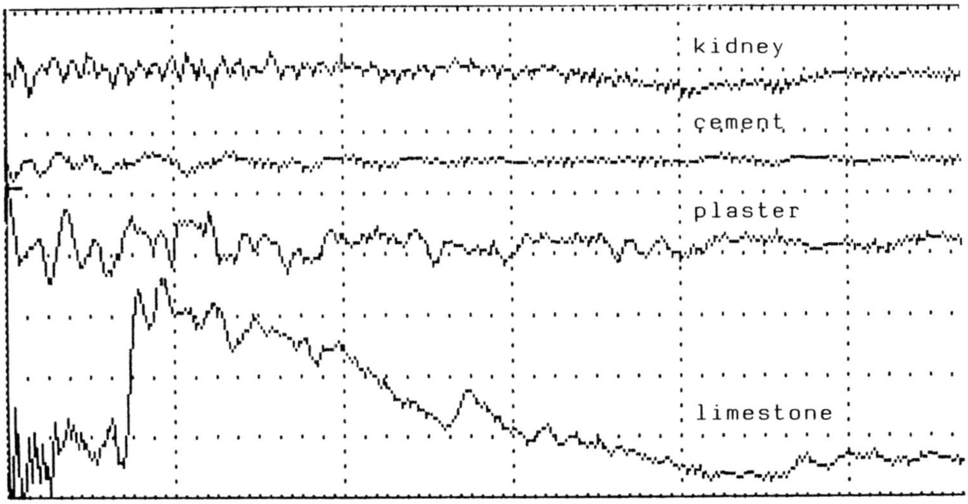

Fig. 5. Shock waves measured inside of stones. In "soft stones," there is no shock wave detectable, whereas in crystalline stones the shock wave can penetrate the material

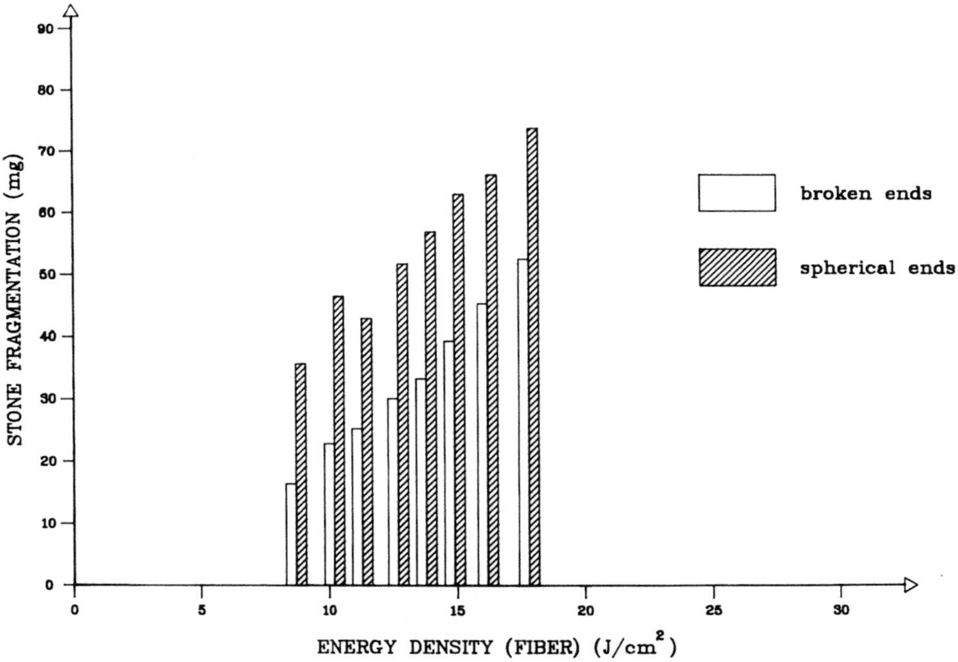

Fig. 6. Stone fragmentation relative to the energy density through PCS (plastic clad silica) fibers. The fragmentation rates with spherically shaped fiber ends are significantly higher than those with fibers with only broken ends

The reaction mechanism of the dye laser and Alexandrite laser pulses is quite different. Three phases can be distinguished:

1. The fiber tip touches the stone; the laser pulse starts to heat up the stone surface.
2. A hot plasma is created which absorbes the rest of the energy of the laser pulse. The emitted light from the plasma can be analyzed by an optical multichannel analyzer.
3. A cavitation bubble is formed at the stone surface which produces a pressure wave responsible for the disintegration of the stone.

In another approach, the spectral analysis of the plasma can be used to control the laser application interrupting the laser pulse if the fiber is not directed to the stone surface. This may be important for safety in the use of such a system.

If absorption of the laser light is primarily responsible for the process, one should examine the wavelength dependence to optimize the reaction; it is the case, however, that the wave-length selectivity is not very pronounced. Even in the deep red region of the spectrum the fragmentation rate of the stones is still at a maximum level. This was the motivation to study the application of the Alexandrite laser.

Of some importance are the transmission systems, especially the quartz fibers. Fibers with different diameters and spherically shaped ends were used in comparison to nicely cleaved ends. Using the Nd:YAG laser a fiber with spherical ends must refocus the laser pulse to give an optical breakdown. Another possibility is to use an optical-mechanical coupler, however, this device has a much larger diameter than the bare fiber. In our experience, the fiber must be rinsed to be protected from mechanical damage. Working in contact with cleaved fiber ends under X-ray or endoscopic control is clinically more practicable and simpler.

The fragmentation rate of the spherically shaped fiber tip is more efficient (Fig. 6). Here a 600-μm PCS (plastic clad silica) fiber has been used with increasing radiation exposure. Comparing the dye laser and the Nd:YAG laser under the same experimental conditions leads to a result slightly favoring the Nd:YAG laser (Fig. 7).

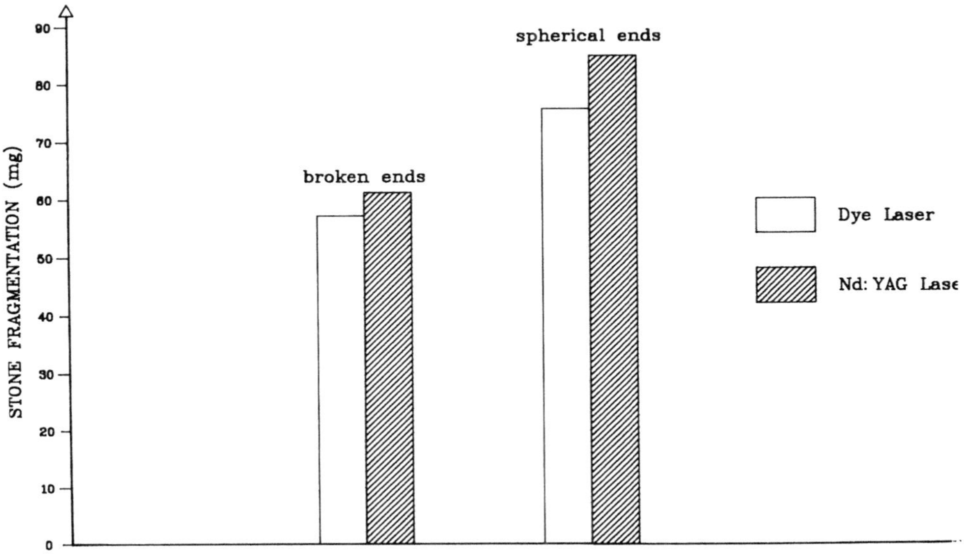

Fig. 7. Comparison of the efficiency of dye lasers and Nd : YAG lasers in lithotripsy. The ND : YAG laser has slightly higher fragmentation rates, but this depends on the stone material (32 J/cm^2; 400 μm Quartz/Quartz fiber)

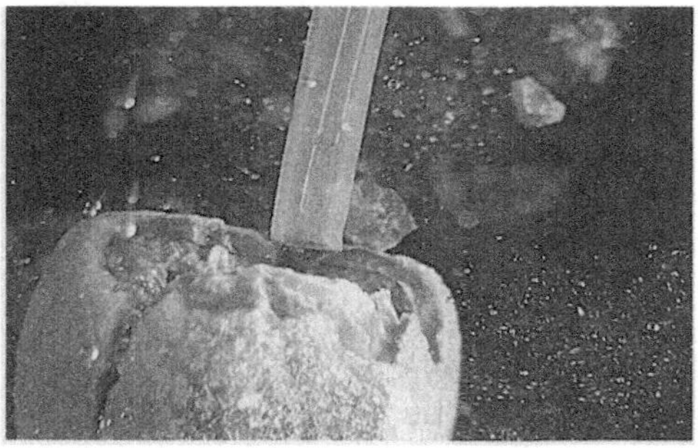

Fig. 8. Gallstone lithotripsy with a Nd:YAG laser. In 2 min the stone was completely disaggregated

The fragmentation of gall stones demonstrated in in vitro experiments (Fig. 8) seems very encouraging, and applications in the biliary duct and gall bladder are clinically possible.

Laser Lithotripsy: Clinical Applications

C. Ell, J. Hochberger, E. G. Hahn, and L. Demling

Department of Medicine, University of Erlangen-Nuremberg, D-8520 Erlangen, FRG

Since the early 1980s several teams have worked on the problem of fragmenting gallstones by laser [1–6]. The first successful endoscopic-retrograde laser fragmentation of a bile duct stone was reported in 1986 [7]. In the meantime, experiences by other teams in clinical laser lithotripsy of bile duct stones have been published [8–10] or reported on (N. Marcon and C. Haber 1989, M. Haws 1989, A.R.W. Hatfield 1989, and T. Ponchon 1989, personnal communications). However, to date, only about 50 patients have been treated with this new therapy method worldwide. The success rate (complete/partial stone removal) is estimated at 50%–80%. Complications after laser lithotripsy have so far not been reported.

In contrast to extracorporeal shock-wave lithotripsy of giant stones in the common bile duct, laser lithotripsy has not yet established itself clinically and is still in its experimental clinical stage. This is due to a number of problems concerning the lithotriptor itself, the safe application of laser energy in the bile duct and the safe endoscopic approach.

Laser Technology

At present there are two laser systems available for clinical application: pulsed Nd-YAG lasers and dye lasers, the Nd-YAG laser offering two pulse qualities for fragmentation. The main properties of the respective pulse qualities are shown in Table 1. It is important to note, however, that the flashlamp-pulsed free running mode laser can be used only for the fragmentation of gallstones, not for that of kidney stones. Of the three Nd-YAG laser systems currently used in clinical tests (LASAG, Thun, Switzerland; Litholas, MBB, FRG; Calculas I, Storz, FRG) only that of LASAG offers the possibility to combine

Table 1. Comparison of different pulsed lasers

	Flash lamp pulsed Nd:YAG	Flash lamp pulsed Dye	Q-switched Nd:YAG
Pulse duration	Milli-s	Micro-s	Nano-s
Nature of fragmentation	Thermal	Thermal (non-c) Mechanical (c)	Mechanical
Quality of fragmentation	Large fragments	Small	Small
Time required for lithotripsy	Seconds	Minutes	Minutes
Suited for	Gallstones	Gallstones + kidneystones	Gallstones + kidneystones

these two pulse qualities. A further advantage of the LASAG system is the possibility to transmit the Q-switched pulses via a 300-µm flexible glass fibre 0.3 mm thick. With the other systems the light can be applied only via 600-µm fibres, rendering the endoscopic-retrograde approach impossible. While the free running mode Nd-YAG laser does not present any problems concerning energy coupling and outcoupling and does not require a special focussing system, this is not the case for the Q-switched Nd-YAG laser; since the energy density can be greater by a factor up to 10^6, the exact energy coupling is of far greater importance. Moreover, since such immense energy densities are necessary to produce a plasma and the following local shock wave, the distal fibre end must be equipped with a focussing unit. Semispheric polishing of the fibre end seems to be the simplest and also a highly practical solution [11]. The 200 µm-diameter quartz fibre is sufficient for light transmission both in the dye laser and in the Nd-YAG laser in the free running mode, making both laser systems ideal for the endoscopic retrograde approach. The technical problems affecting routine clinical use of dye lasers include those of dye stability, easy handling of waste disposal, and dye change (M. Haws 1989 and T. Ponchon 1989, personal communications).

Clinical Application and Safety

While thermal lesions in the area of the choledochal wall are not to be expected if the Q-switched Nd-YAG laser is not used properly, this is not true for the free running mode Nd-YAG laser [6]. However, septic or peritoneal complications have not occurred in animal experiments or in clinical use. In the case of the dye laser, however, thermal and mechanical lesions must be expected if the laser is not applied properly. The Q-switched laser leads only to mechanical lesions, although they have not caused any perforations in our preclinical studies (unpublished data). The endoscopic application of laser energy, working with the dye laser and the free running mode Nd-YAG laser presents the least difficulties. In the Q-switched Nd-YAG laser, a distance of 1–3 mm from fibre end to stone must be exactly and strictly observed, and this may not always be guaranteed in clinical application.

Quite often anatomical changes (previous operation stenoses/strictures) may make a safe endoscopic-retrograde approach impossible, and this represents a major problem for the clinical application of laser lithotripsy.

If the stone can be caught in a special laser lithotriptor basket, it can be fragmented under X-ray control only; the fibre can be placed precisely at the middle of the stone via a central duct in the basket, and there is no danger of applying the energy unintentionally to surrounding tissue. A similar idea is pursued with the use of a balloon catheter with a central hole in the cases of impacted stones (Figs. 1, 2). Since X-ray control is usually possible only in two planes, some uncertainty will remain concerning the correct energy application even if balloon catheters are developed which are better adapted to the anatomical situation.

The safest approach for fragmentation is undoubtedly the use of a baby or mini-endoscope which is inserted into the bile duct via a motherscope (Fig. 3). Mini-endoscopes of an improved standard may be expected in the near future.

Whether laser lithotripsy can become a real alternative to extracorporeal shock-wave lithotripsy for the treatment of stones depends on two factors: early improvement of the laser systems, which are at present not completely satisfactory, and further development of the technolgy of current endoscopes. The argument favouring laser lithotripsy is that laser fragmentation can be executed in the scope of a usually necessary endoscopic pretreatment (papillotomy, contrast X ray, insertion of naso-biliary probe) and does not

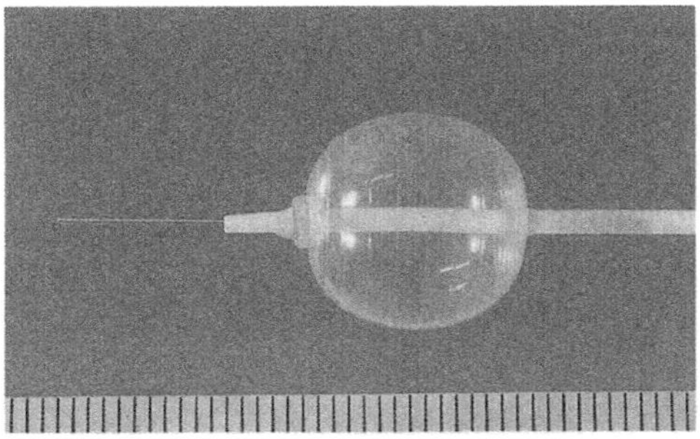

Fig. 1. Balloon catheter (diameter 2.4 mm) with 0.2 mm laser fibre

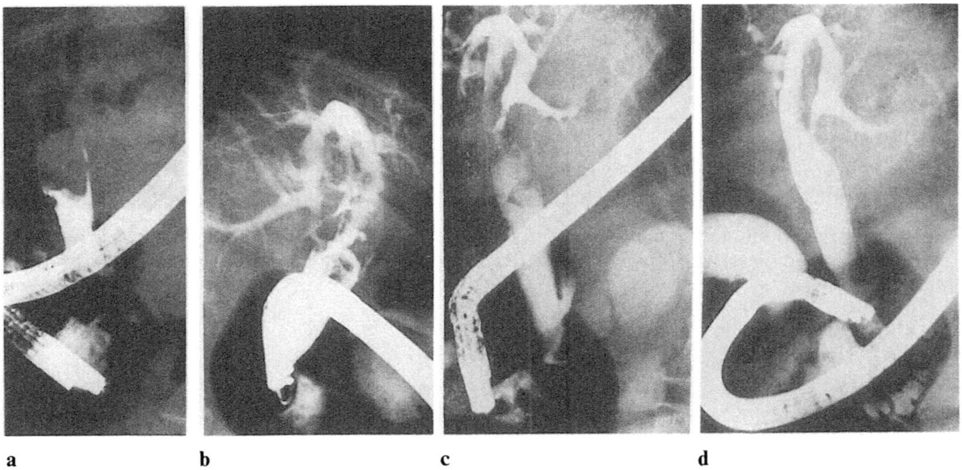

Fig. 2. Impacted common bile duct stone prior to **a** and during (**b**, **c**) lithotripsy via a balloon catheter (seen in **b**) After laser lithotripsy all fragments were removed from the bile duct (**d**)

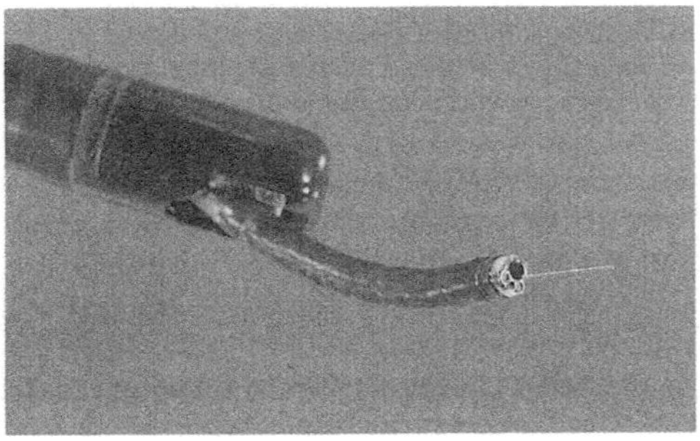

Fig. 3. Mother-babyscope system (Olympus) with the laser fibre (0.2 mm) moved through the instrumental channel (1.7 mm) of the babyscope

require any additional apparatus and organizational preparation beyond the endoscopy equipment. Moreover, laser application in vivo is painless and therefore does not require any additional medication or premedication. If executed under endoscopic vision, the method appears free of any major risks regardless of the laser system used.

a 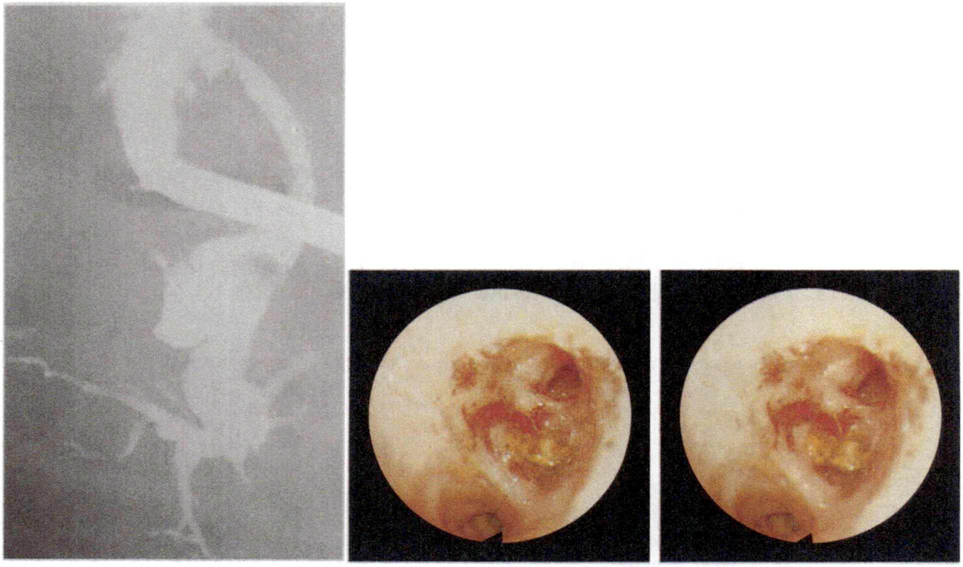 b

Fig. 4. a Large common bile duct stone prior to laser lithotripsy via the babyscope. **b** After laser lithotripsy under direct endoscopic vision the common bile is almost completely free of stone material

References

1. Orii K, Nakahara A, Takase Y, Ozaki A, Sakita T, Iwasaki Y (1981) Choledocholithomy by YAG laser with a cholodechofiberscope; case reports of two patients. Surgery 90:120
2. Mills T, Swain P, Warson G, Bown SG, Salmon PR (1983) Comparison of thermal and photoacoustic fragmentation of biliary calculi using continuous wave and giant pulse lasers. Lasers Surg Med 3:156
3. Bown SG, Mills TN, Watson GN, Swain P, Wickham JE, Salmon PR (1984) Laser fragmentation of biliary calculi. XIIth International Congress of Gastroenterology, Lisbon, Portugal, September 16–22, 1984
4. Ell C, Hochberger J, Müller D, Giedl J, Lux G, Demling L (1986) Laserlithotripsy of gallstones by means of a pulsed neodymium YAG laser in in vitro and animal experiments. Endoscopy 18:95
5. Nishioka NS, Levins PC, Murray SC, Parrish JA, Anderson RR (1987) Fragmentation of biliary calculi with tunable dye laser. Gastroenterology 93:250
6. Ell C (1988) Laserlithotripsie von Gallensteinen. Enke, Stuttgart
7. Lux G, Ell C, Hochberger J, Müller D, Demling L (1986) The first successful endoscopic retrograde laser lithotripsy of common bile duct stones in man using a pulsed neodymium YAG laser. Endoscopy 18:144
8. Ell C, Lux G, Hochberger J, Müller D, Demling L (1988) Laserlithotripsy of common bile duct stones. Gut 29:746
9. Cotton PB, Kozarek RA (1988) Laser lithotripsy of large bile duct stones under direct vision via peroral choledochoscopy. Gut 29:A 1496
10. Kozarek RA (1988) Laserlithotripsy of large bile duct stones. Gastrointest Endosc 28:456
11. Hochberger J, Gruber E, Wirtz K, Wessels G, Dürr D, Hahn EG, Ell C. Laser induced shockwave lithotripsy of gallstones by means of a giant pulse Nd:YAG laser. In preparation

Local Lithology

Local Litholytic Agents: Dissolution of Cholesterol Biliary Tract Stones with Methyl *Tert*-Butyl Ether

J. L. Thistle, B. T. Petersen, J. E. McCullough, C. E. Bender, and A. J. LeRoy

Division of Gastroenterology, Mayo Clinic, Rochester, MN 55905, USA

An estimated 20 million persons in the United States have or have had gallstones, and 80% of these stones are composed predominantly of cholesterol. Efforts to dissolve gallstones with cholesterol solvents are predicated on the premise that removal of the cholesterol will allow the remaining stone components, primarily calcium bilirubinate and calcium carbonate, to be aspirated from the gallbladder or passed spontaneously. Rapidly effective cholesterol solvents have been utilized in the laboratory for decades but have been too toxic or impractical for clinical use. Diethyl ether, for example, rapidly dissolves cholesterol but has a boiling point of 35 °C and expands 225-fold when introduced into the body.

Methyl *tert*-butyl ether (MTBE) is an alkyl ether which is liquid at body temperature (boiling point 55 °C) and has a high capacity for dissolving cholesterol (14 g/dL) [1, 2]. Acute toxicity studies of MTBE when administered topically or parenterally to several animal species have demonstrated tolerance similar to that of diethyl (anesthetic) ether. In sufficient dosage, both ethers can induce general anesthesia and have the potential for inducing intravascular hemolysis. Both ethers are flammable and potentially explosive above 1.5 volume percent in air. MTBE is more stable and less volatile than diethyl ether, however.

The use of MTBE in the United States is investigational, and human studies require Federal Food and Drug Administration (FDA) permission. Delivery of MTBE by percutaneous transhepatic catheter has been easily and safely accomplished utilizing a computed tomographic scan to assess the hepatic-gallbladder interface and plan the

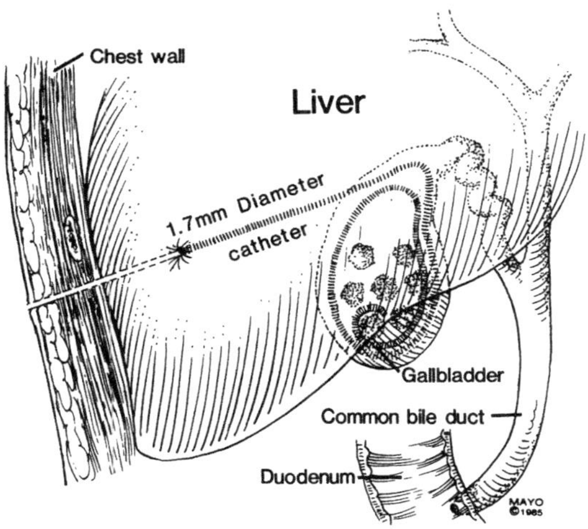

Fig. 1. Placement of percutaneous transhepatic catheter through the gallbladder-hepatic interface with 1.5 loops of catheter in the gallbladder and pigtail located in the fundus

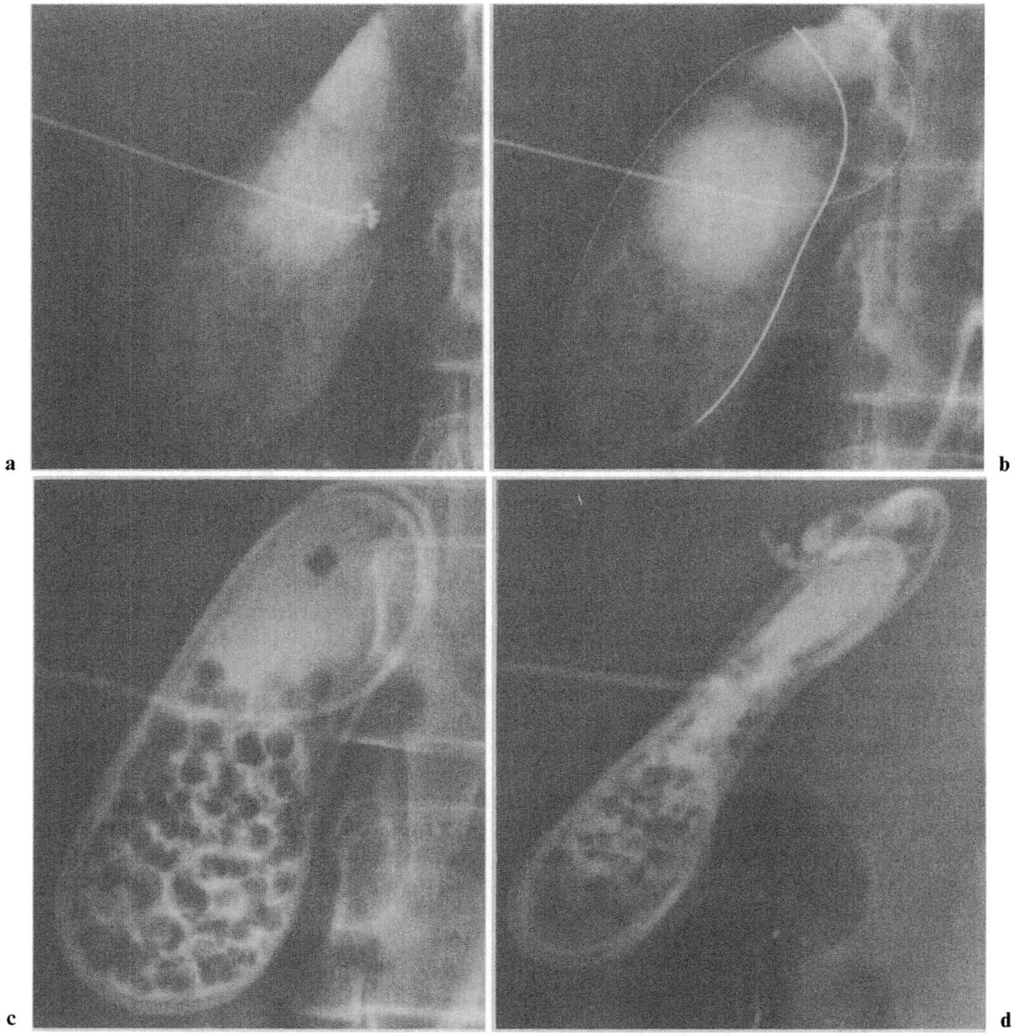

Fig. 2. **a** Needle (22 gauge) placed under fluoroscopic control after opacification of gallbladder by oral iopanoic acid. **b** Guidewire placed through the needle. **c** Catheter (5F) has been placed over a 0.035-inch guidewire (exchanged for the initial guidewire). **d** Stones partially dissolved. **e** Stones completely dissolved and free drainage into duodenum demonstrated

optimal gallbladder entry route. Placement of a 5F (1.7 mm) catheter (Cook Inc., Indianapolis, IN) under fluoroscopic guidance has been accomplished using local and intravenous analgesia in 94 consecutive patients (Figs. 1, 2) [3, 4]. Patients with cirrhosis or coagulopathies have not been treated.

Patients studied have had biliary symptoms, a patent cystic duct, and a high probability of soluble cholesterol stones. Soluble cholesterol stones obstructing the gallbladder neck or cystic duct could be dissolved, but these cannot be clearly differentiated from a fibrotic occlusion secondary to chronic cholecystitis which would leave the patient with

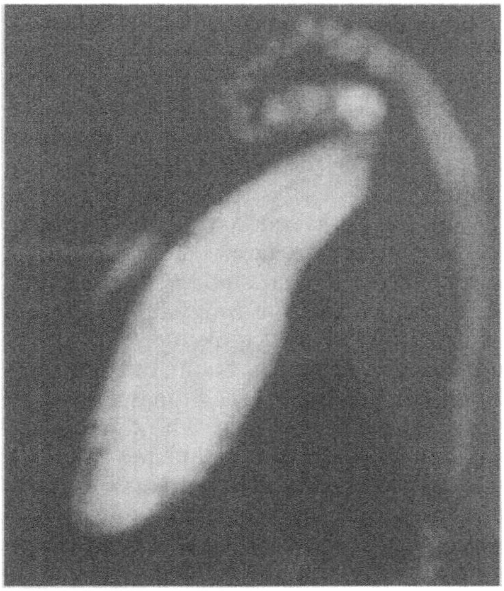

Fig. 2 e

a hydrops. Methods for completely ablating both the cystic duct and the secretory gallbladder mucosa are under investigation but have not yet been shown to be safe and effective. We have not used MTBE in patients with acute cholecystitis or pancreatitis, and no animal data relevant to MTBE use under these circumstances are available. MTBE is available as a high-performance liquid chromatography (HPLC) laboratory solvent which we have redistilled, gas chromatographed to confirm purity, and millipore filtered (0.22 μm) under sterile conditions for investigational use.

Dissolution treatment can be initiated immediately after catheter placement, provided extravasation of radiopaque contrast media at the catheter entry site is not apparent using anticipated treatment volumes. This treatment volume of MTBE is determined fluoroscopically by infusing contrast medium sufficient to envelope the stones, then adding contrast until it begins to enter the cystic duct (the overflow volume). Usually 3–5 ml is an effective treatment volume, and 10–20 ml or more is required to exceed the gallbladder capacity. Overflow does not grossly appear to correlate with infusion pressure since it often occurs well before complete gallbladder filling.

After complete aspiration of bile, continuous cycling of the treatment volume of MTBE can be initiated starting with 1–2 ml and increasing as tolerated to the prescribed treatment volume. Patients often notice discomfort when MTBE is first introduced. Although usually transient and tolerable, patient comfort is optimized by administering an analgesic, e.g., butorphanol 0.5–1 mg intravenously. Butorphanol, in contrast to meperidine or morphine, does not significantly elevate biliary pressure [5]. Sedation is minimized so that development of any anesthetic effect from MTBE is not masked. Nausea and emesis are infrequent and have responded to prochlorperazine suppositories.

Once a comfortable exchange volume and rate of infusion and aspiration of MTBE is established, this regimen is continued using glass syringes and materials stable in MTBE. This procedure may be easily performed by a well-trained and supervised clinical assistant. Complete evacuation of the gallbladder of bile and MTBE after each aspiration stroke and avoidance of reinfusion of bile, stone debris, or infusion of air optimize efficacy and provide complete control over the intragallbladder volume and thus risk of overflow. Acute or persistent overflow or extravasation of an excessive volume of MTBE from the gallbladder could induce intravascular hemolysis, general anesthesia, and possibly duodenitis. This is easily avoided but must not be neglected. Fail-safe pump systems to administer and stir carefully controlled volumes of MTBE are under development [6].

To assure optimal stone and catheter positioning, fluoroscopic assessment should be performed every 2–4 h. Dissolution of stones encircled by the catheter pigtail is much more rapid than at the opposite end of the gallbladder (Fig. 2). Stones can usually be corralled or floated into the newly emptied fundus, but occasionally the pigtail must be repositioned to accommodate to the location of the residual stones. If the pigtail is positioned in the fundus rather than the proximal end of the gallbladder, a large treatment volume can be instilled without overflow. This also avoids infusing MTBE adjacent to the catheter entry site, usually in the upper one-third of the gallbladder.

Solitary stones radiolucent by computed tomographic scan can usually be completely dissolved in 1 day leaving no ultrasonically detectable residual debris. Stones up to 4 cm in diameter may no longer be detectable fluoroscopically after only 3 h of treatment. Large numbers of stones usually require 2–3 days to clear them completely from the gallbladder. Because they often contain substantial amounts of noncholesterol material a few tiny fragments can often be detected ultrasonically in spite of treating the patient for 1–2 h after no debris can be seen fluoroscopically. The natural history of this slight amount of noncholesterol sludge remains to be established, but it has not caused clinical cholecystitis, biliary obstruction, or pancreatitis.

Once stone dissolution is complete, the catheter can be removed using a guidewire and fluoroscopy. This may be accomplished the same day the catheter was placed if dissolution has been completed. Leakage of bile after catheter removal has been infrequent, and only one patient has required replacement of the catheter for this purpose. We have had no symptoms or signs of leakage since initiating placement of Gelfoam in the transhepatic tract at the time of catheter removal.

The morning following catheter removal, a gallbladder ultrasound examination determines most accurately whether radiologically inapparent debris remains. Patients can then resume a normal diet and activity as tolerated, usually returning home that day and to work the following day or week. We are monitoring patients by ultrasound after 6 and 12 months and then annually, to define the incidence of stone recurrence and to assess postdissolution natural history.

Cholesterol stones with one or more radiopaque layers of noncholesterol material may be difficult to dissolve with MTBE using just gentle stirring. Lithotripsy should allow the ether access to the cholesterol and fragment the residual material to fine debris which may be aspirated, passed spontaneously, or more easily dissolved by solvents for calcium, bilirubin, and glycoproteins. Rapid dissolution of stone fragments following extracorporeal shock wave lithotripsy would also eliminate the frequent biliary colic and occasional, more persistent duct obstruction or pancreatitis. Our preliminary experience combining these two techniques in dogs and then in humans with partially calcified cholesterol stones suggests that this approach is feasible and potentially safe and effective [7–10].

References

1. Allen MJ, Borody TJ, Bugliosi TF, May GR, LaRusso NF, Thistle JL (1985) Cholelitholysis using methyl tertiary butyl ether. Gastroenterology 88:122–125
2. Allen MJ, Borody TJ, Thistle JL (1985) In vitro dissolution of cholesterol gallstones: a study of factors influencing rate and a comparison of solvents. Gastroenterology 89:1097–1103
3. Allen MJ, Borody TJ, Bugliosi TF, May GR, LaRusso NF, Thistle JL (1985) Rapid dissolution of gallstones by methyl *tert*-butyl ether. N Engl J Med 312:217–220

4. Thistle JL, May GR, Bender CE, Williams HJ, LeRoy AJ, Nelson PE, Peine CJ, Petersen BT, McCullough JE (1989) Dissolution of cholesterol gallbladder stones using methyl *tert*-butyl ether. N Engl J Med 320:633–639
5. Radnay PA, Duncalf D, Novakovic M, Lesser ML (1984) Common bile duct pressure changes after fentanyl, morphine, meperidine, butorphanol, and naloxone. Anesth Analg 63:441–444
6. McCullough JE, Lesma A, Thistle JL (1989) A rapid stirring automatic pump system for dissolving gallstones using methyl *tert*-butyl ether (MTBE): in vitro comparison with the manual syringe method. Gastroenterology 96:A629
7. Peine CJ, May GR, Nagorney DM, Patterson DE, Segura JW, Thistle JL (1986) Same day sequential extracorporeal shock wave lithotripsy and methyl tert-butyl ether dissolution of gallstones in dogs: effect on gallbladder mucosa and MTBE absorption. Hepatology 6:1206
8. Petersen BT, Segura JW, Thistle JL (1988) Gallstone lithotripsy: in vitro comparison of four different shock wave generators. Gastroenterology 94:A581
9. McCullough JE, Petersen BT, Soper NJ, Bender CE, LeRoy AJ, Thistle JT (1988) Daily electromagnetic shock wave lithotripsy (ESL) and methyl tert-butyl ether (MTBE) dissolution of gallstones (GS) in dogs. Hepatology 8:1255
10. Peine CJ, Petersen BT, Williams HJ, Bender CE, Patterson DE, Segura JW, Nagorney DM, Warner MA, Thistle JL (1989) Extracorporeal shock wave lithotripsy and methyl *tert*-butyl ether for partially calcified gallstones. Gastroenterology 97:1229–1235

Local Litholysis of Calcified Pigment Stones

W. Swobodnik

Department of Internal Medicine II, University Clinic Ulm, Robert-Koch-Str. 8, D-7900 Ulm, FRG

Therapeutic Alternatives in Gallstone Disease

Therapeutic regimens in gallstone disease depend mainly on the composition of the stone. Most conservative approaches are restricted to cholesterol concrements. Systemic litholysis using chenodeoxycholic and ursodeoxycholic acids [1–3] and extracorporeal shock-wave lithotripsy (ESWL; [4, 5]) exhibit high success rates only in cases of small and (in ESWL) preferably single cholesterol stones. Local litholysis, which was performed initially in cholesterol stone disease with ether preparations [6], is the only non-operative therapy which can also be applied in pigment stone disease, provided the proper solvents are used. Furthermore, stone size and stone number do not play a role in the selection of patients for this form of treatment [7, 8]. In complicated gallstone disease, for example, cholecystitis and gallstone ileus, cholecystectomy has been the preferred form of therapy since its introduction in 1882 by Langenbuch [9]. An operative procedure must also be performed in end-stage gallstone disease, especially when the lack of a lumen in chronic cholecystitis prohibits percutaneous puncture. Cholecystectomy is also the procedure of choice in patients with a chronically inflamed, thickened gallbladder wall due the motility defect which would inevitably lead to stone recurrence after successful conservative treatment. A conservative approach in symptomatic but uncomplicated gallstone patients with calcified pigment gallbladder stones is lacking. The development of an alternate technique for local litholysis of this type of stone is demonstrated in this chapter.

Development of Solvents

The development of gallstone-dissolving agents has long been of interest to physicians. As early as 1891 Walker [10], a surgeon, introduced di-ethyl-ether as a cholesterol solvent for the treatment of gallstones. Toxic side effects, however, prohibited the further administration of this drug. In 1953 Best and colleagues [11] applied chloroform to dissolve bile duct stones; Gardner and colleagues [12] in 1975 used heparin preparations to treat residual choledochal calculi postoperatively. This approach was altered by the introduction of chenodeoxycholate mixtures for the dissolution of intra- and extrahepatic concretions [13]. Glyceromono-octanoate (GMOC) and Capmul, a mixture of glyceromono-, glycerodi- and glycerotrioctanoate, showed better results due to its increased cholesterol-dissolving capacity [14]. However, the therapeutic efficacy of all these cholesterol solvents was low due to their slow cholesterol-dissolution kinetics and the restriction of their use to common bile duct stones, which consist mainly of pigment compounds [15, 16].

Therapeutic success rates above 60% were first achieved after the introduction of ethylene-diamine-tetraacetic acid (EDTA) by Leuschner und Baumgärtel [17], enabling the physician to disaggregate bilirubinate and calcium stones as well. The dissolution approach was, at that time, restricted mainly to bile duct stones because they could be easily accessed by endoscopic manoeuvres such as nasobiliary tubing [18] or the surgical T-tube approach.

With the introduction of gallbladder catheterization either under sonographic or radiographic surveillance [19], further improvement in rapid cholesterol-dissolving agents was necessary because most gallstones were thought to consist mainly of cholesterol [20]. GMOC was found to be inadequate for the rapid gallstone dissolution regimens. Therefore, ethers, especially methyl-*tert*-butyl ether (MTBE), a rapid and potent cholesterol solvent, was applied for the contact dissolution of cholesterol gallstones by Thistle's group at the Mayo Clinic [7]. Polyethylene-glycol and di-methyl-sulphoxide are experimental drugs, at least at the present.

Besides dissolution capacity and kinetics, the choice of solvent is dependent on the composition of the stone. Therefore, it is of the utmost importance to determine the structure and consistency of the gallstones which are to be dissolved.

Gallstone Composition

It is widely assumed that in the industrialized Western world of North America, Australia and Europe most gallstones are cholesterol stones. The data reported by Thistle et al. [7] indicate, however, that there must also be other stone components, because in 70% of their carefully selected patients residual stone material was present in the gallbladder lumen after ether administration. This residual debris is thought to consist of pigment stone material. Pigment stones are defined by their chemical composition: the cholesterol content is less than 50%, the calcium exceeds 10%, and the bilirubinate lies above 25%. Most pigment stones are so called "mixed-type" stones, that is, they contain varying amounts of cholesterol.

To determine which solvents should be administered during gallstone dissolution therapy, we examined the composition of 108 gallstones obtained consecutively at cholecystectomy. These were analysed by the micromethod of Nakayama [21]. The results were the following:

- Only two were of the pure cholesterol type.
- Of the "cholesterol mixed-type" there were 76; cholesterol concentration exceeded 75%, but pigment compounds accounted for more than 15% of the dry volume weight.
- The "non-cholesterol mixed type" accounted for 30; by definition the cholesterol concentration was below 50%, calcium concentration above 10% and/or bilirubinate concentration above 25%.

The percentage of gallstones containing pigment materials which cannot be completely dissolved by ethers is higher than had previously been assumed. Therefore, a combination of cholesterol and pigment solvents is essential for efficient gallstone dissolution therapy.

Clinical Applications in the Disaggregation of Calcium Bilirubinate Stones

Solvent Composition

Despite its therapeutic efficacy in cholesterol solubilization MTBE entails a number of major disadvantages in routine clinical applications due to its physico-chemical properties. For example, the boiling point of MTBE is 55 °C, which corresponds to a vapour pressure of 398 mmHg at body temperature (37 °C). One must also anticipate local resorption along with spillover into the systemic circulation, causing severe neurological

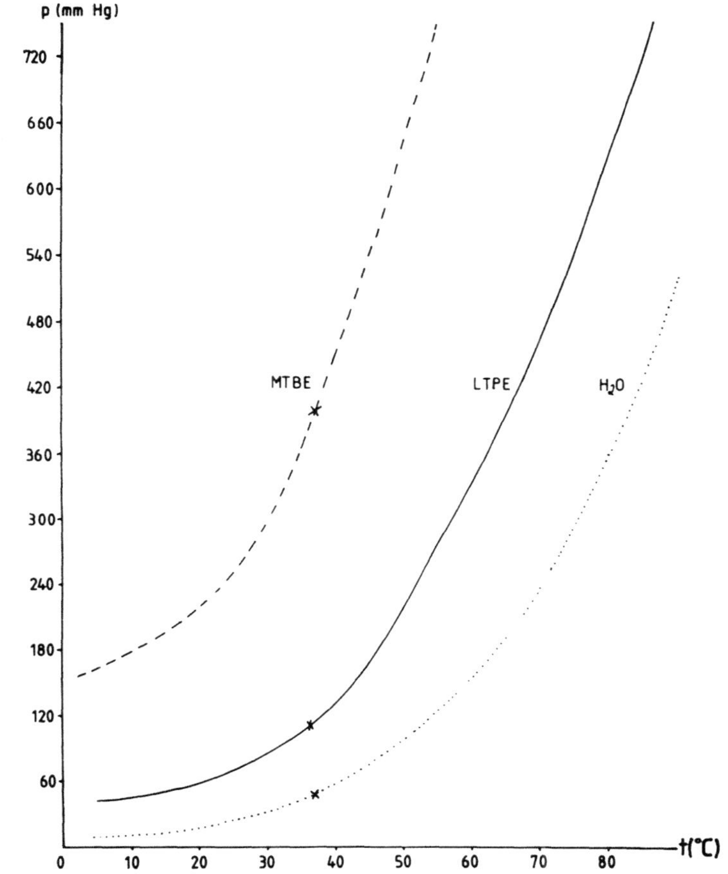

Fig. 1. Vapour pressure of methyl-*tert*-butyl ether (*MTBE*) and lecithin-terpene-pentyl-ether (*LTPE*) at increasing temperature. The vapour pressures of the different solutions at body temperature are cross-marked. Water is included for comparison

and metabolic side effects, as well as an increase in intraluminal gallbladder pressure, with the possible complication of organ disruption. Furthermore, pigmented gallstones are resistant to this drug.

To avoid these possible side effects we developed lecithin-terpene-pentyl-ether (LTPE), which has a boiling point of 87 °C, resulting in a vapour pressure at body temperature of 107 mmHg (Fig. 1). Resorption and spillover into the systemic circulation are therefore minimized. In fact, we observed no neurological deficits in any of our treated patients. The cholesterol-dissolving capacities are comparable to those of MTBE (24.4 versus 26.2 g/100 ml). However pigment compounds still cannot be dissolved.

Consequently we combined LTPE with EDTA in a regimen of alternating administration. EDTA is clinically known from bile duct stone dissolution therapy to have a high calcium-chelating capacity. Severe side effects from EDTA have not been observed, even though it has been administered intravenously for the decorporation of radioactive heavy metals. We observed in vitro that the addition of urea increased the calcium-chelating capacity of EDTA (U-EDTA). This was the reason for the introduction of modified EDTA preparations into clinical use.

Technical Approach

A catheter was introduced into the gallbladder by the Seldinger technique, as described by Thistle (this volume). In contrast to Thistle's approach, the initial puncture of the gallbladder with a 23-gauge fine needle was performed under continuous ultrasound guidance. Opacification of the gallbladder by contrast media was not necessary for organ puncture. Thus, analysis of the non-contaminated bile aspirate could be performed without interference by contrast material.

Clinical Data

Over the period of 1 year we administered LTPE and U-EDTA to 11 patients with calcified gallstones. The results of computed tomography and ultrasonography on the gallstones treated are as follows: two patients had large (>2 cm) gallstones with intense rim calcifications, two exhibited homogeneous calcifications 1.5–2 cm in size; six had multiple stones with a diameter of less than 0.5 cm but homogeneous calcifications throughout the concrement; and one had a stone with a diameter of 1 cm with rim calcifications, as demonstrated on plain abdominal X-ray.

The initially aspirated and analysed gallbladder bile exhibited a cholesterol saturation index of 0.95 ± 0.39 in terms of Carey's critical tables [22]. In combination with a prolonged nucleation time of 9.2 ± 3.8 days these laboratory findings give further evidence of pigmented gallstones, as already determined by sonography and computed tomography. Only three patients showed cholesterol crystals in the native bile, suggesting a rim of cholesterol around the calcified stone centre. The bile acid pattern, determined by high-performance liquid chromatography [23] showed a slight increase in taurine conjugates.

Except in those three patients who had cholesterol crystals in their native bile samples, U-EDTA was administered initially for 1–5 h at 15-min intervals, depending on the calcifications, as demonstrated by computed tomography. In patients with native bile cholesterol crystals the alternating therapeutic regimen was started with the cholesterol solvent (see below). The injection volume of U-EDTA, determined by previous radiographic studies (for reference see Chapter 24), was 5–15 ml. The cholesterol solvent LTPE was then given over the course of 1–3 h at 5-min intervals with injection volumes of 2–12 ml. The alternating administration scheme was maintained until the stones were disaggregated but was limited to a maximum of up to 72 h. The therapy was terminated after this time regardless of the stone condition.

Results

A total volume of 359 ± 316 ml U-EDTA and 214 ± 117 ml LTPE was administered. This resulted in 11.9 ± 8.9 h of effective litholysis with the calcium-chelating agent and 5.1 ± 1.9 h of effective litholysis with the cholesterol solvent. The total dissolution time ranged from 10 to 25 h (average, 17 ± 7.9). One should note that the catheter remained in place between 1 and 3 days. Eight of 11 calcified stones could be disaggregated completely without major side effects (Figs. 2, 3), one greater than 2 cm with rim calcifications, one with homogeneous calcifications, five out of six homogeneous calcified

2 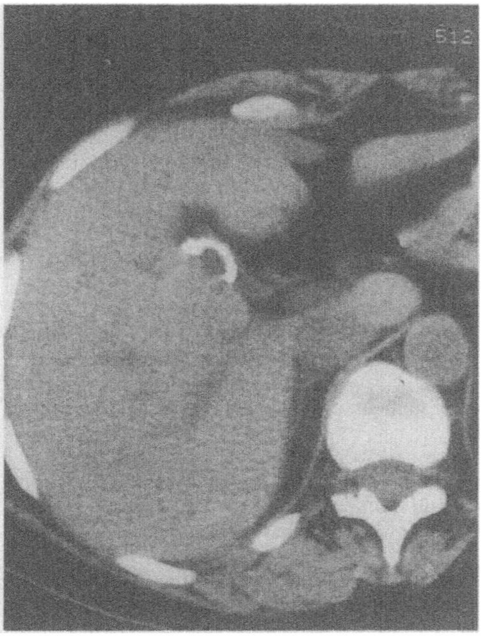
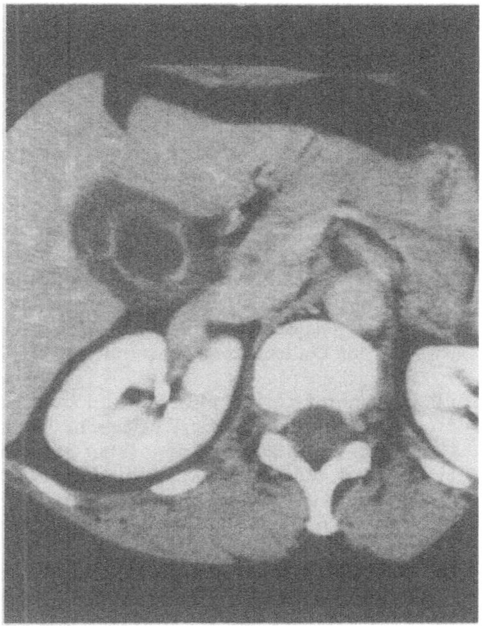 3

Fig. 2. Computed tomographic examination of a patient with a rim-calcified gallstone before treatment with MTBE and U-EDTA

Fig. 3. Control computed tomography after a successful 48-h treatment of the same patient as in Fig. 2. The gallstone has vanished completely, a result which could be confirmed by high-resolution sonography. Note the increased thickness of the gallbladder wall after the treatment

small stones, and one stone 1 cm in diameter with rim calcifications. One of the remaining 11 represented incomplete dissolution, and the remaining two were dissolution failures.

Conclusions

From these preliminary data we conclude that local litholysis of calcium-containing gallstones with U-EDTA and LTPE may provide a therapeutic alternative to cholecystectomy in selected patients.

References

1. Danzinger RG, Hoffmann AF, Schoenfield LJ, Thistle JL (1972) Dissolution of cholesterol gallstones by chenodeoxycholic acid. N Engl J Med 286:1–8
2. Nakagawa S, Makino J, Ishizaki T, Dohi L (1977) Dissolution of cholesterol gallstones by ursodeoxycholic acid. Lancet II:367–369

3. Podda M, Zuin M, Battezzatti M, Ghezzi C, deFazio D, Dioguardi ML (1989) Efficacy and safety of a combination of chenodeoxycholic acid and ursodeoxycholic acid for gallstone dissolution: a comparison with ursodeoxycholic acid alone. Gastroenterology 96:222–229
4. Sauerbruch T, Delius M, Paumgartner G, Holl J, Wess O, Weber W, Hepp W, Brendel W (1986) Fragmentation of gallstones by extracorporeal shock waves. N Engl J Med 314:818–822
5. Sackmann M, Delius M, Sauerbruch T, Holl J, Weber W, Ippisch E, Hagelhauer V, Wess O, Hepp W, Brendel W, Paumgartner G (1988) Shock-wave lithotripsy of gallbladder stones. N Engl J Med 318:393–397
6. Allen MJ, Borody TJ, Bugliosi TF, May GR, LaRusso NF, Thistle JL (1985) Cholelitholysis using methyl tertiary butyl ether. Gastroenterology 88:122–125
7. Thistle JL, May GR, Bender CE, Williams HJ, LeRoy AJ, Nelson PE, Peine CJ, Petersen BT, McCollough JE (1989) Dissolution of cholesterol gallbladder stones by methyl *tert*-butyl ether administered by percutaneous transhepatic catheter. N Engl J Med 320:633–639
8. Hellstern A, Leuschner V, Fischer H, Leuschner M, Caspary W (1988) Percutan-transhepatische Lyse von Gallenblasensteinen mit Methyl-Tert-Butyl Ether. Dtsch Med Wochenschr 113:506–510
9. Langenbuch C (1882) Ein Fall von Exstirpation der Gallenblase wegen chronischer Cholelithiasis: Heilung. Berl Klin Wochenschr 19:725–727
10. Walker JW (1891) The removal of gallstones. Lancet I:874–879
11. Best RR, Rasmusen JA, Wilson CE (1953) An evaluation of solutions for fragmentation and dissolution of gallstones and their effect on liver and ductal tissue. Ann Surg 138:570–577
12. Gardner B, Dennis CR, Patti J (1975) Current status of heparin dissolution of gallstones. Am J Surg 130:293–299
13. Way LW, Motson RW (1976) Dissolution of retained common duct stones. Advanc Surg 10:99–103
14. Thistle JL, Carlson GL, Hoffmann AR, LaRusso NF, McCarthy RL, Flynn GL, Higuchi WJ, Bubayan VK (1980) Monooctanoin, a dissolution agent for retained cholesterol gallstones: physical properties and clinical application. Gastroenterology 68:1016–1020
15. Mok HYI, Bell GD, Whitney B, Dowling RH (1974) Stones in common bile duct: non operative management. Proc Roy Soc Med 67:658–666
16. Wosiewitz V, Schenk J, Sabinski T, Schmack B (1983) Investigation on common bile duct stones. Digestion 26:43–47
17. Leuschner U, Wurbs D, Baumgärtel H, Helm EB, Classen M (1981) Alternating treatment of common bile duct stones with a modified GMOC and BA-EDTA solution by nasobiliary tube. Scand J Gastroenterol 16:497–503
18. Swobodnik W, Wechsler JG, Klüppelberg U, Wenzel H, Faulhaber JD, Junge U, Ditschuneit H (1984) Auflösung von Rezidivsteinen im Choledochus durch modifizierte Spülbehandlung über eine nasobiliäre Verweilsonde. Dtsch med Wochenschr 109:1232–1236
19. Allen MJ, Borody TJ, Bugliosi TG, May GR, LaRusso NF, Thistle JL (1985) Rapid dissolution of gallstones by methyl *tert*-butyl ether. N Engl J Med 312:217–220
20. Sutor BJ, Wooley SE (1971) A statistical survey of the composition of gallstones in eight countries. Gut 12:55–64
21. Nakayama F (1968) Quantitative microanalysis of gallstones. J Lab Clin Med 72:602–611
22. Carey MC (1978) Critical tables for calculating the cholesterol saturation of native bile. J Lipid Res 19:945–955
23. Swobodnik W, Klüppelberg U, Wechsler JG, Volz M, Normandin G, Ditschuneit H (1985) Rapid and accurate reversed-phase high performance liquid chromatographic determination of conjugated bile acids in human bile for routine clinical applications. J Chromatogr 339:263–271

Local Litholysis of Intrahepatic Calculi

K. Draese, J. Schopohl, C.E. Zöckler, and S. Martin

Chirurgische Klinik, Zweckverbandkrankenhaus, Wielandstr. 28, D-4970 Bad Oeynhausen, FRG

Introduction

The prevalence of gallstones is about 15% in adults in the Western world. Cholecystectomy is the most frequently performed abdominal operation. Introduction of the intraoperative diagnosis with radiomanometry, debimetry, and cholangioscopy has reduced the incidence of intraoperative and postoperative complications of surgery, but retained bile duct calculi still represent the most frequent cause of complication. Retained or recurring bile duct calculi absolutely require therapy [18]. Dislocated calculi neglected at surgery are treated according to a plan of treatment in the following order:

1. Attempt at litholysis via T-tube that is left in place.
2. If litholysis is unsuccessful, Burhenne's technique can be used to extract the stone through the T-tube tract.
3. If Burhenne's technique is unsuccessful, or if there is no T-tube, litholysis may be attempted via an endoscopically placed nasobiliary tube.
4. A further possibility is endoscopical sphincterotomy and extraction of intrahepatic calculi with the Dormia basket.
5. A second operation.

Even today surgical removal has its place in therapy along with the endoscopical methods; in treating intrahepatic calculus formation it competes with transhepatic lithotripsy and litholysis [2, 5, 6, 9, 10, 12, 13]. Surgical removal should be performed if all nonsurgical methods have failed. It should always be performed in patients with high, intrahepatic, and difficult strictures of the biliary system or if the diameter of the calculus exceeds 2 cm in diameter.

According to their origin, three types of intrahepatic biliary calculi are distinguished:

1. *Dislocated calculi*. These originate in the gallbladder and are found in the intrahepatic bile ducts, most frequently in the left duct. They are prone to escape detection since they are not palpable and can easily be overlooked at intraoperative radiomanometry. They are often associated with extrahepatic stones. Panlithiasis is a special variety; a continuous gallstone column reaches from Vater's papilla to the intrahepatic biliary tree [7].
2. *Prestenotic calculi*. Suprastenotic stones form proximal to an obstruction of the biliary flow; usually this is a stenosis following bile duct surgery or the stricture of a bilioenteric anastomosis. If the condition persists a long time, the calculi can accumulate and lead to formation of cementlike columns that are almost irremovable.
3. *Calculi associated with intrahepatic bile duct cysts*. These calculi originate from biliary retention in bile duct cysts that function as siphons or in clusters of intrahepatic bile duct cysts.

The complete intrahepatic biliary tree must be demonstrated at intraoperative bile duct cholangiogram as to show intrahepatic calculi or obstructed segmental ducts. The extraction of calculi may be performed with a Fogarty catheter or a lavage catheter. Multiple calculi are removed by irrigation after dilatation or surgical management of the stenosis. If a stenosis is high and cannot be dilated, it must be removed surgically [3, 7, 8].

There will always be stones that cannot be extracted. A wide bilioenteric anastomosis that enables the passage of the stones should be sought if the complete extraction of the calculi is not possible at surgery. Direct extraction of the stone is rarely necessary and is possible only in the left intrahepatic bile duct system. In autonomous bile calculus formation, therapy of the involved part of the biliary tract is a bilioenteric anastomosis or the resection of the calculus forming bile ducts, especially if there is a stenosis of the duct. Resection is no longer possible if all intrahepatic ducts are involved. In this case therapy is limited to retracting as many calculi as possible and to a bilioenteric anastomosis [7, 8, 14].

Results

Calculi in the intrahepatic biliary tract are still among the major problems of biliary tract surgery. After several preceding operations a renewed operation is technically difficult, especially if there is extensive scarring, and if the bile ducts are hidden deep in the altered hepatic tissue [3, 15, 18]. If nonsurgical methods are unsuccessful, we consider a hepaticojejunostomy with or without segment resection to be indicated in the following cases:

1. Stenosis of the common bile duct and its branches
2. Trauma of the biliary tract and biliary fistulas
3. Anatomical disorders of the biliary tract (e.g., cysts)
4. Intrahepatic gallstones if the diameter of the calculus exceeds 2 cm
5. Nonextractable recurring or persisting calculi after preceding operations

In the past 15 years we have treated 52 patients with intrahepatic calculi that had not been completely removed at the primary operation, or that could not be extracted. Of these, 13 patients were treated by reoperation. Among a total of 286 patients with a bilioenteric anastomosis, 39 (13.7%) required hepaticojejunostomy for intrahepatic calculi. The mechanisms that we found to cause intrahepatic bile calculus formation are: dislocated calculi (80% cholesterol gallstones) in 22, prestenotic calculi (pigment gallstones) in 19, and calculi associated with intrahepatic bile duct cysts in 11.

The following concept of treatment for intrahepatic bile calculi has been successfully used in our clinic.

Extraction with Fogarty Catheter Under Cholangioscopic Visualization and Irrigation

Intraoperative cholangiography of the complete intrahepatic biliary tree is necessary since the calculi may present as filling defects. Extraction is performed with a Fogarty catheter under cholangioscopic visualization or with a lavage catheter. The rigid choledochoscope is more useful than the flexible scope because the tip can be directed. Attachments to the scope permit extraction of stones, biopsy of lesions, and cauterization of bleeding points.

We use glycero-octanoate and bile salt EDTA in postoperative litholysis. At first these substances were instilled consecutively; later they were used concurrently in order also to include calcium bilirubinate calculi. An infusion pump set to a rate of 5–10 ml/h was

Table 1. Local litholytic agents for intrahepatic calculi

Cholesterol gallstones: glycero-octanoate (hydrophilic) and 20% methylhexyl ether (130 ml)[a]
Glycero-octanoate (49.0 g)
Polyethylenglukol-6-capryl or capric acid glyceride (34.0 g)
Polyethylenglukol-20-sorbitan mono-oleate (14.0 g)
Polyethylenglukol-20-sorbitan monolaurate (5.5 g)
Methylhexyl ether (26.0 g)
Aqua ad injectabilia (ad 130.0 g)
Ethanolamine (ad pH 78–8.0 g)
Pigment gallstones: bile salts and ethylenediamine-tetraacetate, buffer augmented (300 ml)[b]
Sodium tauroursodeoxycholate (0.9 g)
Sodium ursodexycholate (0.7 g)
Sodium chenodeoxycholate (0.4 g)
Trisodium ethylenediaminetetraacetate (3.2 g)
Trisodium citrate (0.7 g)
Allantoin (0.4 g)
L-Carnosine (0.7 g)
L-Arginine (0.6 g)
L-Lysine (1.2 g)
Glyceromonocaprylate (3.0 g)
Poloxalene (Pluronic F 68; 15.0 g)
Ethanolamine (ad pH 9.5)

[a] Dose: 5–10 ml/h or 0.815–1.63 g/h
[b] Dose: 0.0535–0.107 g/h

used for instillation through a lavage catheter that had been placed intra- or postoperatively (Table 1). The mean duration of instillation was 2.5 weeks [9–11, 13].

In three patients dissolution or reduction in size of the calculi was attained so that they were either passed spontaneously or could be passed mechanically through irrigation. In a fourth patient we discontinued litholysis after vomiting and diarrhea had occurred as side effects. A second operation was performed at which the calculus was extracted.

Bilioenteric Anastomosis

Hepaticojejunostomy Without Segment Resection

The calculi were not completely extractable in 48% of our patients. If it was not possible to remove all calculi from the intrahepatic biliary tree, we performed a hepaticojejunostomy. Remaining calculi could then fall into the isolated Roux-en-Y jejunal loop through the anastomosis. U-tubes combined with lavage catheters that had been placed intraoperatively using Burhenne's technique enabled local chemical litholysis postoperatively. This procedure has proven successful in our clinic. These U-tubes are placed in the affected segments of the biliary tract transhepatically and drain externally, the distal segment being placed percutaneously through a jejunal Witzel's fistula. The replacement of these catheters at roughly 6-week intervals ensures continued patency of the hepaticojejunostomy and prevents the accumulation of bile sludge in the catheter, which would occlude the anastomosis. Lavage catheters for local litholysis were placed in a total of 25 patients [1, 3, 16–18].

Hepaticojejunostomy with Segment Resection

If peripheral biliary tree segments are involved in cholelithiasis, a partial hepatectomy may have to be considered. Partial resection of the right hepatic lobe, especially in the major hepatic segments 3 and 4, poses more problems than resection within the left hepatic lobe. Calculi in the distal caudal segments can also be treated using Longmire's technique for hepatojejunostomy. In this procedure the involved bile duct is attained through incision of the hepatic tissue and the Roux-en-Y jejunal segment is anastomosed directly with the lowest area of the involved duct (Figs. 1, 2).

The procedure is more complicated if there is a stenosis of the intrahepatic bile ducts or of a biliary-intestinal anastomosis. Liver function tests are not always reliable in the preoperative evaluation of a bilioenteric anastomosis. Even if the anastomosis is wide, a slightly elevated level of serum alkaline phosphatase is often found. This is probably caused by the stagnation of bile in the efferent loop or bacterial colonization of the biliary tract. Depending on the type of anastomosis, bacteriobilia is reported in about 70% of operated patients [3, 4]. Bacteriobilia does not in itself lead to symptomatic cholangitis; in order for this to occur there must also be obstruction of the bile flow that may be caused by calculi. In 31 patients with intrahepatic calculi we found the following bacterial colonization in bile: *Escherichia coli* in 100%, enterococci (*Streptococcus faecalis*) in 89%, *Klebsiella* in 56%, anaerobic bacteria (*Bacteroides fragilis*) in 55% and *Pseudomonas aeruginosa* in 45%.

If there are calculi proximal to a stenosis, these are irrigated out after the stenosis has been either removed surgically or dilated. Pneumatic dilation should be attempted first; the stenosis is intubated and then dilated over a period of several minutes. If the stenosis is high and solid and cannot be dilated, it must be removed surgically. The question concerning autonomous intrahepatic calculus formation such as that described by Caroli

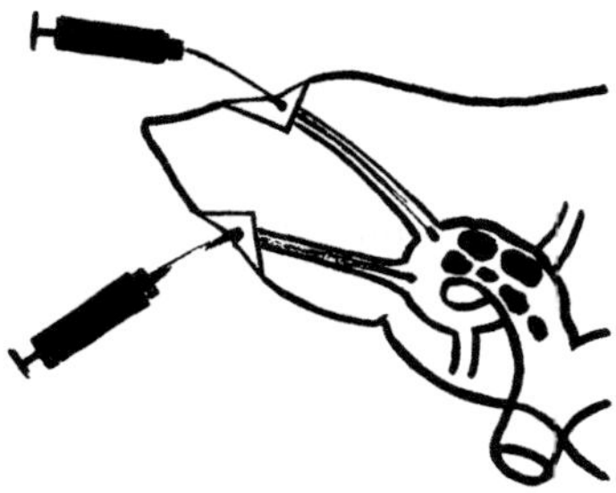

Fig. 1. Incision of the hepatic tissue. Lavage catheter placed intraoperatively

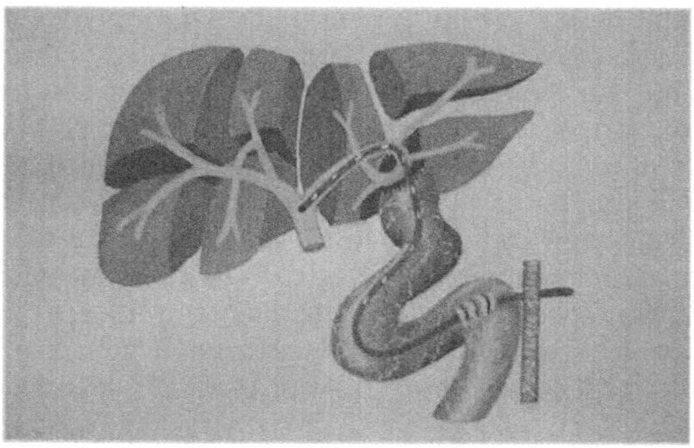

Fig. 2. Hepaticojejunostomy with segment resection. Lavage catheter and U-tube placed using Burhenne's technique

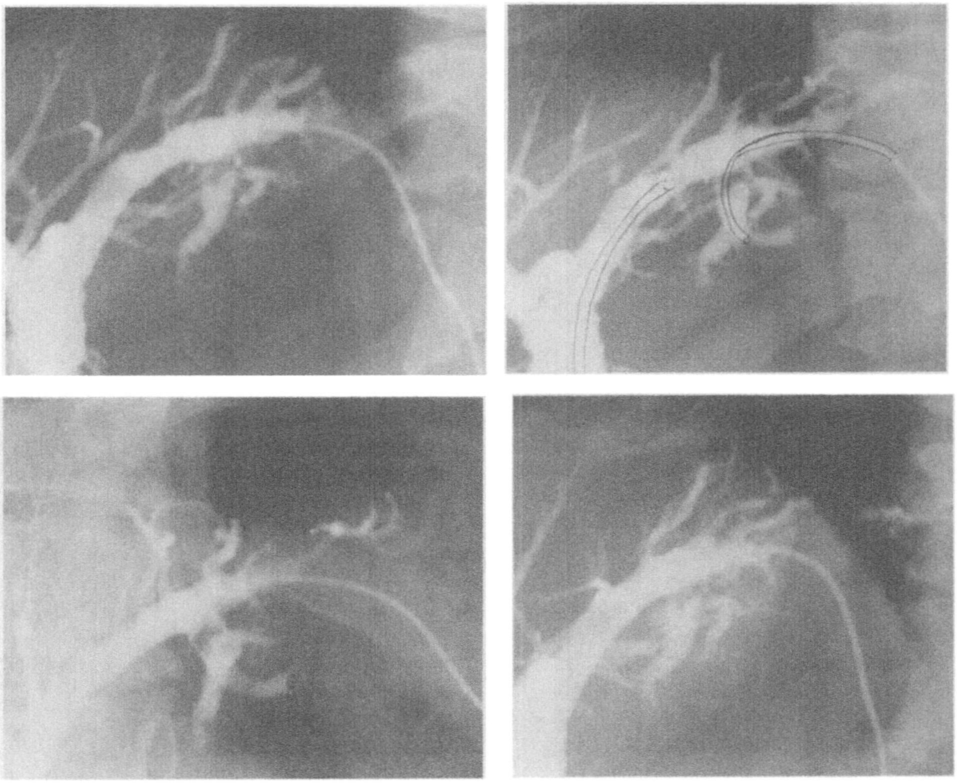

Fig. 3. Intrahepatic calculi; lavage catheter placed using Burhenne's technique

still remains unsolved. Since a stenosis of the intrahepatic bile ducts was also reported in several cases, there can be no certain proof as to whether these calculi had been caused by an obstruction of the bile flow or not. We resected the left hepatic lobe in two of our patients with Caroli's syndrome.

In three other patients we continued to find calculi in the intrahepatic bile ducts after several operations when we later saw them as outpatients. In spite of a hepaticojejunostomy with a sufficiently wide anastomosis there was recurring calculus formation in every case. Through postoperative litholysis and irrigation of the bile ducts concerned, a calculus-free state could be attained in two of these patients (Figs. 3, 4). In one patient new calculi continued to develop in spite of intermittant litholysis and irrigation. Spectrographic analysis showed them to be bilirubinate calculi. The tricoordinate graph did not prove effective in analyzing the relative composition of bile lipids. Autonomous calculus formation must be considered certain in this patient.

The assessment of early and late results (Figs. 5, 6) shows that the combination of surgical treatment and postoperative local litholysis has led to long-term freedom from biliary calculi in 23 out of 25 patients. In one patient the calculi had to be extracted surgically because litholysis had been unsuccessful. In another patient a satisfying result could not yet be attained because of autonomous calculus formation. When seen for follow-up, 18 patients (72%) stated that they were free of complaints; normal liver function tests were found in 20 patients (80%).

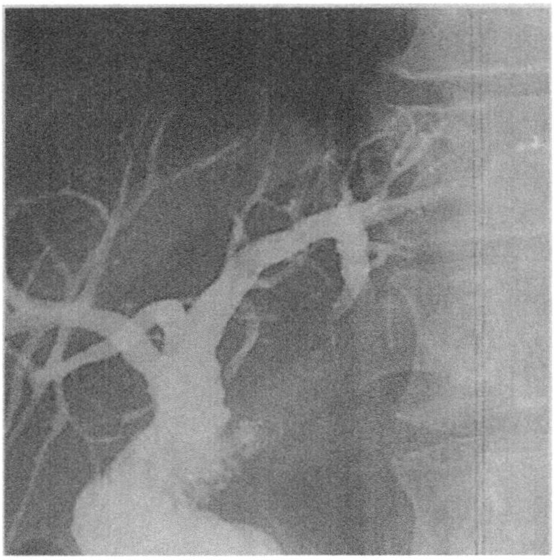

Fig. 4. Results: the combination of surgical treatment and local letholysis led to freedom from biliary calculi

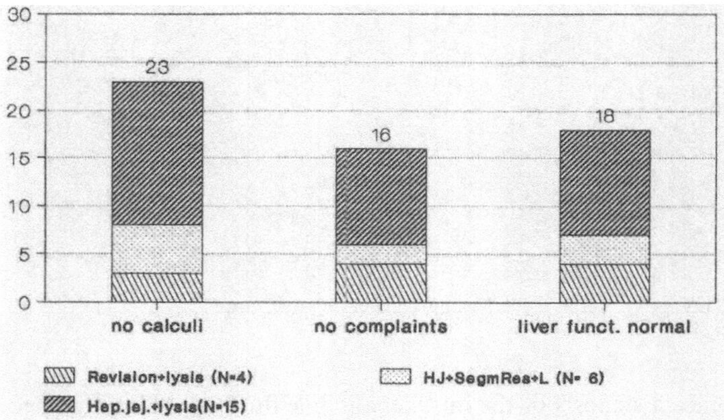

Fig. 5. Intrahepatic calculi following local litholysis: early results ($n=25$)

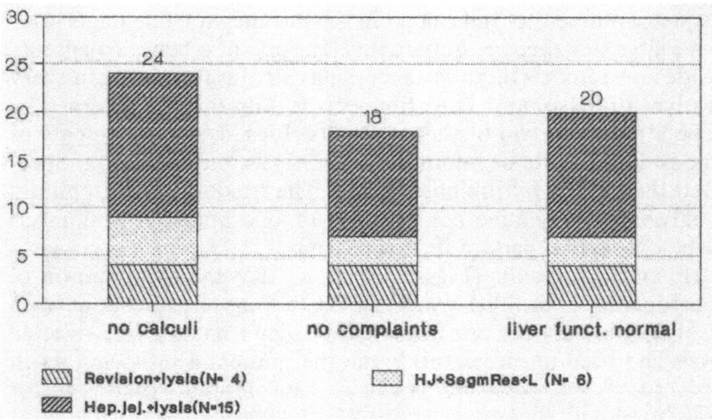

Fig. 6. Intrahepatic calculi following local litholysis: follow-up results ($n=25$)

Summary

The bilioenteric anastomosis combined with postoperative local litholysis has proven successful in treating nonextractable intrahepatic calculi in our clinic. The feasibility of local intrahepatic litholysis and the low rate of side effects if the dosage of the irrigation fluid is individually adjusted allow therapy even if bile ducts are filled with stone columns. Lavage catheters can be placed intraoperatively using Burhenne's technique or postoperatively through drains.

References

1. Burhenne HJ (1972) Extraktion von Residualsteinen der Gallenwege ohne Reoperation. Fortschr Geb Röntgenstr 117(4):425–428
2. Dotter CT, Bilbao MK, Katon RM (1979) Percutaneous transhepatic gallstone removal by needle tract. Radiology 133:242–243
3. Draese K, Schopohl J, Zöckler CE (1988) Restenosierung nach Hepatico-Jejunostomie: Pathogenese, Diagnostik, Therapie. In: Häring R (ed) Postoperative Folgezustände: Pathogenese, Diagnostik, Therapie. Überreuter Wissenschaft, Vienna, p 282
4. Farthmann EH, Lausen M, Rädecke J (1988) Postoperative Folgezustände und Syndrome nach Cholecystektomie und Gallengangseingriffen. In: Häring R (ed) Postoperative Folgezustände: Pathogenese, Diagnostik, Therapie. Überreuter Wissenschaft, Vienna, p 255
5. Günther R, Schmidt HD, Braun B (1981) Perkutane transhepatische Gallensteinextraktion. Dtsch Med Wochenschr 106:615–617
6. Günther R, Klose K, Schmidt HD, Staritz M (1983) Perkutane transhepatische Zertrümmerung von Gallensteinen und Fragmentextraktion. Fortschr Geb Röntgenstr 139(3):256–260
7. Hess W (1977) Nachoperationen an den Gallenwegen. Enke, Stuttgart
8. Hess W (1986) Postoperative Beschwerden. In: Hess W, Cireni A, Rohner A, Akovbiantz A (ed) Die Erkrankungen der Gallenwege und des Pankreas, vol II. Piccin Nuova Libraria, Padua, p 2377
9. Husen van N (1988) Alte und neue Techniken der endoskopischen Steinzertrümmerung. Med Klin 83(6):214–218
10. Leuschner U (1986) Chemische Behandlung von Gallenblase- und Gallengangssteinen. Aktueller Stand und kritische Stellungnahme. Med Klin 81(6):217–222
11. Leuschner U, Baumgärtel H, Phillip J, Jessen K, Hagenmüller F, Trüber E, Classen M (1982) Spülbehandlung und Endoskopie im kombinierten Einsatz bei der Therapie von Gallengangssteinen. Dtsch Med Wochenschr 107:285–290
12. Molnar W, Stockum AE (1978) Transhepatic dilatation of choledochoenterostomy strictures. Radiology 129:59–64
13. Paumgartner G, Sauerbruch T (1988) Heutiger Stand von Litholyse und Lithotripsie von Gallensteinen. Chirurg 59:190–196
14. Peiper HJ (1980) Wiederholungseingriffe an den Gallenwegen einschließlich rekonstruktiver Operationsverfahren. Internist 21:597
15. Schopohl J, Zöckler CE, Draese K (1987) Hepatico-Jejunostomie. Besondere Techniken und Ergebnisse. Chir Praxis 37:593
16. Schriefers KH, Gerometta R (1982) Sekundäreingriffe an den Gallenwegen. Chirurg 53:766–772
17. Steinbrecher P, Becerra VM (1981) Fragen zur Reoperation an den Gallenwegen. Med Welt 32:288
18. Zöckler CE, Draese K (1980) Rezidiv-Eingriffe an den Gallenwegen und biliodigestive Anastomosen. Aktuelle Chirurgie 15:313–334

Reduction of Biliary Cholesterol Saturation by Inhibition of Cholesterol Synthesis: New Therapeutic Consequences?

K. von Bergmann, T. Heinemann, and D. Lütjohann

Department of Medicine, Division of Clinical Pharmacology, University of Bonn, Sigmund-Freud-Straße 25, 5300 Bonn 1, FRG

Introduction

Large epidemiological studies have clearly demonstrated that hypercholesterolemia is a major risk factor for coronary heart disease. Dietary and/or drug treatment to reduce elevated serum cholesterol reduces the incidence of cardiac events. At least two placebo-controlled prospective studies revealed a reduction in the incidence of cardiac events [1, 2]. Drug treatment of hyperlipoproteinemia also influences biliary lipid metabolism; for example, in the Coronary Drug Project [3] and the World Health Organization trial [4], treatment of hyperlipoproteinemia was associated with an increased incidence of gallstone formation and cholecystectomies. This side effect of clofibrate had been predicted by measurement of biliary cholesterol output [5]. During treatment with clofibrate the output of biliary cholesterol was higher than without drug treatment. This change in cholesterol secretion was followed by an increase in biliary cholesterol saturation. Other fibric acid derivatives also increase biliary cholesterol saturation by elevation of hepatic output of cholesterol [6–8]. In addition, all fibric acid derivatives studied so far diminished bile acid synthesis, and at least one analogue also decreased hepatic bile acid output [8]. Although fibric acid derivatives are very safe drugs, and at least one derivative reduces the event of cardiac disease [2], the formation of gallstones may be a possible side effect. This is especially a problem in subjects with a higher risk for gallstone formation.

An interesting new class of drugs for treatment of hypercholesterolemia are competitive inhibitors of 3-hydroxy-3-methylglutaryl coenzyme A reductase (HMG-CoA reductase), the rate-limiting enzyme in cholesterol synthesis. These compounds reduce cholesterol synthesis in cultured cells in vitro and total body cholesterol in man in vivo [9, 10].

The reduction in total body cholesterol synthesis must ultimately affect biliary lipid metabolism. Indeed, Duane et al. [11] have demonstrated that treatment of patients with hypercholesterolemia with simvastatin decreases biliary cholesterol saturation. Athough it might be anticipated that the reduction in biliary cholesterol saturation is due to a decrease in hepatic output of cholesterol, measurements of biliary lipid secretion before and during treatment with an HMG-CoA reductase inhibitor have not been performed so far. To elucidate the mechanism by which HMG-CoA reductase inhibitors decrease biliary cholesterol saturation in man, biliary lipid secretion, total cholesterol, and bile acid synthesis were measured in two male subjects with familial hypercholesterolemia before and 6 weeks after treatment with simvastatin (40 mg/day).

Methods and Materials

Patients

Two patients with familial hypercholesterolemia participated in the study; their clinical data are given in Table 1. Both patients had normal liver function, and neither showed

Table 1. Patients' clinical data

Patient no.	Age (years)	Weight (kg)	Height (cm)	Clinical diagnosis
1	30	81	182	Heterozygous FH, xanthomas, MI (28 years); father MI†
2	34	78	182	Heterozygous FH, xanthomas, arcus lipoides; father MI†

FH, familial hypercholesterolemia; MI, myocardial infarction

signs of renal disease, thyroid dysfunction, or diabetes mellitus. Patient 1 had a history of myocardial infarction, and an aneurysmectomy had been performed 1 year previously. He was under continuous treatment with triamterene (50 mg/day), hydrochlorothiazide (25 mg/day), and amiodarone HCL (2 × 150 mg/day). Before treatment patients were instructed to keep a dietary record for 1 week in order to calculate dietary cholesterol intake. At this time fecal balance and biliary lipid secretion studies were performed. Thereafter both patients received simvastatin in a daily dose of 40 mg once at night, and the study was repeated after 6 weeks. This investigation was conducted in accordance with the principles of the Helsinki Declaration, and written informed consent was obtained from both subjects.

Serum Lipids

Total serum cholesterol, triglycerides, and high-density lipoprotein (HDL) cholesterol were measured enzymatically [12, 13]. Very low density lipoprotein was separated by ultracentrifugation at density 1.006 g/ml on each sample. Cholesterol was measured on the infranatant both before and after precipitation of low-density lipoprotein (LDL) with heparin manganese [14].

Fecal Excretion of Neutral and Acidic Sterols

Fecal excretion of neutral and acidic steroids was estimated by chemical analysis [15]. Before administration of β-sitosterol and chromic oxide as fecal markers, all stools of both patients were collected for 3 days. Baseline levels of β-sitosterol and its metabolites were quantified in these samples by gas liquid chromatography (GLC) [16]. Daily excretion of these plant sterols averaged 120 mg/day and 132 mg/day in patients 1 and 2, respectively. At the end of both periods β-sitosterol (100 mg t.i.d.) and chromic oxide (60 mg t.i.d.) were administered in capsules for 1 week. After subtracting the baseline levels of the previously quantified plant sterols, the recovery of total plant sterols averaged 95% ± 5% and 97% ± 7% in patients 1 and 2, respectively. These results indicate that the recovery of orally administered β-sitosterol was complete, and that fecal excretion of neutral steroid could be measured and calculated on an outpatient basis.

During the study, stools were collected during the last 3 days of each period in portable deep-freeze boxes (Engel 10, Model MHFD-010-A, Sawafuji Electric Co., Tokyo, Japan). Neutral and acidic fecal steroids were isolated separately, and their masses were determined by GLC [16].

Biliary Lipid Secretion

Lipid composition of gallbladder bile and biliary lipid secretion rates were measured by the intestinal perfusion technique of Grundy and Metzger [17]. The evening before the study the subjects were admitted to the Metabolic Ward where they swallowed a triple-lumen tube. After an overnight fast the tube was positioned with two proximal outlets adjacent to the ampulla of Vater and a third outlet 10 cm distally just beyond the ligamentum of Treitz. Cholecystokinin (0.5 IU/kg body weight; Kabi Diagnostica, Studsvik, Sweden) was injected intravenously. Thereafter dark gallbladder bile was obtained (approximately 20 ml) and shaken vigorously; 3 ml bile was mixed immediately with chloroform/methanol (2/1, vol/vol), and the rest was returned to the duodenum through the most proximal outlet of the triple-lumen tube.

A liquid-formula diet (1.42 cal/kg per hour) containing 36% of calories as fat, 16% as protein, and 48% as carbohydrates (Nutrodrip, Wander GmbH, Osthofen, FRG) together with β-sitosterol (Delalande, Cologne, FRG) as a nonabsorbable marker was infused constantly through the most proximal outlet. After allowing 4 h for stabilization of hepatic bile secretion, hourly samples were obtained for 6 h from the second proximal outlet and the distal port by continuous aspiration. Storage of gallbladder bile and samples from the proximal outlet, and separation of bile acids from cholesterol and phospholipids were performed as described in the National Cooperative Gallstone Study [18]. The distal samples were added to 10 ml ethanol. In every sample, cholesterol and β-sitosterol were measured by GLC as trimethylsilylethers using 5-α-cholestane as an internal standard. In gallbladder bile and every sample from the proximal outlet, bile acids were determined enzymatically [19] and phospholipids by the method of Bartlett [20]. Hourly outputs of cholesterol, bile acids and phospholipids were then calculated according to the formula of Grundy and Metzger [17]. Biliary lipid composition was expressed as molar percent for each lipid component, and cholesterol saturation of bile was expressed as lithogenic index according to Hegard and Dam [21] and Holzbach et al. [22].

Statistics

The results are expressed as the mean $\pm$ standard deviation. Statistically significant differences were calculated using Wilcoxon's signed ranks test for paired observations.

Results

Administration of simvastatin (40 mg) once at night resulted in a marked reduction in total and LDL cholesterol in both patients (Table 2). The reduction in LDL cholesterol in patients 1 and 2 averaged 56% and 40%, respectively, indicating good compliance. HLD cholesterol was increased in patient 1 by 14%. Table 3 summarizes the results on fecal excretion of endogenous neutral and acidic sterols. The results clearly demonstrate that administration of synvinolin decreased both bile acid and total cholesterol synthesis in the two patients with familial hypercholesterolemia. On the average, bile acid and total cholesterol synthesis were reduced by 39% and 41%, and 29% and 33% in patients 1 and 2, respectively. The results of biliary lipid secretion in patients 1 and 2 before and during simvastatin treatment are given in Table 4. Biliary cholesterol secretion was significantly reduced in both patients, while bile acid and phospholipid output was not altered by administration of simvastatin. The reduction in biliary cholesterol output was followed by a significant reduction in cholesterol saturation of hepatic bile.

Table 2. Serum lipids and lipoproteins (mg/dl) in two patients with familial hypercholesterolemia before and after 6 weeks of treatment with simvastatin (40 mg/day)

	Cholesterol	Triglycerides	LDL cholesterol	HDL cholesterol
Patient 1				
Control	419±17	79±27	354±10	49±4
Simvastatin	228±17[a]	83±34	156±15[a]	56±3[a]
Patient 2				
Control	397±18	151±22	340±18	31±6
Simvastatin	263± 3[a]	100±12[a]	205±12[a]	30±5

$n=3$; mean ± SD
[a] $p<0.05$ compared to control value

Table 3. Cholesterol and bile acid synthesis (mg/day) in two patients with familial hypercholesterolemia before and after 6 weeks of treatment with simvastatin (40 mg/day)

	Endogenous neutral sterols	Bile acid synthesis	Cholesterol synthesis
Patient 1			
Control	638±134	372±64	1010±184
Simvastatin	494±127[a]	226±57[a]	720±123[a]
Patient 2			
Control	583±53[a]	321±61	904±107
Simvastatin	420±82[a]	189±37[a]	609±125[a]

$n=4$; mean ± SD
Dietary intake of cholesterol in patient 1 and 2 averaged 300 and 265 mg/day; these values were already substrated from the results of endogenous neutral sterols.
[a] $p<0.05$ compared to control value

Table 4. Hepatic output (mg/h) of biliary lipids and cholesterol saturation of hepatic bile in two patients with familial hypercholesterolemia before and after 6 weeks of treatment with simvastatin (40 mg/day)

	Cholesterol	Bile acid	Phospholipids	Cholesterol saturation
Patient 1				
Control	54±1	988±202	282±65	118±26
Simvastatin	31±4[a]	879±169	265±86	74±21[a]
Patient 2				
Control	40±4	914±214	384±79	72±12
Simvastatin	25±4[a]	1026± 90	239±72	60±11[a]

$n=6$; mean ± SD
[a] $p<0.05$ compared to control value

Discussion

The present data confirm the results of Duane et al. [11] that administration of simvastatin to patients with primary hypercholesterolemia reduces cholesterol saturation of bile. Thus, in contrast to clofibrate and its derivatives, simvastatin, lovastatin, and probably other HMG-CoA reductase inhibitors possibly do not increase the risk of gallstone formation. This is important because HMG-CoA reductase inhibitors are extremely effective agents in reducing serum cholesterol in patients with primary hypercholesterolemia, and a recent survey in the United States revealed that one million patients are already taking lovastatin for elevated serum cholesterol (E. Grundy, S.M., personal communication). From the specific inhibition of the rate-limiting enzyme in cholesterol synthesis and from studies with isolated perfused rat livers [23] it could be anticipated that these drugs reduce the available cellular cholesterol for biliary secretion. Indeed, in the present study a marked reduction in biliary cholesterol output was observed. The reduction in intracellular free cholesterol may also reduce available cholesterol for bile acid synthesis. From the results of the present study in two patients with familial hypercholesterolemia there is no doubt that at least simvastatin also reduces bile acid synthesis.

To our surprise, the reduction in bile acid synthesis was not accompanied by diminished hepatic output of bile acids. However, the reduction in bile acid synthesis in our patients may also have reduced bile acid pool size, and in a previous study we have shown that a smaller pool of bile acids is followed by an increased cycling frequency [26]. The present data and the results of Duane et al. [11] clearly indicate that simvastatin reduces biliary cholesterol saturation significantly; therefore, it is postulated that treatment with HMG-CoA reductase inhibitors do not increase the risk of gallstone formation. Will these drugs, in addition to chenodeoxycholic and ursodeoxycholic acids, prove new agents for cholesterol gallstone dissolution? The respective mechanisms in reduction of biliary cholesterol saturation with simvastatin and chenodeoxycholic acid are quite similar. Both agents reduce biliary cholesterol secretion and inhibit endogenous bile acid synthesis and HMG-CoA reductase. However, in contrast to simvastatin, chenodeoxycholic acid may increase serum cholesterol [24]. In addition, in at least one study it could be shown that bile acid output increases during oral administration with chenodeoxycholic acid [16]. On the other hand, several studies have shown that patients with cholesterol gallstones have elevated hepatic output of cholesterol. Thus, administration of simvastatin may alter the underlying metabolic disorder in patients with cholesterol gallstones.

The recent development of extracorporeal shock-wave lithotripsy for cholesterol gallstones, with subsequent complete dissolution of the fragments by a combination therapy with chenodeoxycholic and ursodeoxycholic acids [25, 26], may provide a possible indication of HMG-CoA reductase inhibitors for prevention of recurrence in patients with hypercholesterolemia. However, only well-controlled studies will show whether treatment with HMG-CoA reductase inhibitors can prevent recurrence of cholesterol gallstones after complete dissolution.

References

1. Lipid Research Clinics Program. The Lipid Research Clinics Coronary Primary Prevention Trial Results. I. (1984) Reduction in incidence of coronary heart disease. JAMA 251:351–374
2. Frick MH, Elo O, Haapa K, et al. (1987) Helsinki Heart Study: primary-prevention trial with gemfibrozil in middle-aged men with dyslipidemia: safety of treatment, changes in risk factors, and incidence of coronary heart disease. New Engl J Med 317:1237–1245

3. The Coronary Drug Project Group Research (1975) Clofibrate and niacin in coronary heart disease. JAMA 231:360–381
4. Committee of Principal Investigators (1978) A co-operative trial in the primary prevention of ischaemic heart disease using clofibrate. Br Heart J 40:1069–1118
5. Grundy SM, Ahrens EH, Salen G, et al. (1972) Mechanism of action of clofibrate on cholesterol metabolism in patients with hyperlipidemia. J Lipid Res 13:531–551
6. von Bergmann K, Leiss O (1984) Effect of short-term treatment with bezafibrate and fenofibrate on biliary lipid metabolism in patients with hyperlipoproteinaemia. Eur J Clin Invest 14:150–154
7. Leiss O, von Bergmann K, Gnasso A, Augustin J (1985) Effect of gemfibrozil on biliary lipid metabolism in normolipemic subjects. Metabolism 34:74–82
8. Leiss O, Meyer-Krahmer K, von Bergmann K (1986) Biliary lipid secretion in patients with heterozygous familial hypercholesterolemia and combined hyperlipidemia. Influence of bezafibrate and fenofibrate. J Lipid Res 27:713–723
9. Endo A, Kuroda M, Tanzawa K (1976) Competitive inhibition of 3-hydroxy-3-methyl-glutaryl coenzyme A reductase by ML-236A and ML236B fungal metabolites, having hypocholesterolemic activity. FEBS Lett 72:323–326
10. Grundy SM, Bilheimer DW (1984) Inhibition of 3-hydroxy-3-methylglutaryl-CoA reductase by mevinolin in familial hypercholesterolemia heterozygotes: effects on cholesterol balance. Proc Natl Acad Sci USA 81:2538–2542
11. Duane WC, Hunninghake DB, Freeman ML. Pooler PE, Schlasner LA; Gebhard RL (1988) Simvastatin, a competitive inhibitor of HMG-CoA-reductase lowers cholesterol saturation index of gallbladder bile. Hepatology 8:147–150
12. Roeschlau P, Bernt E, Gruber W (1974) Enzymatische Bestimmung des Gesamt-Cholesterins im Serum. Z Klin Chem Klin Biochem 12:226–231
13. Eggstein M, Kreutz FH (1966) Eine neue Bestimmung der Neutralfette im Blutserum und Gewebe. Klin Wochenschr 44:262–266
14. Lipid Research Clinic Program Manual of Laboratory Operations (1975) Department of Health, Education of Welfare Publication, NIH, pp 75–628
15. von Bergmann K, Mok HYI, Hardison M, Grundy SM (1979) Cholesterol and bile acid metabolism in moderately advanced, stable cirrhosis of the liver. Gastroenterology 77:1183–1192
16. von Bergmann K, Gutsfeld-Epple M, Leiss O (1984) Different mechanisms of chenodeoxycholic and ursodeoxycholic acid on biliary lipid metabolism in patients with gallstones. Gastroenterology 87:136–144
17. Grundy SM, Metzger AL (1972) A physiological method for estimation of hepatic secretion of biliary lipids. Gastroenterology 62:1200–1217
18. Hofmann AF, Grundy SM, Lachin JM, et al. (1982) Pretreatment biliary lipid composition in white patients with radiolucent gallstones in the National Cooperative Gallstone Study. Gastroenterology 83:738–752
19. Paumgartner G, Horak W, Probst P, et al. (1971) Effect of phenobarbital on bile flow and bile salt excretion in the rat. Naunyn Schmiedebergs Arch Pharmacol 270:98–102
20. Bartlett GR (1959) Phosphorous assay in column chromatography. J Biol Chem 234:446–468
21. Hegardt FG, Dam H (1971) The solubility of cholesterol in aqueous solution of bile salts and lecithin. Z Ernaehrungswiss 10:228–233
22. Holzbach RT, Marsh M, Olszewski M, Holan K (1973) Cholesterol solubility in bile. Evidence that supersaturated bile is frequent in healthy man. J Clin Invest 52:1467–1479
23. Stone BG, Erickson SK, Craig WY, et al. (1985) Regulation of rat biliary cholesterol secretion by agents that alter intrahepatic cholesterol metabolism: evidence for a distinct biliary precursor pool. J Clin Invest 76:1773–1781
24. Sauerbruch T, Delius M, Paumgartner G, et al. (1986) Fragmentation of gallstones by extracorporeal shock waves. N Engl J Med 14:818–822
25. Sackmann M, Delius M, Sauerbruch T, et al. (1988) Shock-wave lithotrypsy of gallbladder stones: the first 175 patients. N Engl J Med 318:393–397
26. Mok HYI, von Bergmann K, Grundy SM (1977) Regulation of pool size of bile acids in man. Gastroenterology 73:684–690

Gallstone Prevention by Alteration of Gallbladder Mucin Secretion via Prostaglandin Synthesis Inhibition *

B. F. Smith and J. T. LaMont

Section of Gastroenterology and Hepatology, Boston City Hospital, and Section of Gastroenterology, University Hospital, Boston University Medical Center, Boston, MA 02118, USA

Regulation of Mucin Secretion in the Gastrointestinal Tract and Gallbladder

Very little is known regarding the physiologic control of mucus secretion in the gastrointestinal tract and gallbladder. Two types of mucus secretion have been identified: slow basal secretion which appears to maintain the mucus gel on the epithelial surface in the unstimulated state and rapid secretion in response to physiologic neural, hormonal, and noxious stimuli [1]. Several mediators have been identified which stimulate mucus secretion in different epithelia. In the stomach, small intestine, and colon the vagus nerve and its specific neurotransmitter acetylcholine have been identified as potent stimulants for mucus secretion. Prostaglandins also stimulate mucus secretion in the gut as well as modulate multiple other mucosal functions such as blood flow and acid secretion [2]. Whether the cytoprotective effect of prostaglandins for the gastric mucosa is mediated in part by stimulation of mucus secretion remains unclear. Other substances such as dibutyl cyclic AMP, histamine, secretin, bile salts, cholera toxin, and cysteamine have been shown to stimulate mucus secretion in the stomach, small intestine, and colon. The role that these substances play in the normal physiology of mucus secretion or in the pathophysiology of disease states has not been established.

Cholecystokinin produces a potent stimulus for gallbladder mucus secretion when infused intravenously or released by the small intestine in response to a fatty meal. No information is currently available regarding the factors which modulate basal secretion of mucus by the gallbladder epithelium. From a teleologic point of view, maximum protection of the gallbladder epithelium should be required during periods of fasting when the highest concentrations of bile are achieved within the gallbladder lumen. The role which meal-stimulated mucus secretion, mediated through cholecystokinin release, plays in normal mucosal protection has not been defined. The remainder of this chapter focuses on the pathologic hypersecretion of mucus which occurs during gallstone formation and the potential for gallstone prevention by pharmacologic inhibition of mucus secretion.

Aspirin Inhibits Mucin Secretion and Gallstone Formation in the Cholesterol-Fed Prairie Dog

Hypersecretion of mucus has been documented to occur in several animal models of gallstone formation prior to cholesterol crystal nucleation and gallstone formation [3–5]. Accumulation of mucus gel in the gallbladder of human patients can be identified by ultrasonography and has been termed biliary sludge [6, 7]. In selected patient populations

---

* B.F.S. was supported by NIH Resarch Grant DK39017 and J.T.L. by NIH Research Grant DK28195

at high risk for gallstone formation, biliary sludge accumulates in the gallbladder prior to the formation of gallstones [8]. As discussed in an earlier chapter (Smith), convincing evidence exists to indicate that mucin, the principle organic constituent of mucus, is a critical element in gallstone formation and may provide the nidus for heterogeneous nucleation of cholesterol monohydrate crystals from cholesterol-supersaturated bile [9, 10].

Lee et al. used aspirin, a known inhibitor of mucin secretion in the gut, to pharmacologically block mucin hypersecretion in the gallbladder during gallstone formation in the cholesterol-fed prairie dog [11]. These investigators used ex vivo gallbladder organ culture to quantitate the effect of aspirin on mucin synthesis. Aspirin, at a concentration of 25 mM, inhibited basal mucin secretion in control gallbladder explants by 80% and caused a dose-dependent inhibition of mucin synthesis and secretion in the gallbladders from cholesterol-fed animals. Concomittant administration of cholesterol and aspirin (100 mg/kg body weight) in the diet caused a highly significant inhibition of mucin secretion by the gallbladder epithelium, but aspirin did not alter the time course or degree of cholesterol supersaturation of gallbladder bile. Aspirin prevented the visible accumulation of mucus gel in the gallbladder lumen and completely inhibited the appearance of cholesterol crystals and gallstones in these animals. These results suggested that hypersecretion of mucin was critical for gallstone formation, and that pharmacologic inhibition of mucin secretion effectively prevented cholesterol gallstone formation in this model. These studies represented the initial demonstration that pharmacologic therapy could prevent gallstone formation despite the presence of cholesterol supersaturation in bile. Furthermore, the ability of aspirin to inhibit mucin secretion strongly indicated that prostaglandins may mediate mucin secretion by the gallbladder epithelium and were at least partially responsible for the hypersecretion of mucin which occurs in response to cholesterol feeding in these animals.

Potential Mediators of Mucin Hypersecretion During Gallstone Formation

Several lines of evidence indicate that the stimulus for mucus hypersecretion by the gallbladder in response to a lithogenic diet is delivered to the gallbladder epithelium through the bile [3, 5]. Mucin hypersecretion occurs only in the gallbladder during gallstone formation in experimental animals, and not in the stomach or colon. This observation suggests that mucin hypersecretion is not a generalized phenomenon which occurs in response to the hypercholesterolemia which develops in the cholesterol-fed animals. Furthermore, ligation of the cystic duct prevents contact of bile with the gallbladder epithelium and also prevents mucin hypersecretion in the gallbladder in response to the lithogenic diet. Recent studies have sought to identify the possible mediators of mucin hypersecretion in the cholesterol-supersaturated bile of experimental animals.

Since aspirin inhibits mucin secretion both in organ culture and in vivo, it seemed reasonable to test the hypothesis that prostaglandins could directly stimulate mucin secretion. The effect of arachidonic acid, the immediate precursor for prostaglandin synthesis, on mucin secretion in gallbladder organ culture was examined [12]. Arachidonic acid caused a dose-dependent stimulation of mucin synthesis and secretion by gallbladder explants in vitro. Furthermore, indomethacin, an inhibitor of the prostaglandin synthetic enzyme cyclo-oxygenase, inhibited prostaglandin synthesis in gallbladder explants and also inhibited arachidonic acid mediated stimulation of mucin synthesis and secretion. Arachidonic acid was exclusively metabolized by the gallbladder epithelium into 6-keto-prostaglandin F^{1a}, the stable metabolic byproduct of prostacyclin. These studies confirmed the apparently important role of prostaglandins as mediators of mucin secretion by the gallbladder epithelium.

LaMont and his coworkers next investigated the effect of hydrocortisone, a known inhibitor of phospholipase A_2 activity, on mucin secretion by gallbladder explants in organ culture [13]. In several model systems, the rate-limiting reaction in prostaglandin synthesis is hydrolysis of membrane phospholipids by phospholipase A_2 with resultant release of free arachidonic acid as substrate for prostaglandin synthesis. Hydrocortisone, a known inhibitor of phospholipase A_2 activity, reversibly inhibited mucin secretion by gallbladder explants in a dose-dependent fashion and also inhibited arachidonic acid stimulated mucin secretion. Furthermore, hydrocortisone inhibited the production of 6-keto-prostaglandin F^{1a}, the stable metabolite of prostacyclin, under both basal and arachidonic acid stimulated conditions. These findings suggest that arachidonic acid is incorporated into membrane phospholipids in the gallbladder epithelium and subsequently cleaved by phospholipase A_2 prior to serving as substrate for prostaglandin synthesis.

Increased activity of phospholipase A_2 in the gallbladder epithelium could potentially increase the availability of arachidonic acid for prostaglandin synthesis and would also result in increased generation of lysophosphatidylcholine (LPC), the other metabolic product following fatty acid hydrolysis from phosphatidylcholine. LPC has been suggested as a potential mucin secretagogue in the gallbladder and is present in increased concentrations in the gallbladder bile of cholesterol-fed prairie dogs. LaMorte et al. demonstrated an increase in prostaglandin synthesis in the gallbladder and an increase in LPC concentration in the gallbladder bile of cholesterol-fed prairie dogs [14]. These increases occurred prior to mucin hypersecretion which in turn occurred prior to cholesterol crystal nucleation and gallstone formation. In addition, LPC caused a dose-dependent increase in mucin secretion by gallbladder epithelium incubated in organ culture. The increase in mucin secretion caused by LPC was not felt to be secondary to the detergent properties of LPC since LPC did not cause a significant increase in the leakage of lactate dehydrogenase from the epithelial cells. Furthermore, LPC concentrations in hepatic bile remained unchanged during gallstone formation in the prairie dog, suggesting that LPC was generated in the gallbladder. The time course of the increase in prostaglandin synthesis and LPC generation during cholesterol feeding was identical, which suggests that both these substances arose from a common source.

A current working hypothesis regarding mucin hypersecretion in the gallbladder during cholesterol gallstone formation in the prairie dog includes the following sequential steps:

1. The molecular species of phospholipid secreted into bile, particularly those of phosphatidylcholine, undergo an alteration in their fatty acid composition in response to cholesterol feeding.
2. The percentage of biliary phospholipids containing arachidonic acid at the sn-2 position is increased in response to cholesterol feeding.
3. Biliary phospholipids in gallbladder bile are incorporated into the plasma membrane of the gallbladder epithelial cell where they undergo hydrolysis by phospholipase A_2.
4. Hydrolysis of the sn-2 arachidonyl-phospholipids in the plasma membrane of the gallbladder epithelium generates free arachidonic acid which stimulates prostaglandin synthesis.
5. Increased prostaglandin synthesis stimulates mucin synthesis and secretion.
6. LPC, which also results from hydrolysis of membrane phospholipids, is released from the gallbladder epithelial cell accounting for the increased concentrations of LPC in gallbladder bile.
7. LPC in gallbladder bile further stimulates mucin secretion by the gallbladder epithelium.

Several studies of the phospholipid species present in the bile of patients with gallstones support the central arm of this hypothesis, that increased cholesterol secretion in bile alters the fatty acid conjugates of biliary phospholipids. In addition, preliminary studies in the prairie dog have demonstrated an increase in biliary arachidonyl-phospholipids in response to cholesterol feeding [15]. Further elucidation of the stimulus in bile for mucin hypersecretion during cholesterol gallstone formation will require detailed analyses of the multitude of phospholipids species in bile and will also require direct demonstration that appreciable quantities of biliary phospholipids are absorbed into and metabolized by the gallbladder epithelium.

Implications for Prevention of Gallstone Formation in Selected Patients

Pharmacologic doses of aspirin can prevent gallstone formation in the cholesterol-fed prairie dog by inhibiting prostaglandin-mediated mucin hypersecretion. Further delineation of the mediators of mucin hypersecretion and the metabolic pathways responsible for their effects should lead to novel therapeutic strategies for gallstone prevention in this model. However, the acute introduction of cholesterol into the diet of herbivorous rodents is not physiologically similar to the chronic increase in cholesterol of the Western human diet.

Are the insights regarding the pathophysiology of cholesterol cholelithiasis in these animal models relevant to gallstone formation and prevention in man? A recent study of obese patients entering a rapid weight loss program evaluated the potential for pharmacologic inhibition of gallstone formation in this very select group of patients [16]. Obese patients who experience rapid weight loss have an increased risk for the development of biliary sludge and gallstones. Based on the natural history of gallstone formation during weight loss, patients were treated at entry into a supervised weight loss program with either placebo, ursodeoxycholic acid, or aspirin. Ursodeoxycholic acid was administered at a dose of 1200 mg/day, and aspirin was administered at a dose of 1300 mg/day (four standard tablets; approximately 13 mg/kg body weight). In the patients receiving ursodeoxycholic acid, the cholesterol saturation index of bile fell during therapy and gallstones did not develop in any patients. Among the placebo group, gallstones had formed in 5 of 19 patients 3 weeks after completion of therapy. In the aspirin-treated group, only two patients developed gallstones, and both these patients had only trace amounts of aspirin in their serum during treatment, suggesting noncompliance with aspirin therapy. Aspirin also significantly decreased the levels of glycoproteins and prostaglandin E_2 in bile. The placebo patients, on the other hand, had a highly significant increase in the concentration of biliary glycoproteins associated with their increased risk for cholesterol crystal nucleation and gallstone formation.

These findings strongly support the proposed importance of gallbladder mucin in gallstone formation in humans. Furthermore, prevention of gallbladder mucin hypersecretion with modest doses of aspirin is not only feasible but may have a therapeutic role in prevention of gallstone formation in selected patients. Future research will need accurately to define populations at high risk for gallstone formation and extend these preliminary observations on the potential for the safe pharmacologic prevention of cholelithiasis in man.

References

1. Whalin T, Bloom GD, Danielsson A (1976) Effect of cholecystokinin-pancreozymin (CCK-PZ) on glycoprotein secretion from mouse gallbladder epithelium. Cell Tissue Res 171:425–435
2. Miller TA, Jacobson ED (1979) Gastrointestinal cytoprotection by prostaglandins. Gut 20: 75–87
3. Freston JW, Bouchier IA, Newman J (1969) Biliary mucous substances in dihydrocholesterol-induced cholelithiasis. Gastroenterology 57:670–678
4. Womack NA (1971) The development of gallstones. Surg Gynecol Obstet 133:937–945
5. Lee SP, LaMont JT, Carey MC (1981) Role of gallbladder mucus hypersecretion in the evolution of cholesterol gallstones. Studies in the prairie dog. J Clin Invest 67:1712–1723
6. Lee SP, Nichols JF (1986) Nature and composition of biliary sludge. Gastroenterology 90:677–686
7. Allen B, Bernhoft R, Blankaert N et al. (1981) Sludge is calcium bilirubinate associated with bile stasis. Am J Surg 141:51–56
8. Messing B, Bories L, Kuntslinger F, Bernier J (1983) Does total parenteral nutrition induce gallbladder sludge formation and lithiasis? Gastroenterology 84:1012–1019
9. Levy PF, Smith BF, LaMont JT (1984) Human gallbladder mucin accelerates nucleation of cholesterol in artifical bile. Gastroenterology 87:270–275
10. Smith BF (1987) Human gallbladder mucin binds biliary lipids and promotes cholesterol crystal nucleation in model bile. J Lipid Res 28:1088–1097
11. Lee SP, Carey MC, LaMont JT (1981) Aspirin prevention of cholesterol gallstone formation in prairie dogs. Science 211:1429–1432
12. LaMont JT, Turner BS, DiBenedetto D, Handin R, Schafer AI (1983) Arachidonic acid stimulates mucin secretion in prairie dog gallbladder. Am J Physiol 245:G92–G98
13. Moore JRL, Turner BS, LaMont JT (1984) Hydrocortisone inhibits mucin secretion from guinea pig gallbladder. Am J Physiol 247:G427–G431
14. LaMorte WW, LaMont JT, Hale W, Booker ML, Scott TE, Turner BS (1986) Gallbladder prostaglandins and lysophospholipids as mediators of mucin secretion during cholelithiasis. Am J Physiol 251:G701–G709
15. Booker M, Scott T, LaMorte W (1988) Cholesterol feeding increases arachidonate in biliary phospholipids. Gastroenterology 94:A527
16. Broomfield PH, Chopra R, Scheinbaum RC, Bonorris GG, Silverman A, Schoenfield LJ, Marks JW (1988) Effects of ursodeoxycholic acid and aspirin on the formation of lithogenic bile and gallstones during loss of weight. New Engl J Med 319:1567–1572

Gallstone Prevention After Successful Treatment

R. H. Dowling

Gastroenterology Unit, Guy's Hospital, Guy's Tower, London SE1 9RT, U.K.

In patients with symptomatic gallstones, four types of non-surgical treatment may leave the patient free of stones and symptoms but with an intact gallbladder in which stones may reform: (a) oral bile acids [1, 2], (b) direct dissolution with methyl *tert*-butyl ether (MTBE) [3], (c) extracorporeal shock-wave lithotripsy (ESWL) with or without oral bile acids [4] or MTBE [5], and (d) percutaneous cholecystolithotomy [6]. The timing and frequency of gallstone recurrence have been well documented after oral bile acids [7], and preliminary results on recurrence rates are starting to appear after ESWL [8] and MTBE [9]. However, as yet there are no data after minimal scar surgery (percutaneous cholecystolithotomy).

Ultrasound is more sensitive than cholecystography in detecting gallstone recurrence [10], and after oral treatment there is a linear increase in cumulative recurrence rates (10%–15% per annum by actuarial analysis) which may reach a plateau of 30%–60% after 3.5–6.0 years [7, 11–13]. Most instances of gallstone recurrence are silent or asymptomatic.

Risk factors predicting gallstone recurrence include pre-treatment stone number, the stone-free interval between "clearance" of the gallbladder and the start of preventive treatment, non-steroidal anti-inflammatory drug (NSAID) ingestion [14] and, in some studies, the patient's sex and age [7, 11]. Thus, in the British-Belgian study [11] the cumulative recurrence rates at 3.5 years were $42 \pm 9\%$ in patients who originally had multiple stones versus only $15 \pm 10\%$ in those with solitary stones. Patients who had been stone free for at least 9 months before starting post-dissolution treatment (the median stone-free interval), constituted a low-risk group ($13 \pm 6\%$ recurrence) compared with those who had been stone free for less than 9 months ($55 \pm 12\%$) [11].

As in primary gallstone formation, at least three pathogenetic factors contribute to recurrence: (a) supersaturated bile, (b) nucleation defects and (c) gallbladder motor dysfunction. Until now, treatments to prevent recurrence have been based mainly on reducing biliary cholesterol saturation with small doses of ursodeoxycholic acid ranging from 3 mg/kg per day [11] up to 300 mg/kg per day [12, 15] or diets high in fibre (> 30 g per day) and low in refined carbohydrate (< 15 g per day) [11]. Results from one prospective, random-allocation trial [11] and from two non-randomised trials [12, 15] show that low-dose ursodeoxycholic acid reduces (by approximately 50%) and delays, but does not prevent, gallstone recurrence. The high-fibre, low-refined carbohydrate diet had no protective effect.

Four lines of evidence suggest that after stone clearance, manipulation of nucleating factors may be more important in preventing recurrence than inhibition of the invariable recurrence/persistence of biliary cholesterol supersaturation: (a) Aspirin prevents cholesterol micro-crystal and primary gallstone formation in prairie dogs fed a lithogenic diet [16], probably by inhibiting gallbladder mucosal prostaglandin synthesis, mucus glycoprotein production and nucleation [17]. (b) In the British-Belgian study [14], regular NSAID ingestion completely prevented gallstone recurrence (no recurrences in 12 NSAID users versus 20 recurrences in 63 non-users; $p < 0.02$). (c) Aspirin ingestion significantly reduced biliary crystal, micro-stone and gallstone formation in obese patients undergoing weight reduction [18]. (d) The higher recurrence rate in patients who initially had multiple, rather than single, gallstones [11, 12] suggests that those forming multiple stones have a more severe nucleation defect with many "seeding" agents than in those developing single stones. If similar nucleation defects persist after stone clearance, this may explain the low (10% – 15%) overall recurrence after ESWL [8] for which patients with solitary stones are selected.

Gallbladder motor dysfunction seems to persist after stone clearance [19], but there are no data as yet to suggest that pro-cholecystokinetic agents expel sludge/crystals and prevent gallstone recurrence.

References

1. Danzinger RG, Hofmann AF, Schoenfield LJ, Thistle JL (1972) Dissolution of cholesterol gallstones by chenodeoxycholic acid. N Engl J Med 286:1–8
2. Bell GD, Whitney B, Dowling RH (1972) Gallstone dissolution in man using chenodeoxycholic acid. Lancet 2:1213–1216
3. Allen MJ, Borody TJ, Bugliosi TF et al. (1985) Rapid dissolution of gallstones by methyl *tert*-butyl ether. N Engl J Med 312:217–220
4. Sackmann M, Delius M, Sauerbruch T et al. (1988) Shock wave lithotripsy of gallbladder stones: the first 175 patients. N Engl J Med 318:393–397
5. Peine CJ, Petersen BT, Williams HJ et al. (1989) Extracorporeal shock-wave lithotripsy and methyl *tert*-butyl ether for partially calcified gallstones. Gastroenterology 97:1229–1235
6. Kellett MJ, Wickham JEA, Russell RCG (1988) Percutaneous cholecystolithotomy. Br Med J 296:453–455
7. Dowling RH, Gleeson DC, Hood KA, Ruppin DC, the British/Belgian Gallstone Study Group (1987) Gallstone recurrence and postdissolution management. In: Paumgartner G, Stiehl A, Gerok W (eds) Bile acids and the liver. MTP Press, Lancaster, pp 355–367
8. Sackmann M, Ippisch E, Sauerbruch T, Holl J, Paumgartner G (1988) Early gallstone recurrence after successful shock-wave therapy. Hepatology 8:1221
9. Scholz DG, McCullough, Petersen BT, Thistle JL (1988) Gallstone recurrence following complete dissolution with oral bile acid therapy or methyl *tert*-butyl ether. Hepatology 8:1372
10. Gleeson D, Ruppin DC, the British Gallstone Study Group (1985) Discrepancies between cholecystography and ultrasonography in the detection of recurrent gallstones. J Hepatology 1:597–607
11. Hood K, Gleeson D, Ruppin DC, Dowling RH, the BBGSG (1988) The British/Belgian Gallstone Group: Can gallstone recurrent be prevented? The British/Belgian postdissolution trial. Gastroenterology 94:A548
12. Villanova N, Bazzoli F, Taroni F et al. (1989) Gallstone recurrence after successful oral bile acid treatment. Gastroenterology 97:726–731
13. O'Donnell LDJ, Heaton KW (1988) Recurrence and re-recurrence of gallstones after medical dissolution: a long term follow up. Gut 29:655–658
14. Hood K, Gleeson D, Ruppin DC, Dowling RH, the BBGSG (1988) Prevention of gallstone recurrence by non-steroidal anti-inflammatory drugs. Lancet ii:1223–1225
15. Perez-Aquilar F, Breto M, Alfonso V, Martinez-Silvestre M, Berenguer J (1986) Gallstone recurrence following cessation of dissolving treatment and during prophylactic administration of either low-dose chenodeoxycholic acid (CDCA) or medium-dose ursodeoxycholic acid (UDCA). J Hepatology 1:S305
16. Lee SP, Carey MC, LaMont JT (1981) Aspirin prevention of cholesterol gallstone formation in prairie dogs. Science 211:1429–1430
17. LaMont JT, Turner BS, Di Benedetto D, Handin R, Schafer AI (1983) Arachidonic acid stimulates mucin secretion in prairie dog gallbladder. Am J Physiol 245:G92–G98
18. Broomfield PH, Chopra R, Sheinbaum RC, Bonorris GG, Silverman A, Schoenfield LI, Marks JW (1988) Effects of ursodeoxycholic acid and aspirin on the formation of lithogenic bile and gallstones during loss of weight. N Engl J Med 319:1567–1572
19. Sylvestrowicz TA, Shaffer EA (1988) Gallbladder function during gallstone dissolution. Effect of bile acid therapy in patients with gallstones. Gastroenterology 95:740–748

Intermittent Bile Acid Therapy as an Alternative Therapeutic Strategy

T.C. Northfield and R.P. Jazrawi

Division of Biochemical Medicine, St. George's Hospital Medical School, London SW17 ORE, U.K.

Introduction

Since this meeting is being held in Germany, and since the subject concerns the war against gallstone disease, we have consulted the writings of a famous German military strategist – von Clausewitz. He states that "die Strategie ist der Gebrauch des Gefechts zum Zweck des Krieges", which can be translated into English as "strategy is the use of battles for the objectives of the war". Thus, strategy consists of relating methods to clearly defined objectives. The objective of the war against gallstone disease is to maintain the vast majority of gallstone patients gallstone free in the long term. Our thesis is that intermittent bile acid therapy constitutes the best long-term strategy for achieving this objective by non-surgical means.

The specific questions that we plan to address are as follows:

1. What proportion of gallstone patients is potentially suitable for non-surgical treatment?
2. What is the role of bile acid therapy in relation to the new non-surgical therapies?
3. How can the efficacy of bile acid therapy be enhanced?
4. Is intermittent bile acid therapy a realistic long-term strategy?

Proportion of Patients Suitable for Non-surgical Therapy

Selection criteria for all forms of non-surgical treatment must consider the gallstones, the gallbladder and the patient. The gallstones must be non-calcified, although according to Swobodnik (see this volume) dissolution of calcified stones may become a possibility in the future. The diagnostic criteria for calcification are changing since it is now known that CT scanning is a more sensitive method of detection. CT scanning is now recommended before attempting treatment with extracorporeal shock-wave lithotripsy (ESWL) or methyl-tert-butyl ether (MTBE). Theoretically, the same approach should be applied also before embarking on bile acid therapy, but no information is available on whether patients who are resistant to treatment with bile acids can be identified more readily by this method than by oral cholecystogram. The gallbladder must opacify on an oral cholecystogram. Failure to do this may indicate blockage of the cystic duct by a gallstone, and this would make all current forms of non-surgical treatment ineffective and/or dangerous. The patient must have biliary symptoms, emphasised already by Paumgartner (see this volume). These three criteria (radiolucent gallstones in a functioning gallbladder in a symptomatic patient) are currently prerequisites for considering non-surgical treatment.

If the patient fulfils these prerequisites, then the actual decision on whether to adopt a non-surgical or a surgical approach will have to be made in the light of other considerations. Age and the presence of coexisting medical disease will tip the balance in favour of non-surgical treatment. The personal preference of the patient is also of great importance in making the decision. Some patients are afraid of surgery, or are reluctant to accept it for cosmetic reasons, or cannot afford the length of time off work that would follow a surgical operation. On the other hand, some patients prefer surgery as a definitive act that does not carry a long-term risk of gallstone recurrence.

Table 1 derives figures for the proportion of gallstone patients potentially suitable for surgery and for the three non-surgical therapies under discussion (bile acid therapy, ESWL and MTBE), based on the above selection criteria as applied to the gallstone population described in the Italian epidemiological study from Rome [1]. According to this study, approximately 33% of the gallstone population identified on ultrasound examination have symptoms, 70% have radiolucent stones, of which 70% are in gallbladders that opacify on oral cholecystography. An additional criterion to be taken into account in deciding the form of non-surgical therapy is gallstone size. Bile acid therapy is most suitable for small stones (<6 mm in diameter, constituting 10% of the total), although it can also be considered for medium-sized stones (6–15 mm in diameter, 25% of the total). By contrast, ESWL is only considered suitable for stones 8–30 mm in diameter (80% of the total). In this respect, therefore, these two methods of treatment are complementary, and, indeed, the object of ESWL is to convert large stones into small fragments that can then be more rapidly dissolved by bile acids. MTBE can be applied to any stone size.

The only selection criterion that limits suitability for surgical treatment is the requirement for biliary symptoms (33%), so that when all these criteria are considered, surgical treatment can be considered potentially suitable for 33% of patients. The proportion potentially suitable for non-surgical treatment varies from 6% for bile acid therapy alone to 13% if it follows ESWL and 15% for MTBE. Thus, almost half of the patients who are suitable for surgical treatment are now potentially suitable for non-surgical treatment using these new approaches. Nevertheless, the proportion of patients being treated by non-surgical methods in the United Kingdom is currently only about one thirtieth of that being treated by surgery. Inpatient hospital statistics [2] indicate that 1% per annum of the gallstone population is being treated by cholecystectomy, whereas data based on prescription charges for bile acid therapy indicate that only 0.03% of the gallstone population is being treated by this method at present. The main reason for this large discrepancy is that general practitioners, whom the patient sees first, traditionally think of gallstones as a surgical disease. This situation is likely to change if the introduction of ESWL has the effect of popularizing non-surgical treatment.

Table 1. Percentage of gallstone patients potentially suitable for different therapies [after 3]

Criteria	BA therapy	Fragmentation	MTBE	Surgery
Symptoms	33	33	33	33
Radiolucent	70	70	70	100
GB visualisation	70	70	70	100
Diameter <6 mm	10	–	10	
6–15 mm	25 } 35	25 } 80	25 } 90	100
5–30 mm	–	55	55	
All criteria	6	13	15	33
In therapy in UK	0.03 per annum	–	–	1 per annum

BA, bile acid; MTBE, methyl-tert-butylether

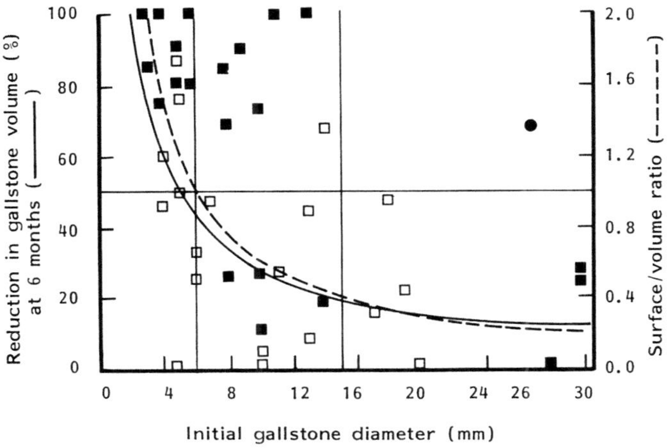

Fig. 1. Relationship between gallstone size and gallstone dissolution rate. *Solid squares*, UDCA; *open squares*, CDCA (after [3])

Central Role of Bile Acid Therapy in Strategy

Bile acid therapy is at its most effective for small gallstones. Figure 1 relates initial gallstone diameter to gallstone dissolution rate expressed as reduction in gallstone volume at 6 months by carefully standardised and validated oral cholecystography [3]. The continuous line shows the relationship between these two measurements, whereas the discontinuous line shows the theoretical relationship between the surface area and volume of a sphere. The close correspondence between these two curves suggest that in this group of patients the rapid dissolution rate found with small stones is due to the fact that these have a larger surface area : volume ratio than large stones. In the case of the small stones (< 6 mm diameter), almost all achieved 50% dissolution or more in the first 6 months using either ursodeoxycholic acid (UDCA) or chenodeoxycholic acid (CDCA). By contrast, none of the large stones (> 15 mm diameter) achieved this degree of dissolution.

It is this basic fact that bile acids dissolve small stones more rapidly than large stones that gives bile acid therapy its central role in the strategy outlined in this chapter (Fig. 2). It can be used in three different situations: (1) Following ESWL. The object of ESWL is to convert large stones into small ones that can then be dissolved much more rapidly by bile acid therapy; (2) For initial treatment of small stones. These stones are not suitable for ESWL because of the problem of focussing the shock waves on a small target, and can be treated from the start by bile acid therapy with good prospects for rapid dissolution. Even more rapid dissolution can of course be achieved by MTBE, but the fact that this is an invasive procedure is likely to deter some of the patients who have a personal preference for non-surgical treatment; (3) Following gallstone recurrence. If these patients who have achieved complete gallstone dissolution are followed by regular ultrasound examination at 6–12 monthly intervals, the recurrence is likely to be detected at an early stage when rapid redissolution can be expected.

Tactics for Enhancing Bile Acid Therapy

Tactics for enhancing bile acid therapy can be considered for all three situations where bile acid therapy still has a role. An understanding of the mechanism of action of bile acid

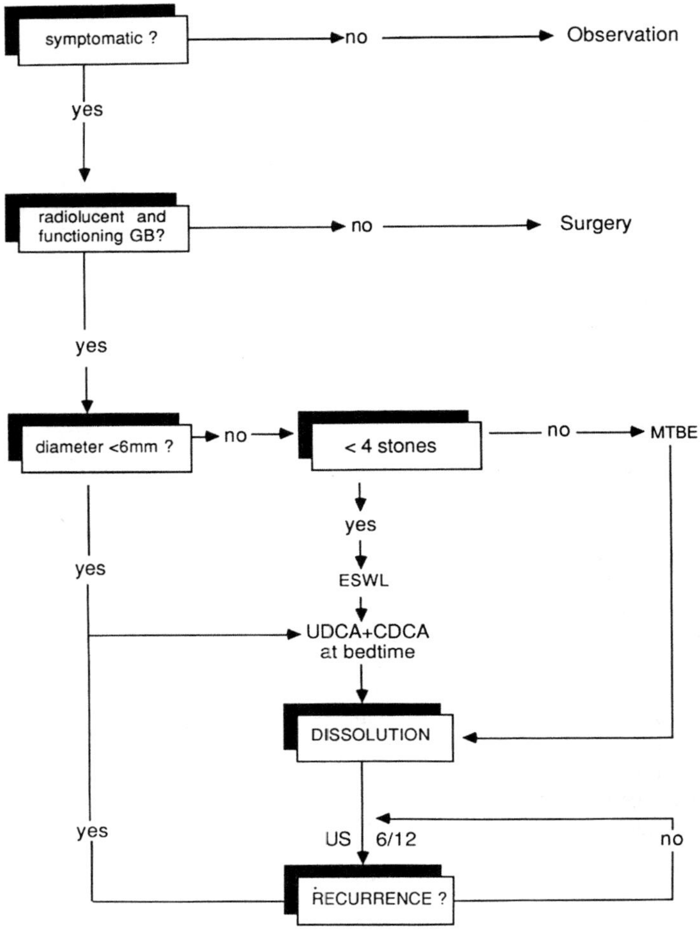

Fig. 2. Overall strategy for gallstone management

therapy is of help in pointing the way to potential methods of enhancing their action. In the case of both CDCA and UDCA, the mechanism of action involves a reduction in hepatic cholesterol secretion, but the cause of this reduction appears to be different for the two bile acids. Stiehl (this volume) has already pointed out that in the case of CDCA, cholesterol synthesis is inhibited; whereas in the case of UDCA cholesterol absorption from the intestine is inhibited. CDCA mobilizes cholesterol from the gallstone surface purely by micellar solubilization, but in the case of UDCA liquid crystal formation is also involved. These facts suggest that UDCA might be more effective than CDCA, and this has been shown to be the case, as discussed in the chapters and by Stiehl and Kurtz (this volume). It also suggests that a combination of the two bile acids might be more effective than either bile acid alone, and Podda (this volume) has shown data confirming this.

We as a group have also been interested in the effect of dose timing and of diet in enhancing the effect of bile acid therapy. In our studies on the effect of CDCA and of UDCA on biliary lipid secretion we have found that, although these bile acids make hepatic bile more unsaturated with cholesterol at high bile acid secretion rates, bile is still

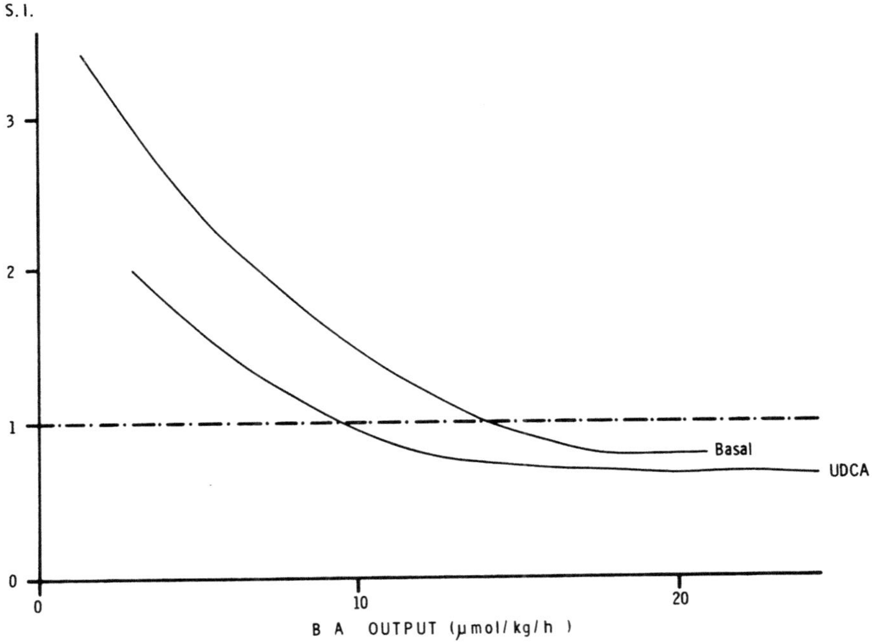

Fig. 3. Effect of UDCA on relationship between bile acid (*BA*) secretion rate and SI of hepatic bile (after [12])

supersaturated with cholesterol at the low bile acid secretion rates found during overnight fasting (Fig. 3). This is due to nocturnal interruption of the enterohepatic circulation of bile acids. We have therefore put forward the hypothesis that, if the whole dose of bile acid were given at bedtime, it should prevent this nocturnal interruption of the enterohepatic circulation, thus preventing the secretion of supersaturated bile. We have recently tested this hypothesis in duodenal perfusion studies [4]. As shown in Fig. 4, hepatic bile acid secretion rate rises after an evening meal and then falls during overnight fasting if the patient is not on bile acid therapy. Secretion rates of less than 10 μg/kg per day are accompanied by secretion of supersaturated hepatic bile. If UDCA is given at bedtime, it prevents the reduction in hepatic bile acid secretion rate and the associated secretion of supersaturated hepatic bile. We have also noted during our duodenal perfusion studies that, although hepatic cholesterol secretion is reduced during treatment with CDCA and UDCA, cholesterol continues to be secreted, despite the fact that cholesterol synthesis has been inhibited during CDCA. This led us to the hypothesis that the continued cholesterol secretion might be due to exogenous cholesterol, and that if we were to reduce exogenous dietary intake of cholesterol in addition to inhibiting endogenous synthesis, then we might be able to enhance the effect of CDCA. We now realise that this hypothesis is unlikely to be valid for UDCA because this does not inhibit exogenous synthesis.

Bedtime administration of both CDCA [5] and UDCA [6] does indeed produce a further significant reduction in saturation index (SI) of gallbladder bile by comparison with mealtime administration of the same total daily dose of the two bile acids (Fig. 5). As predicted above, a further significant reduction in SI (Fig. 6) can be obtained by adding a low cholesterol diet to bedtime administration of CDCA [7], but not UDCA [6]. The

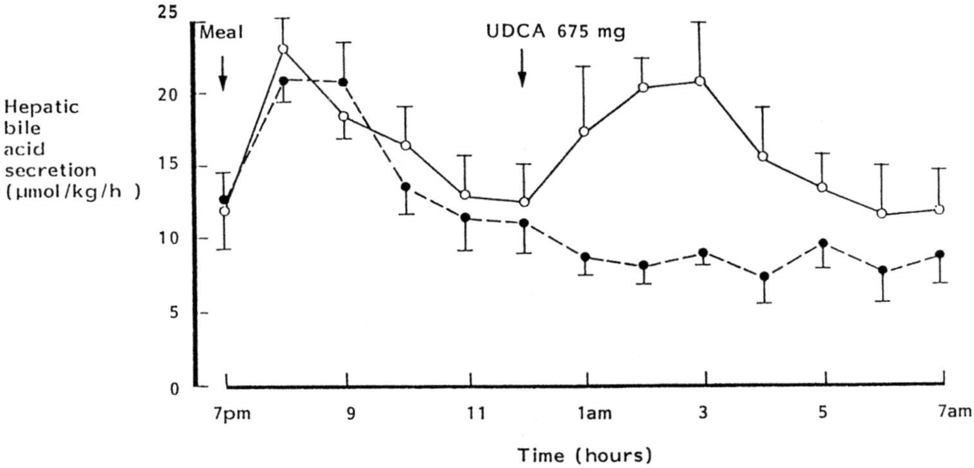

Fig. 4. Effect of bedtime UDCA on overnight hepatic bile acid secretion rate. *Open circles*, bedtime UDCA; *solid circles*, pre-treatment (after [4])

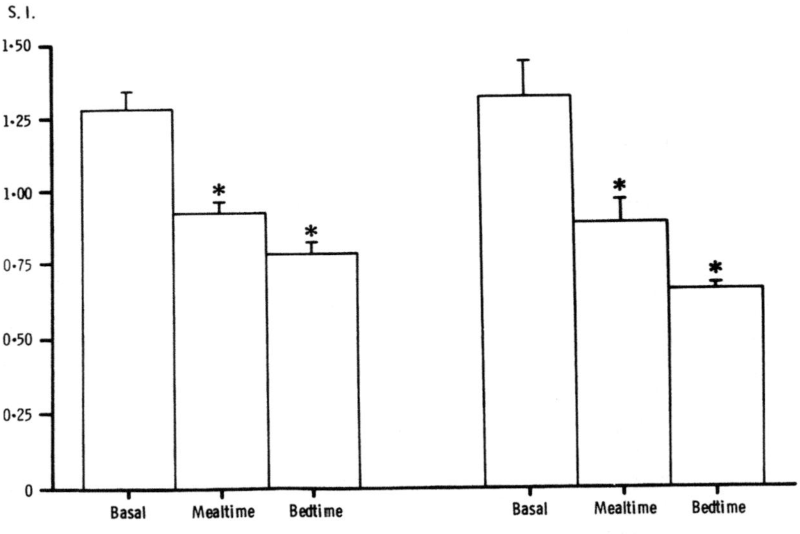

Fig. 5. Effect of bedtime administration of CDCA (15 mg/kg per day; *left*) and UDCA (12 mg/kg per day; *right*) on cholesterol SI of galbladder bile. Asterisks indicate significant differences from previous values (after [5, 6])

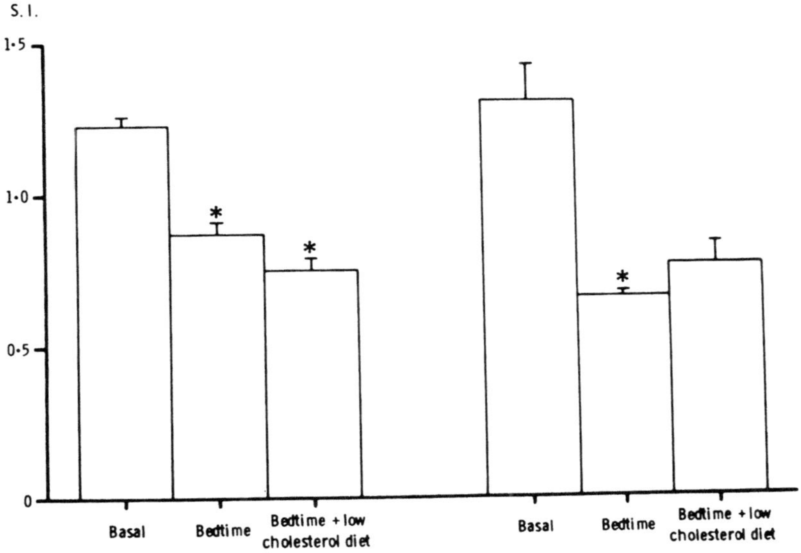

Fig. 6. Effect on SI of adding a low cholesterol diet to bedtime CDCA (15 mg/kg per day; *left*) and UDCA (12 mg/kg per day; *right*). Asterisks indicate significant differences from previous values (after [6, 7])

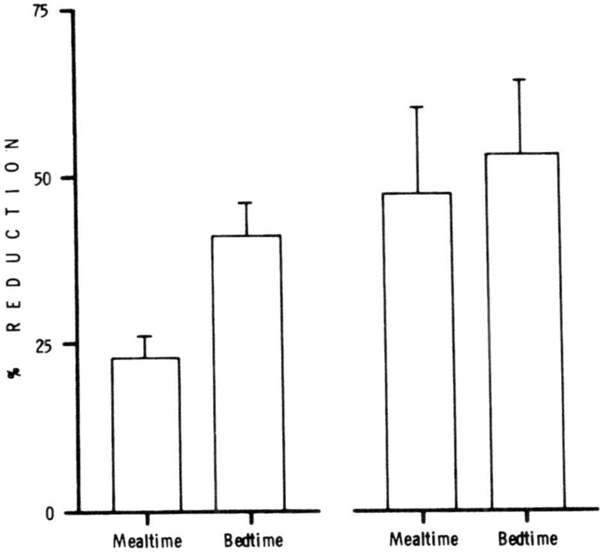

Fig. 7. Comparison between effect of CDCA (*left*) and UDCA (*right*), 12.5 mg/kg at bedtime, on percentage reduction in gallstone volume at 6 months as an index of gallstone dissolution rate (after [6])

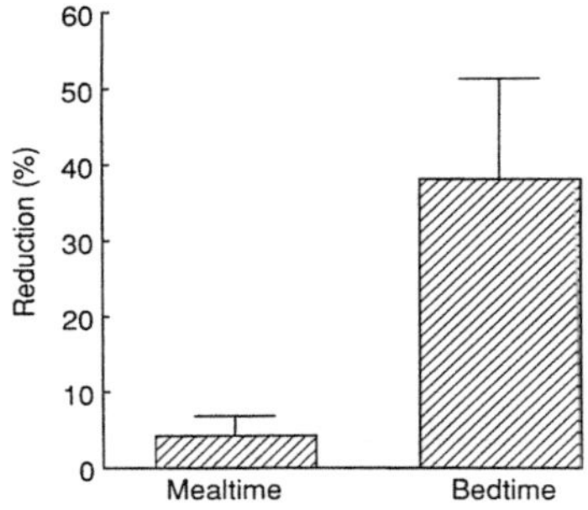

Fig. 8. Effect of UDCA (4 mg/kg per day at bedtime) on gallstone dissolution rate

reduction in SI during bedtime administration of CDCA is accompanied by a significant increase in gallstone dissolution rate [6], but this is not the case for UDCA at this particular dose (12 mg/kg per day; Fig. 7). The dose used in this study was higher than the recommended dose of UDCA because we wanted to use the same dose as for CDCA. Studies by Erlinger and colleagues [8] have suggested that a dose of 8 mg/kg per day is optimal for UDCA and that a further increase in dose may actually reduce gallstone dissolution rate. We therefore repeated our experiment with a suboptimal dose of UDCA (4 mg/kg per day) and found a significant increase in gallstone dissolution rate with bedtime administration (Fig. 8). We therefore predict that the effect of combination therapy, using a reduced dose of both UDCA and CDCA, should also be enhanced by bedtime administration.

Intermittent Bile Acid Therapy as a Long-Term Strategy

The advantage of surgery over all forms of non-surgical treatment is that it does not carry the risk of gallstone recurrence. It is therefore very important to asses this risk for non-surgical therapies. In an early study, Professor Dowling's group [9] asked the question "Is gallstone recurrence inevitable after bile acid therapy?". This question arose in these early studies because results were analysed in terms of cumulative recurrence rate. More recent studies have been based on an actuarial method to correct the recurrence rates for different lengths of follow-up, and these studies are in agreement in showing that the recurrence rate is about 10%–15% per year and that it plateaus off at about 50% at 5 years onwards [10, 11]. Thus, it seems that half of the gallstone population is not at risk of recurrence following bile acid therapy.

A viable strategy is needed for the 50% of patients who are liable to develop gallstone recurrence. As reported in the previous chapter by Professor Dowling (see this volume), the prospective British/Belgian Gallstone Study did not show a clear-cut advantage for low dose bedtime UDCA or for a diet high in fibre and low in refined carbohydrate. Retrospective analysis suggested that non-steroidal anti-inflammatory drugs (NSAIDS) might be of benefit in prevention, but this needs testing in a prospective controlled trial.

An alternative strategy is intermittent bile acid therapy. This would entail ultrasound monitoring at regular intervals of 6–12 months following successful non-surgical treatment of gallstones, in order to detect recurrent stones at an early stage while they are still small and susceptible to rapid dissolution by bile acid therapy. We have constructed a mathematical model to provide a theoretical test of this strategy. Figure 9 shows the mathematical model as applied to a cohort of 100 gallstone-free patients following non-surgical treatment. If one takes a pessimistic figure of 20% for gallstone recurrence,

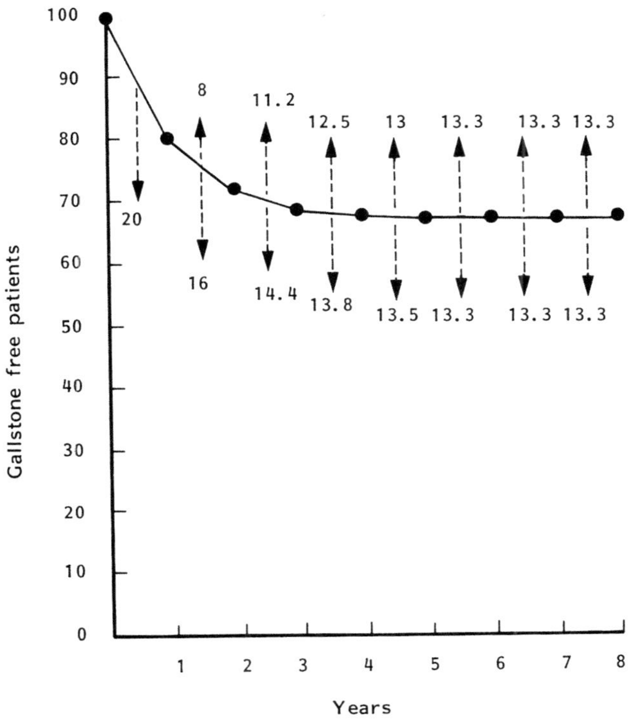

Fig. 9. Complete gallstone redissolution (*upper values*) and recurrence (*lower values*). A mathematical model for intermittent bile acid therapy, assuming a recurrence rate of 20% per annum and a redissolution rate of 40% per annum (after [3])

then 20 patients will have a recurrence in the 1st year; and if one also takes a pessimistic figure of 40% for gallstone redissolution, then eight of these patients will have redissolution in the 2nd year. Eventually, a steady state situation will be reached with an equal number of patients having gallstone recurrence and gallstone redissolution in any given year; the proportion of gallstone free patients even with the above pessimistic figures is 70% when this steady state situation is reached. If a more optimistic figure is taken of 10% for recurrence rate and 80% for redissolution rate, then 90% of the patients should be gallstone free in the long term. The true figure probably lies somewhere between 70% and 90%. In any case, this therapeutic approach would achieve the stated objective of our strategy in maintaining the vast majority of gallstone patients gallstone free in the long term. This approach needs to be tested prospectively, and this is now being done in a collaborative trial involving two British and three Italian centres.

Conclusions

Up to 15% of the gallstone population is now potentially suitable for non-surgical treatment, i.e. almost half the proportion that is suitable for surgical treatment. Bile acid therapy still has a central role in a non-surgical strategy for the initial treatment of small stones, for the treatment of larger stones that have been converted into small fragments by ESWL, and for recurrent stones detected by ultrasonography during routine follow-up. UDCA is more effective than CDCA, and a combination of the two bile acids is probably more effective than either bile acid alone. Bedtime administration is more effective than mealtime administration for CDCA and also for UDCA at a suboptimal dose. The recommended regimen is therefore a combination of a reduced dose of both CDCA and UDCA at bedtime. Intermittent bile acid therapy should prove to be a realistic long-term strategy following all forms of non-surgical treatment, maintaining the vast majority of the gallstone population gallstone free in the long term.

References

1. Attili AF (1986) Natural history and prevention. In: Bateson M (ed) Gallstone disease and its management. MTP Press, Lancaster, pp 57–70
2. Hospital In-Patient Enquiry, 1985 (1987) Series HB4 No. 27. DHSS Office of Population Censuses and Surveys. HMSO London
3. Northfield TC, Jazrawi RP (1988) Non-surgical treatment of gallstones: overall strategy. In: Northfield TC, Jazrawi RP, Zentler-Munro P (eds) Bile acids in health and disease. Kluwer, Dordrecht, pp 205–213
4. Lanzini A, Facchinetti D, Northfield TC (1988) Maintenance of hepatic bile acid secretion rate during overnight fasting by bedtime bile acid administration. Gastroenterology 95:1029–1035
5. Maudgal DP, Bird R, Northfield TC (1979) Optimal timing of doses of chenic acid in patients with gallstones. Br Med J 1:922–923
6. Northfield TC, Lanzini A, Jazrawi R, Kupfer R, Maudgal DP (1985) Gallstone dissolution rate and recurrence rate during and after bile acid therapy. In: Barbara L, Dowling RH, Hofman AF, Roda E (eds) Recent advances in bile acid research. Raven Press, New York, pp 289–302
7. Maudgal DP, Bird R, Blackwood WS, Northfield TC (1978) Low cholesterol diet: enhancement of effect of CDCA in patients with gallstones. Br Med J 2:851–853
8. Erlinger S, Go AL, Hussen JM, Fevery J (1984) Franco-Belgian cooperative study of ursodeoxycholic acid in the medical dissolution of gallstones: a double-blind randomised, dose-response study, and comparison with chenodeoxycholic acid. Hepatology 4:308–314
9. Ruppin DC, Dowling RH (1982) Is recurrence inevitable after gallstone dissolution by bile acid treatment? Lancet 1:181–185
10. Lanzini A, Jazrawi RP, Northfield TC (1986) Gallstone recurrence after medical dissolution an overestimated threat? Hepatology 3:241–246
11. O'Donnell LDJ, Heaton KW (1988) Recurrence and recurrence of gallstones after medical dissolution: a longterm followup. Gut 29:655–658
12. Northfield TC, Lanzini A, Jazrawi R, Maudgal DP, Kupfer R (1985) Methods of improving the efficacy of litholytic therapy. In: Paumgartner G, Stiehl A, Gerok W (eds) Enterohepatic circulation of bile acids and sterol metabolism. MTB Press, Lancaster, pp 335–350

Subject Index

GPSR Compliance

The European Union's (EU) General Product Safety Regulation (GPSR) is a set of rules that requires consumer products to be safe and our obligations to ensure this.

If you have any concerns about our products, you can contact us on ProductSafety@springernature.com

In case Publisher is established outside the EU, the EU authorized representative is:

Springer Nature Customer Service Center GmbH
Europaplatz 3
69115 Heidelberg, Germany

Batch number: 10704713

Printed by Printforce, the Netherlands